Management in Physical Therapy Practic

DATE			

Management in Physical Therapy Practices

Catherine G. Page, PT, MPH, PhD

Professor
School of Physical Therapy and
   Rehabilitation Sciences
University of South Florida
Tampa, Florida

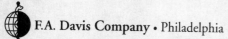 F.A. Davis Company • Philadelphia

F. A. Davis Company
1915 Arch Street
Philadelphia, PA 19103
www.fadavis.com

Copyright © 2010 by F. A. Davis Company

Printed in the United States of America

Last digit indicates print number: 10 9 8 7 6 5 4 3 2 1

Acquisitions Editor: Margaret Biblis
Developmental Editor: Keith Donnellan
Manager of Content Development: George W. Lang
Art and Design Manager: Carolyn O'Brien

As new scientific information becomes available through basic and clinical research, recommended treatments and drug therapies undergo changes. The author(s) and publisher have done everything possible to make this book accurate, up to date, and in accord with accepted standards at the time of publication. The author(s), editors, and publisher are not responsible for errors or omissions or for consequences from application of the book, and make no warranty, expressed or implied, in regard to the contents of the book. Any practice described in this book should be applied by the reader in accordance with professional standards of care used in regard to the unique circumstances that may apply in each situation. The reader is advised always to check product information (package inserts) for changes and new information regarding dose and contraindications before administering any drug. Caution is especially urged when using new or infrequently ordered drugs.

Library of Congress Cataloging-in-Publication Data

Page, Catherine G.
 Management in physical therapy practices / Catherine G. Page.
   p. ; cm.
Includes bibliographical references.
 ISBN-13: 978-0-8036-1872-5
 ISBN-10: 0-8036-1872-7
 1. Physical therapy—Practice. 2. Physical therapy services—Management. I. Title.
 [DNLM: 1. Physical Therapy (Specialty)—organization & administration—United States. 2. Delivery of Health Care—organization & administration—United States. 3. Practice Management—organization & administration—United States. WB 460 P132m 2010]
 RM705.P34 2010
 615.8'2—dc22

                                                                              2009016748

I read once that writing a book is like having a crazy uncle who comes for dinner and never leaves. This book seems to have affected my family that way. So, thank you to my husband Jack, my sister Valeria, and my mother Louise for their support and forbearance during the intrusion of this book in our lives. The crazy uncle has finally moved on.

Preface

Books are the bees, which carry the quickening pollen from one to another mind.

James Russell Lowell

Like many textbook authors, I was driven by my professional experiences to write this book. These range from clinical experiences as a physical therapist and department head, through academic appointments as a teacher and program director. The early managerial responsibilities I held as a young physical therapist and in my first job in education presented many challenges and offered many triumphs. Equally challenging has been teaching management courses to physical therapy students, since such courses are rarely considered the highlight of one's professional education.

I came to realize two things through my teaching and professional practice. Many physical therapists make the transition from clinical to managerial responsibilities easily and successfully, without much preparation or concern about their new responsibilities. More often than not, however, physical therapists (and many students) seem to avoid management opportunities because of their commitment to and interest in direct patient care, or perhaps out of a fear of the unknown.

Management in Physical Therapy Practices is for both groups. It provides an introduction for those whose career plans involve seeking management positions in any health-care setting. It also offers reluctant managers and students an opportunity to view a broad range of possibilities for physical therapists as managers that they might not otherwise consider. Physical therapists who come to the United States from other countries well prepared for direct patient care but unprepared for the system in which they will now practice also can use this text to better understand their profession, whether they are in management positions or not. Physical therapist assistants who aspire to management positions and the faculty who teach them also will find value in this text.

This book is intended to serve as a springboard for discussion of the physical therapist as manager across all health-care settings rather than being a how-to text on management. Ideally, it will provoke conflicting opinions and opposing views so that readers can practice making important management decisions in the absence of clear, straightforward guidelines. The management activities are based on my own work experiences and those of other managers in a wide variety of health-care settings. Through discussions with others while working on these activities, readers have the opportunity to reflect on the decisions they would make in these situations from different perspectives. There are no hard and fast correct answers. The objective is to develop the ability the weigh the pros and cons of important managerial decisions that affect the care of patients in physical therapy practices.

Other activities in the book lead readers to delve more deeply into certain topics, and frequent sidebars offer clarification of key points and guide readers to online resources and other information so they can remain current with issues and policies affecting the profession and their professional roles. Because health-care policy and professions are evolving, these resources have the potential to serve as ongoing resources for readers.

The four chapters in Section 1, Introduction to Management and Physical Therapy in Health Care, consider the culture and business of health care, the complexity of these organizations, and the role of managers and leaders. Selected contemporary health-care issues are presented, including workforce diversity, the culture of physical therapy, the leadership-management continuum, and health insurance for physical therapy. Readers are asked to examine their current views on management as a career goal.

Chapters 5 to 13 in Section 2, Responsibilities of the Physical Therapy Manager, address each of the core responsibilities of health-care management: vision, mission, and goals; policies and procedures; marketing; staffing; patient care; fiscal; legal and ethical; risk management; and communication. A model for strategic planning is introduced and used throughout the text to encourage development of managerial decision-making skills. The activities in these chapters explore each area of managerial responsibility in more depth. These chapters may stand alone or serve as the foundation for Chapter 14.

Chapter 14, Conducting a Feasibility Study, is the exception to the claim that this is not a how-to text. On completion and collation of all of the activities in Chapter 14, readers will have in hand the final product that Section 2 has been leading toward: a feasibility study for a real-world physical therapy practice. Suggestions for expanding the feasibility study to a business plan also are discussed.

Each chapter in Section 3 addresses management of physical therapy in a different setting: long-term care, outpatient centers, special education units in schools, home health agencies, and hospitals. The importance of the management of multidisciplinary rehabilitation units is addressed. Each chapter in Section 3 has two parts. The first considers contemporary issues in one physical therapy situation. The second focuses on the core responsibilities presented in Section 2, identifying managerial issues relevant

to that chapter's setting. Chapter-ending activities provide the opportunity to develop managerial decision-making skills through classroom discussions and assignments.

The final chapter, Commentary on the Physical Therapist as Manager, discusses what we know about the management of physical therapy practices and what we need to know. The future of the profession and the importance of managerial skills for individual professionals are addressed.

The style of the text is to present complex management concepts in a user-friendly, interactive format that reflects contemporary physical therapy practice through interesting activities. My intent is that this "busy-little-bee" text will excite and stimulate the minds of physical therapists about management, increasing the number eager to seek management positions and to spread the "pollen" of this enthusiasm. It is important to their careers and to our profession that we expand this aspect of professional practice. I have had a wonderful career because I have been a manager, and I wish the same for my readers.

Catherine G. Page, PT, MPH, PhD

Expert Content Reviewers

Lois E. Benedetti, PT, MS, DPT
Instructor
Boston University Sargent College of Health
and Rehabilitation Sciences
Boston, Massachusetts

Diane M. Davis, PT, CLT
Director, Therapy Services
University of Chicago Medical Center
Chicago, Illinois

Lydia M. Gomez-Bamford, DPT, MBA
Vice President, Paradise Rehab Solutions
Adjunct Instructor, University of South Florida
Tampa, Florida

Scott S. Harp, PT, PhD
Executive Director
METT Therapy Services
Joliet, Illinois

Amy Maxeiner
University of Illinois at Chicago
Chicago, Illinois

Gina Maria Musolino, PT, MSEd, EdD
Associate Professor & Director of Clinical Education
School of Physical Therapy & Rehabilitation Sciences
University of South Florida College of Medicine
USF Health
Tampa, Florida

William L. Roberts, PT, PhD
Land O Lakes, Florida

Sharon D. Weil, PTA, MEd
Academic Coordinator of Clinical Education, Physical
Therapist Assistant Program
Indian River Community College
Fort Pierce, Florida

Reviewers

Denise G. Bender, JD, PT, GCS
Associate Professor
Rehabilitation Sciences
University of Oklahoma Health Sciences Center
Oklahoma City, Oklahoma

Suzanne R. Brown, MPH, PT
Consultant
Mesa, Arizona

Susan Callanan, DPT
Instructor
Physical Therapist Assistant
North Iowa Area Community College
Mason City, Iowa

Tracey L. Collins, PT, PhD, MBA, GCS
Assistant Professor
Physical Therapy
University of Scranton
Scranton, Pennsylvania

Linda T. Coultas, PT, MHA
Director
Rehabilitation
Cambridge Health Alliance
Medford, Massachusetts

Jim Dronberger, PT, DPT, OCS, MBA
Associate Professor
Physical Therapy Education
Rockhurst University
Kansas City, Missouri

Charles J. Gulas, PT, PhD, GCS, CWS
Dean, School of Health Professions
Associate Professor, Physical Therapy
Maryville University
St Louis, Missouri

Vicky N. Humphrey, PT, MS
Lecturer
Physical Therapy
The Ohio State University
Columbus, Ohio

Dianne V. Jewell, PT, PhD, DPT, CCS
Assistant Professor
Physical Therapy
Virginia Commonwealth University
Richmond, Virginia

Stephanie Johnson, PT, MBA, EdD
Director, Assistant Professor
Physical Therapy
Simmons College
Boston, Massachusetts

David A. Krause, PT, MBA, DSc, OCS
Instructor
Physical Medicine and Rehabilitation
Mayo Clinic
Rochester, Minnesota

Rosalie B. Lopopolo, PT, PhD, MBA
Professor
Physical Therapy
Arcadia University
Glenside, Pennsylvania

Sandra Marden-Lokken, PT, MA
Assistant Professor
Physical Therapy
College of St. Scholastica
Duluth, Minnesota

Contents

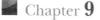

Chapter 9
Responsibility for Patient Care   101

Chapter 10
Fiscal Responsibilities   110

Chapter 11
Responsibility for Risk Management   122

Chapter 12
Legal and Ethical Responsibilities   145

■ Chapter **13**
Communication Responsibilities   153

■ Chapter **14**
Conducting a Feasibility Study   174

■ Section **3**
Management in Specific Physical Therapy Settings   187

■ Chapter **15**
Management Issues in Long-Term Care   188

▪ Chapter 16

Management Issues in Outpatient
Centers   210

▪ Chapter 17

Management Issues in School-Based
Services   232

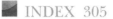 Chapter **20**

Commentary on the Physical Therapist as Manager   297

INDEX 305

Contemporary Issues in Health-Care Management

This section of the text provides an introduction to some of the contemporary challenges facing physical therapists who are managers or who seek to become managers in any type of health-care organization. Potential opportunities and career paths that can lead to mid-level and executive management positions are presented.

With these possibilities in mind, the complex world of health-care organizations is introduced. The role that managers play in the culture and the socialization process of organizations is emphasized. Next, the need for both leaders and managers in health-care organizations is explored in an introduction to the various theories related to these roles in organizations and a discussion of how these roles are changing. Finally, with Figure S1.1 as a model of the major stakeholders in health care, the last chapter introduces health care as a unique business that requires every manager to develop a comprehensive view of the interactions of these players and their influence on the quality of patient care. The types of health insurance policies and regulations are presented. The importance of mid-level managers in ensuring that the relationships in Figure S1.1 are clearly understood is presented.

The ultimate responsibilities of mid-level health-care managers are two: identifying and implementing the means for professionals to provide quality care to each of their patients, and contributing to the goals and protecting the interests of their organizations so that necessary resources for providing that care are available. The balancing and coordinating of these responsibilities rests on the ability to seek managerial opportunities; grasp the fundamentals of organizations, leadership, and management; and appreciate the unique business of health care. The foundations for that understanding begins with this section.

For health professionals who are not managers, this section provides information that may facilitate discussions with people who are their managers as important questions about their work and health-care organizations arise.

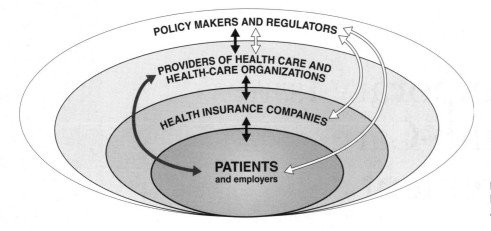

Figure S1.1 ✦ Factors in health-care management and leadership.

Chapter 1

Management in Health Care

Learning Objectives

+ Compare and contrast the qualifications of health-care managers with prior clinical experience to those with academic degrees in management and no clinical experience.
+ Discuss the pros and cons of career ladders that include formal managerial responsibilities.
+ Determine the role of mentoring physical therapists as they transition from clinical to managerial roles.
+ Discuss the relationship of direct patient care skills and management skills of physical therapists, regardless of their job titles.
+ Determine the typical responsibilities of mid-level and executive managers in health-care settings.
+ Determine the types of managerial opportunities across different types of health-care organizations.
+ Discuss the need for new managers to possess communication skills, a sense of perspective, and industriousness.
+ Determine the need for and appropriateness of delegation.
+ Distinguish between a manager's horizontal and vertical communication skills.
+ Discuss contemporary issues presented to health-care mid-level managers including the nature of work, a diverse workforce, planning, and financial reporting that all affect their relationships with patients.

Becoming a Manager

Regardless of the type of health-care organization, physical therapists have many opportunities to pursue management roles at many levels, or they may assume *all* managerial roles in businesses they own. Although many upper-level managers and some mid-level managers may start their careers directly into these positions, some of them are patient care providers who work their way up the corporate health-care ladder. These clinicians often leave behind their professional roles in patient care as they assume new managerial duties. Private practice physical therapists often divide their time between their business and patient care responsibilities.

It is certainly common in many organizations for expert clinicians to evolve into at least supervisory or mid-level manager positions. In fact, many health-care corporations offer in-house training programs or tuition deferment programs to encourage promotion from within their ranks of health-care professionals. Other large health-care organizations often prefer to hire people with degrees in health-care management or health services administration strictly for their managerial expertise, particularly at the executive levels. An example of such decision making about hiring is found in Activity 1.1.

ACTIVITY 1.1
WHOM WOULD YOU HIRE?

Two candidates have applied for the position of Vice-President of Patient Care Services in the Community Health Care System. Shannon Silverman holds a Master's degree in Health Care Administration from UCLA. She has held a similar position in a comparable institution where the quality of care and profits improved dramatically under her direction. Jessie Fowler has held positions as a physical therapy supervisor for 2 years and as a rehabilitation manager for the entire Community Health Care System for 4 years. He has excelled at direct patient care. Under his leadership, rehab services were recognized as the outstanding clinical service in the health-care system for the last 2 years. Role-play a meeting of the executive committee of the Community Health Care System to discuss filling this position. Is Shannon or Jessie the better candidate to manage *all* patient care services? What were the criteria for selection?

Many health professionals ask themselves why anyone would want to be a health-care manager. The complexity and challenges can be daunting, but managers see the rewards in having a positive influence on the lives of many more patients and the community at large. The work of managers is like multiplying the satisfaction of direct patient care a thousand fold. Mid-level managers essentially influence a broader spectrum of patients and patient care as they accomplish the organization's goals through the work of others.

An opportunity to demonstrate that there may be a better way to handle things becomes very motivating to many people who are often mystified by the decisions made by "upper management." Other people may reach a point in their careers where they are ready for new responsibilities and new skill sets. Rather than continuing to narrow their work within a clinical specialization, a transition to management responsibilities presents opportunities in a broader sphere of influence. These mid-level management positions may take a variety of forms in the career ladders of health-care professionals. They may become managers in their own disciplines, leaders of

interdisciplinary programs, or executives in large health-care systems. For many physical therapists, these opportunities evolve from their patient care roles and responsibilities during the course of their careers.

Transitioning From Patient Care to Management

Some health-care professionals find themselves formally and deliberately seeking management positions or independent practices. Others are forced, or coaxed, into managerial roles that they reluctantly accept. They all face the same transitional challenges. Lombardi identifies these transitions as moving from:[1]

+ *Self-direction to selfless service.* Managerial work depends on highly variable and unpredictable factors rather than on the more specific professional needs and desires that drive professional performance.
+ *Autonomous control to circumstantial control.* The work of managers depends on unpredictable circumstances and situations rather than on assigned caseloads and productivity expectations. Flexibility is much more critical.
+ *Quantitative to qualitative outcomes.* The outcomes of the efforts of managers are more dependent on perception than on clearly defined measures. The immediate gratification and rewards for stellar performance found in reaching productivity goals and patient outcome measures as a health-care professional diminish.
+ *Definitive clinical criteria to overall comprehensive goals.* The performance criteria for managers are often gray and flexible as organizations change, and managers' responsibilities fluctuate with the needs of the organization. The clear job descriptions of clinicians are replaced with more ambiguous expectations.

Put another way, health-care professionals focus on making independent decisions about individual patients based on the continued development of their technical skills for quality, direct patient care. As managers, they become more removed from patients and individual outcomes. Instead, their focus is on facilitating others and building networks in the broader health-care organization. The rewards of helping patients accomplish their goals are replaced with the less concrete managerial rewards of helping others achieve their work performance goals.[2]

The transition to management certainly involves exciting opportunities for the acquisition of a new skill set for new duties. At the same time, there is that period of discomfort that comes from leaving behind the structure and familiarity with patient care to take on the uncertainties of management. Managerial opportunities and possibilities to expand upon and enrich a professional career can be intimidating, but it soon grows on people, including some managers who protest too strongly about their new roles.

Whether managing by choice or by fiat, health-care professionals may choose to explore graduate degrees to prepare for management positions, or they may learn the skills by the seat of their pants, or self-study. Typically, it is some combination of all of these strategies. Determining the value of formal programs is an important decision. Activity 1.2 offers some ideas for exploring management degree programs.

ACTIVITY 1.2
MANAGEMENT EDUCATION/PREPARATION

Group Discussion Questions:

1. What should someone look for in a formal management degree program?

2. What are all of the graduate degree possibilities? Is the MBA or master of public administration (MPA) the degree of choice for health-care managers? Are there other choices? Defend your choice.

3. What do the following organizations say about health-care management?
   American College of Health Care Administrators at http://www.achca.org/
   Medical practice management at http://www.mgma.com/about/default.aspx?id=242
   Descriptions of medical and health service managers at http://www.bls.gov/oco/ocos014.htm
   American College of Healthcare Executives at http://www.ache.org/

   Commission on Accreditation of Health Care Management at http://www.cahmeweb.org/
   Association of University Programs in Health Administration at http://www.aupha.org/i4a/pages/ index.cfm?pageid=1

4. Identify at least two graduate programs in management. Compare and contrast their curricula, costs, and graduate placement information. Are they accredited? By whom? Which one is most attractive? Why?

5. Identify a health-care corporation or system that has an internal management development program. Find out about it. Talk to a physical therapist who has experience with one. What is good about the program? What is its downside? Determine if the emphasis of the programs is developing people management skills or financial management skills. Does it matter? Why?

Mentoring

Another important consideration in transitioning from clinical care to management responsibilities is to identify mentors who can help in the process. Morton-Cooper has identified the importance of mentoring in health-care careers and suggests that it should begin with the very first clinical position. In his model, the person who seeks mentoring must initiate it as a long-term intimate, personal, enabling relationship. A mentor does not formally assess the person but rather provides unstructured support for learning and for facilitating access to the important social and political networks needed for continued career socialization.[3]

Mentoring when taking on new managerial responsibilities may be even more critical than having a clinical mentor. Because the roles and expectations of managers are much more unpredictable and dependent on the changing needs of the organization, the support of a mentor or mentors to "think out loud" is a very important asset in long-term career development and in meeting day-to-day managerial challenges.

A different model of mentoring places the responsibility for mentoring on the organization. The organization provides mentors to all new employees. The mentors in this model are responsible for "showing them the ropes" of the technical, functional aspects of their positions, and introducing them to the organizational culture. Such a formalized program is believed to improve the retention of employees because they develop emotional ties to the organization through their mentors. Increased job satisfaction and productivity are the result.[4] However, this model does not preclude a person from personally initiating

Sidebar 1.1

Roles of a Mentor

Particularly in health care, new managers need to identify what they need in a mentor(s) to ensure a smooth transitions to health care from other businesses, or from health professional to manager. Identifying which type of mentor is most important is a critical first step.[2]

✦ Sponsor: to open doors for the new manager

✦ Coach: to show the "the ropes" of the new position

✦ Protector: to buffer negative experiences

✦ Exposer: to create new opportunities

✦ Challenger: to stretch the manager's new skills and their scope of work

✦ Role model: to develop new behaviors by example

✦ Counselor: to accept and confirm efforts, and offer friendship

Sidebar 1.2

Mentoring and the APTA

Explore the mentoring program available through the American Physical Therapy Association at http://www.apta.org/

interaction with upper level management that includes the chief executive officer and a cadre of vice presidents who are responsible for organizational units such as finance, purchasing, human resources, marketing, facilities management, patient care, medical services, etc. The larger the organization becomes, the more divided the executive functions become to conquer the complexity and to keep current with changes in health-care reimbursement, rules and regulations, new technology, and other demands. It often appears that upper management is top-heavy because of the decreasing numbers of mid-level managers in many organizations that have flattened their bureaucratic structures. This will be discussed in the next chapter.

Those mid-level managers remaining in health care have a direct influence on the coordination and delivery of patient care through frequent interactions with the staffs they supervise. This level of management may be organized by departments such as rehabilitation, pharmacy, nursing, housekeeping, dietary, and business office; or they be organized into multidisciplinary teams with a focus on the delivery of specialized patient care such as a heart institute or a stroke team. Many large health-care organizations are a hybrid of the two models, which is discussed later in this chapter.

Management of Other Health-Care Settings

In smaller health-care organizations, all levels of employees may interact with upper level managers almost every day. A long-term care skilled nursing facility is an example. The nursing home administrator is directly responsible for *all* of the organization's functions that would be handled by several people in larger organizations. On one hand, these administrators work in concert with their directors of nursing and rehabilitation, who have responsibility for the patient care clinical services. On the other hand, they work as closely with their business office managers who typically handle human resources, payroll, reimbursement, billing, etc. They all report directly to the administrator, who may have "home office" corporate support if the nursing home is part of a larger chain of many buildings. More likely, the bulk of the management of a nursing home occurs in-house as the direct responsibility of the administrator.

mentoring relationships, from within or beyond their organizations. See Sidebars 1.1 and 1.2 for more information on mentoring.

Transitioning to new roles and mentoring, like most management issues, are found in all types of businesses. The differences in health care that require special skills of managers arise because of the special nature of their business—the provision of efficient, effective health care for the people in their communities while controlling ever-increasing costs with ever-decreasing reimbursement for the services they provide. In any type of organization, management occurs at a variety of levels that are driven by the size and complexity of the organization.

Large Health-Care Organizations

The day-to-day health-care worker in a large health-care organization or system has very little direct

The solo practitioner physical therapist is another kind of health-care manager who wears *all* hats as both the executive and mid-level manager of the business, while concurrently having *all* responsibility for direct patient care. These physical therapists may have other staff to supervise in the provision of physical therapy care to patients, and they may contract services such as billing, accounting, and rembursement contract negotiations. Despite this support, it is basically a one-person show in which the organization begins with, and the results end with, the work of the solo practitioner.

Somewhere in between large health-care systems and solo practitioners lie the other components of health care. Home health agencies, physician practice groups, and special education services in school systems are all examples that have varying levels of managerial responsibilities. For instance, a physical therapist may be either the countywide coordinator for all rehabilitation services in a school system, or the supervisor of an interdisciplinary team that provides rehab services in several schools in a district. The unique challenges for managers in different types of health-care settings are presented in Sections 2 and 3.

Mid-Level Managers

The good news for physical therapists and other health-care professionals is that unlike other businesses, mid-level health-care managers spend a great deal of their time—about 65%—on people management, which is already a strength of successful practitioners. With only about 10% of their time spent on financial analysis, the rest of the time is spent dealing with special projects and "administrivia."[1] The emphasis on people management responsibilities may make a move to a management position more attractive, or less threatening, for many physical therapists. A shift of their already well-developed people skills to a different level of interaction with others often comes naturally.

The challenge, of course, is that most people are very resistant to being managed. The best performers know enough and care enough to manage themselves—especially health-care professionals. We all prefer *not* to be told what to do. In reality, managers cannot force people to care about patients, or expect them to know all there is to know about patient care, or demand that they create new approaches to accomplish patient goals. What managers *can* do is sustain the best interests and qualities of individuals in their work performance so that the organization and its collective purpose are what really matter to everyone. Managers resolve the tension between the needs of the health-care organization as a whole and the needs of the individuals who work within it in order to provide quality patient care. Health care depends on managers to forge these links so that there is a good fit between the organization and its employees, and so that everyone shares the same values.[5]

Mid-level managers are the people in organizations upon whom fall the responsibility for reconciling the personal values and standards of employees with the culture of the organization. All behaviors of managers must be consistent with the attitudes, values, and beliefs of the organization. In other words, managers must "walk the talk" to resolve any differences between employees and the organization. They are the people who ensure that employees are happy and that the organization is happy. Achieving this happiness is dependent upon managers having the following important characteristics and skills:[4]

- ✦ Trustworthiness and trust
- ✦ Empowerment and delegation
- ✦ Consistency in decisions and mentorship

People Management

Aspiring or already-appointed mid-level managers do not lack for a wide range of "how-to" sources to address their underlying ability to manage people and communicate effectively. The following topics provide managers with some food for thought on these important issues. For instance, Magretta and Stone suggest that managers who know what employees really want are at an advantage. They suggest the following hints that appear very much like what health professionals aspire to in their interactions with patients—another form of management after all:[5]

- ✦ Be kind and respectful.
- ✦ Be fair.
- ✦ Do as you say and mean what you say.

✦ Guide and give inspiration to people.

✦ People yearn to be loyal.

✦ People want to be trusted.

✦ Foster "know thyself" so people can self-manage.

✦ Ask this important question often, "Why do you work?"

✦ Focus on the results of work rather than how hard someone is working.

✦ Hang together even if there is disagreement.

✦ Managing is about tradeoffs not compromise.

✦ Managers can't be all things to all people.

✦ Stay the course of the organization.

Lombardi has also given thought to what new managers need and he reminds them that they need only three things—a sense of perspective, industriousness, and communication skills, which are discussed here. Because they are in the spotlight and former colleagues now report to them, he cautions new managers against developing personal relationships and playing psychologist. Lombardi's view is that all employees really want is a fair wage, work direction, respect, and recognition for their level of performance. Managers who can do that for people are bound to be successful and feel good about their managerial efforts.[1] Activity 1.3 provides an opportunity to address some of these managerial challenges.

ACTIVITY 1.3
GIVING THEM WHAT THEY WANT

Sam Thompson is the new manager of rehab services that includes a staff of three physical therapists, three physical therapist assistants, three occupational therapists, three occupational therapy assistants, and one speech language pathologist. There is also a pool of four physical therapists and two occupational therapists who work as contract per diem employees. Because he is new to this health-care system and the person he is replacing was ineffective, Sam wants to wipe the slate clean and get to know his employees. What should be his plan for doing so? How long should it take? What information does he need to gather from his staff? What questions should he expect his staff to ask? What do you think Sam should anticipate as most important to his staff?

A Manager's Sense of Perspective and Industriousness

When problem solving or making decisions, mid-level managers need to consider the points of view of all stakeholders in order to take action that is most likely to be successful. The perspective of patients is foremost in health care and will be discussed in more depth. However, determining the other perspectives on a particular issue—what does the boss think?, what do my team members think?, what do the other managers think?—is a much more important process than determining their self-interest. Effectively synthesizing all of these perspectives is a challenge that is easier said than done. Failure to identify the perspectives is perhaps riskier than failure to reconcile them effectively.

Industriousness is another important characteristic for mid-level managers to have. If for no other reason than managers who are industrious role model the hard-working, conscientious, and energetic behaviors that are desired in the people they supervise to accomplish patient care goals. It also means taking initiative and learning to delegate effectively. It does not mean doing it alone and it does not mean delegating it all. Why and how often tasks are delegated is a major factor in the determination of managerial effectiveness. See Sidebar 1.3 for suggestions on delegation.

Industriousness does not necessarily mean working 80 hours per week to accomplish all of the work for which health-care managers are responsible. Achieving balance through time management and priority setting establishes a model for the people who are supervised to emulate. A sign of effective management is the ability to take a worry-free extended vacation because the acceptance of delegation of responsibilities has been tested, is expected, and is acceptable to subordinates in the absence of the manager. In other words, to use the old cliché—it takes a team that pulls together to accomplish the goals of the organization. None of these goals can be accomplished by, nor should they be dependent on, one person.

It may often seem that the entire weight of the organization falls on mid-level managers caught in the cross hairs of the organization's aim for its vision. The reality is that it is not the amount of work but rather the unpredictable nature of the work that creates stress as managers face the threat of approaching deadlines and multiple alternative actions. It often seems that the best-laid plans for completing

---

Sidebar 1.3

Things to Delegate and Not to Delegate

DELEGATE WHEN...	DO NOT DELEGATE WHEN...

DELEGATE WHEN. . .

✦ All necessary information is available for the task to be delegated.

✦ The responsibilities are more about operations than about planning and organizing.

✦ Others are more qualified or have the necessary skills that are not your strengths.

✦ Responsibilities can be provided that allow people to grow and challenge them.

✦ Assignments require evaluation and recommendations.

✦ The tasks are more routine requiring only minor decisions.

✦ There are clear job descriptions and work expectations.

✦ A follow-up plan upon completion is in place.

DO NOT DELEGATE WHEN. . .

✦ The team needs leadership in determining priorities and setting goals.

✦ The task involves planning and solving new problems.

✦ The task is developing teams.

✦ Coaching and motivating are needed.

✦ Evaluating performance of subordinates.

✦ Rewarding or disciplining personnel.

✦ The assignment was given directly to you to complete.

✦ The work had already been assigned to someone else; do not overlap assignments.

Huffmire, DW, Holmes JD. *Handbook of Effective Management.* Westport, CT: Praeger; 2006, pp. 45–46.

the day's work are sidetracked by an urgent meeting or a new deadline for something that was not even on the radar screen when the manager arrived at work. Often it is not time management that is the issue, it is crisis management. Everything that comes up seems to be someone's crisis. Taking care of "it," the sooner the better, and as simply as possible, often requires time that was intended for anticipated or scheduled work.

Industriousness is more about fitting things in than blocking time out. Avoiding the temptation to continue expanding the time devoted to work rather than fitting the work into a given block of time is perhaps one of the management skills most required for success—and sanity. Communication skills become critical for managers because of the intensity of their interactions with other mid-level managers, upper management, and the people they directly supervise to accomplish the goals of the organization within the time available.

Horizontal Communication

Determination of which other mid-level managers are most important to their work is a concern for new managers. Importance is dependent on the time spent with them, or common management goals to be accomplished, or shared responsibility for a particular patient population.[1] This horizontal interaction also is a way that mid-level managers keep current with news within their organizations and about health-care policy that impacts the work they manage and the people they lead.

In well-designed organizations, mid-level managers have time for planning and thinking because they are not caught up in an ongoing, never-ending eruption of daily brushfires that must be extinguished. Organizations need to find the perfect number of mid-level managers—not so many that communication and coordination among them to accomplish the organization's goals is impossible, but not so few that each one is overwhelmed with responsibilities with very little power to manage them. Without time for planning because they are stretched thin, avoiding brushfires to begin with may be impossible. As a result, crisis management replaces people management. The fewer mid-level management positions there are, the more important it is for those managers to be prepared to, and permitted to, solve problems for themselves and empower their work groups to make decisions for themselves.[6]

In efforts to improve efficiency, health-care systems may take a hybrid approach to mid-level management.

For instance, nonclinical mid-level managers (physical plant, housekeeping, dietary, maintenance, etc.) may have responsibility for services in multiple units or multiple locations of a larger system. Clinical services, at the same time, may appear as more of a matrix structure across the system with a clinical manager from a particular health profession coordinating a team of people from different disciplines who may or may not be in the same location.

As an example, an occupational therapist may be the director of rehabilitation services that include six interdisciplinary teams of therapists to provide services in an inpatient rehabilitation unit, the rest of the hospital, three outpatient centers, and a home care agency. Or clinical services may be organized in a matrix model with a coordinator who pulls together the interdisciplinary team within one particular unit of the system.[7] At the same time, the director of rehabilitation services may rely on a single person in human resources to meet his or her workforce needs throughout the system while communicating with a different housekeeping supervisor in each unit that he or she manages. See Activity 1.4.

ACTIVITY 1.4
HORIZONTAL MANAGEMENT

Rebecca Levin is the manager of rehabilitation services in a Good Shepard Health Care System. She wants to analyze her interactions with all of the other managers in the system to determine if she is concentrating her efforts effectively. Create a list of all of the managers (clinical and support services) with whom Rebecca can expect to interact. Rate her interactions with each manager using the following scale. Discuss what factors determined your weightings. Estimate how much of the expected interactions is face to face. Estimate how much of the interactions are devoted to planning activities and how much are devoted to crisis management. How might she wish to change the rate of these interactions to improve the visibility and success of rehab services?

5 = more than one interaction/day
4 = daily interaction
3 = at least 3 interactions/week
2 = weekly interaction
1 = less than weekly
0 = no interactions

Vertical Communication

Communication vertically also is important to mid-level managers. First of all, communication with their immediate superiors *must* include a clear understanding of responsibilities, priorities, and the level of authority for duties that they are assigned. Establishing the method for and the frequency of communication is vital. Determining what needs to be reported when is critical, and receiving feedback on performance is necessary.

The mid-level manager may have to take the initiative and be persistent for this communication to happen, particularly when numerous people are reporting to the same person, each of whom wants to carve out time with the boss. Consistent communication with upper managers is important because of the volatile nature of health care and the effect that change has on the day-to-day operations of patient care. Constantly clarifying duties and responsibilities and making time for reporting and feedback is essential so that the organization can solve problems quickly and take action proactively in order to ensure its growth and success.

Communication with the people that mid-level managers supervise follows the same cascading principle. Employees need to hear from their direct supervisors about what their responsibilities are, what and when they need to report to their bosses, and how they are performing. They also need consistent communication about the work they are doing, although it tends to be more predictable for longer periods of time.

For instance, the work of the staff physical therapists is the same after their patient care and other assignments are established. The therapists need feedback on productivity and patient outcomes, and they must have clarification when their responsibilities are changed. Unlike the establishment of a routine schedule for communication with their bosses, the frequency of communication that mid-level managers have with each member of their work teams may decrease as that work stabilizes. This may not be the same for all employees or the same over time for each employee. In all cases, again the mid-level manager must assume responsibility for initiating and sustaining this communication.

As the go-between for the organization and the employees they supervise, mid-level managers also are the filter for both formal and informal information about the organization as a whole. Knowing what and when to share this broader information is a delicate process. No one likes to be the last to know, but on the other hand, too much information can be distracting and disruptive. Managers want to avoid the distrust that is driven by suspicions that there are upper management secrets to be learned, and avoid overwhelming employees with so much information that they no longer listen.

At the same time, what and how much information mid-level managers receive from employees should be relayed to their superiors presents similar questions. What are the small issues that a manager has the authority to handle without reporting? What are the big issues that need to be reported? The ability to be selective about what is important is the art of mid-level management. See Activity 1.5 and Sidebar 1.4.

ACTIVITY 1.5
THE PERSON IN THE MIDDLE

Scenario One: Jackie Janowitz is the director of rehabititation services in a large medical center. Jackie has a standing meeting with Paula Johannson, the Vice President for Clinical Services every Monday at 3 p.m. for about 15 minutes. They call it the "debriefing." They consistently devote some of that time each week to discuss patient care and staffing issues. The rest of the time is an opportunity for Paula to notify Jackie of pending projects or reports, and Jackie reports on any "hallway" talk she thinks Paula needs to know about.

This formal weekly process of communication has been effective for the last year or so. However, this is now the third week that Paula has cancelled the meeting because of other things that have come up. Jackie is unsure what to make of this. What do you think? If you were Jackie, what would you have done over the past 3 weeks? What should you do now?

Scenario Two: Jackie has received an unexpected memo by e-mail from the Vice President for Facilities Management. Effective the first of the month, a little more than 2 weeks from now, the staff office for the rehabilitation team is being moved to the basement in order to expand the space for outpatient radiology services. What would be your reaction if you were Jackie? What should she do next?

Scenario Three: Jackie has all of her staff block out 11:30 a.m. to 12:00 p.m. every other Wednesday to hold a staff meeting if necessary. She is very good about communicating items that the staff needs to know and giving them kudos every day. The meetings are for staff input into decisions, projects, etc. She is trying to decide whether the move to a new space, the second time this year, should be communicated by e-mail or whether she should wait until next week's meeting, or whether she should hold an emergency meeting this week. What do you think?

Sidebar 1.4

Six Simple Words

"How can I help you today?" is a question that is key to successful vertical and horizontal management communication as well as patient care success. It gives the person questioned an open-ended chance to define the interaction and its importance. It allows managers to then focus on facilitating the most important work of health care at any moment.[8]

Other Contemporary People Management Issues

Perhaps a reflection of some of the broader changes in the workforce in general, several issues that demand the attention of mid-level, health-care managers more than ever are included here. The way work is scheduled, the diversity of health-care workers, implementation of plans, and the reporting of revenue and expenses all affect the most important responsibility of health-care managers—patient care.

The Nature of Work

The nature of work in health care today presents many opportunities for mid-level managers to hone effective people management and communication skills. There are fewer people who are the traditional full-time employees dedicated to an organization for their entire careers. It is not uncommon to have health-care staffs that include workers who are placed in organizations by temporary employment agencies for brief assignments, or who are independent contractors who accept only assignments attractive to them on a part-time or intermittent basis.

Dependency on this unpredictable and expensive source of workers is one of the major challenges in health-care management that is intensified because of the 24/7 nature of the business. The constant demand for workers is also driven by third-party utilization management demands. For instance, the rehabilitation process for patients cannot be delayed for even a day because of the potential negative affect on discharge plans. The demand for managers to provide 7-day coverage of efficient and effective patient care has significantly increased as a result. It is easy to understand how in times of manpower shortages, the human resources manager is likely to be the most critical horizontal connection for other mid-level managers.

Workforce Diversity

Another consideration in managing workers in health care is the issue of diversity. Although organizations may direct much attention to the need for cultural competency to meet the needs of diverse groups of people, very little is known about the actual effect of a diverse staff on the outputs of health-care organizations. In fact, there is actually some controversy about its value. One view is that a diverse workforce is desirable because a variety of perspectives is invaluable in managerial problem-solving and for meeting the needs of a wide range of cultures represented by the patients served in any community. Not only has this view not been supported, but to the contrary, diverse groups of workers have been found to be less communicative and less integrated. This distancing results in increased levels of conflict among workers.[9]

Racial/Ethnic Diversity

The challenge for predominantly white, male upper management in health-care organizations is to see beyond minority hiring in lower level positions as the answer to diversity challenges. They need to understand that any racial and ethnic tensions in their communities spill over into their organizations. Aries explored these challenges for an understanding of the effect of diversity on health-care workers and the patient populations they serve. The conclusions of this qualitative study included:[9]

- ✦ Different groups viewed cultural competence and the effectiveness of organizational interventions to achieve it differently.
- ✦ The focus of upper level managers was managing diversity at the broadest level rather than at the level of patient care.
- ✦ Mid-level managers had a great deal of freedom to manage diversity at the departmental level, which resulted in a perception of inconsistent and mixed messages among employees and patients about the institution's commitment to cultural competence.
- ✦ Mid-level managers were aware of diversity problems but felt that the problems were those of particular individuals rather than a system-wide issue. They felt that workers should focus on the demands and competence of coworkers rather than these distracting concerns.
- ✦ Frontline workers resented the responsibilities for addressing the needs of diverse patient populations. They feel that cultural stereotyping and racism are embedded in the institution and affect their work.
- ✦ For patients, their impression of the quality of care they received was rooted in the way they were treated as members of racial or ethnic groups. They were not sensitive to the effect of the diversity of the staff who cared for them.
- ✦ Available translation services are inadequate with reliance on informal systems. Bilingual employees are often called upon for translation, taking them away from their assigned duties.
- ✦ Staff and patients see biases embedded in the day-to-day operations regardless of lip service to diversity and cultural competence.

The potential for others to perceive managers as playing favorites with staff who are of the same racial or ethnic group may become an issue if job descriptions, performance criteria, and other decisions are not communicated clearly and consistently to everyone. The more diverse the work group, the more important it becomes to demonstrate actions and decisions that provoke reactions of fairness and trust. Employees need to be reassured that any new emerging group will not threaten established personnel policies. Managers need to spend time observing and discussing coworker interactions to determine whether the inevitable conflicts that arise in any workplace are individual differences or a broader cultural issue that demands broader system-wide attention.[9]

Generation Gaps

Another source of diversity for consideration is the diversity of different generations of workers. Also controversial, generational differences have received a great deal of recent attention in the popular press. For instance, based on the definitions of generations defined by Zemke, Raines, and Filipczak[10] as Veterans, Baby-Boomers, Xers, and Nexters, Arsenault studied how each group viewed the characteristics of leaders. Briefly summarized, the results for each generation were:[11]

- ✦ Veterans (born 1922–1943): Value loyalty; believe in authority and hierarchical relationships. Franklin D. Roosevelt and Dwight D. Eisenhower are their ideals.
- ✦ Baby Boomers (born 1944–1960): Prefer participative, collegial workplace with shared responsibility and respect. John F. Kennedy is their leadership role model.
- ✦ Generation X (born 1961–1980): Expect diversity and change, informality and fun, no respect for authority. Believe in collective action. Ronald Reagan and Bill Gates are examples of leaders respected as change agents.
- ✦ Nexters (born 1981–2000): Prefer a polite relationship with authority and want leaders to pull people together. Believe in collective action and a will to change things. Optimistic and confident with pride in civic duty. Expect ambitious and determined leaders like Tiger Woods and Bill Clinton.

Managers need to determine the potential value of the recognition of generational differences and their effects on work in health care. Identification of ways to build on the strengths of each group may be the key to reducing another source of potential conflict among coworkers. See Activity 1.6.

ACTIVITY 1.6
STAFFING

As the only physical therapist in Shady Pines Nursing Home, Bob Crawford has been called to a meeting by the administrator with the Director of Nursing, the occupational therapist (OT), and the part-time speech-language pathologist. The agenda is to brainstorm ideas to address the increasing tensions among the staff about patient schedules, responsibilities for patient care, cooperation between nursing and rehab, and what are perceived to be unfair management decisions about salaries and scheduling vacations.

About 85% of the certified nursing assistants (CNAs) are Haitian. About 60% of the LPNs are African American, the RNs and all of the therapists and the administrator are white. The PT assistant is Puerto Rican and the two OT assistants are Jamaican. The administrator is in her early 30s but everyone else at the meeting is in their 50s.

The patients who are permanent residents represent a wide range of ethnic groups but less than 10% are people of color and only 1% is Spanish speaking. The short-term residents, who are admitted for rehab and typically discharged in a few weeks, are predominantly of the Jewish faith.

In groups, brainstorm ideas for decreasing the tension in this nursing home.

Financial Issues for Mid-Level Managers

A potential misconception about mid-level managers is that they need a master of business administration (MBA) to function effectively because of their financial responsibilities. It is more likely that their financial responsibilities are limited to completion of reports and requests during the organization's budgeting process. This requires more negotiation than financial skills to influence budget decisions that are not really the responsibility of mid-level managers. Typically, requests for capital equipment, and maybe even supplies, must be approved by, at the least, the next in command.

Perhaps more importantly, mid-level managers *are* expected to track and understand income and expenses for their units. They need a level of proficiency to identify and analyze trends and flukes in daily patient care data that must be explained to their bosses. Justification of bonuses and other performance rewards for their employees may be driven by the ability to translate the numbers into action vertically in both directions. Solo practitioners who also are the executive managers for their own businesses typically rely on accountants or business financial experts to assist them with the money management of their businesses. These practitioners need to know enough to have discussions for decision making with these experts.

Implementation of Plans

The other skill that mid-level managers are held accountable for is the implementation of the many subdecisions that are generated by the plans laid out by executives in upper management. The major reason that these broad plans fail to be implemented is because the implementers are not adequately supervised in the sequence of tasks that must be completed to achieve an outcome.[12]

Organizing these tasks in health care falls to mid-level managers. After clarifying and sequencing the tasks, managers need to guide the implementation process. Adapting modifications necessitated by ongoing change, which seems to be *the* standard operating procedure for health care, is a major challenge for mid-level managers. At the same time, changes such as new community (market) demands, new technology that changes the nature of work, and planning for growth are what make managerial work exciting and unpredictable.

Managers and Patients

The financial bottom line of an organization must be considered in the context of the *real* bottom line—the health and satisfaction of the community it serves. The implementation of plans that managers supervise are all related to the delivery of patient care, the most critical management responsibility in health care.

Most managers in health care are at least one step removed from the direct patient care provided by the practitioners they supervise. This creates an important patient-practitioner-manager triad that may be viewed from Anderson's framework for understanding service organizations.[13] For instance, one of Anderson's propositions is that an employee's perception of being treated unfairly and unjustly may lead to poor work performance, which then leads to less than satisfactory customer satisfaction. When the manager–employee relationship is good, so are work outcomes, and so, it follows, are positive patient outcomes. Any small change in the manager-practitioner relationship may have a huge influence on the employee's relationship with a patient. In other words, the patient-provider relationship mirrors the provider-manager relationship.

When things are not going well, the frustration and dissatisfaction of an employee may be sensed as a discomfort by the patient. Health care is emotional labor in which workers perform the work and manage the work processes as well. Unlike other industries, the patient is part of the production, hence the complex linkage that occurs among patients, providers, and managers.[13]

Although mid-level managers often find their interactions with their staffs positive and rewarding, it is the result of those interactions, their indirect influence on patient care, which remains the true source of their satisfaction. It is with the mid-level manager that all of the communication, coordination, and collaboration efforts come together to provide important services to patients. These services that they receive become the measure of quality for patients.

This manager-practitioner-patient triad makes health-care managers different from managers in other industries. Because they manage services that are intangible, nonstandardized, and produced and consumed simultaneously, it is difficult to measure managerial success. Even determining what is a good day is difficult when there is so much gray rather than black-and-white measures of the results of their efforts. Identification of these measures of success is important to establish. Avoiding the tendency to define the work only by what can be measured demands attention. See Activity 1.7.

Executive Managers in Health Care

Many managers who come from clinical disciplines may feel that mid-level management is as far as they would like to reach beyond patient care. Others may aspire to executive positions but realize that these career moves create such a huge gap between them and patients, that they no longer feel part of their professional disciplines. This reluctance of clinicians to move up in a health-care organization may be the reason that people who hold management degrees but lack patient care experience often hold executive positions in health care.

Typically, the staff in health-care organizations knows who their executives are, although they are not seen on a regular basis. The front office is perceived to be isolated or at least distant from the real work of patient care. Contrary to popular opinion, these hidden executives are not the ultimate decision makers. Rather, they are the agents of their governing boards. They design the structures and implement the processes needed to support decisions that are made by all stakeholders in the organization.

Perhaps an even more important executive responsibility is running the collateral organization—that group of task forces, committees, and ad hoc groups that are formed to bring to the table different perspectives on issues for discussion. The purpose of this organization within an organization is to address common problems in the accountability chains so that conflict and confusion are diffused. Some of them are formed to address a particular problem and others are formed as long-standing committees. Executives are responsible for identifying membership in these groups to work out the details of implementing strategic decisions.[14]

The challenges for many executives in health care is that they are typically *not* health professionals who are managing health professionals who have their own ideas of how health care should be run from a clinical rather than business perspective. Clinicians may become resentful because of their perception that nonhealth-professional bosses do not know how patient care works, although the ability of executives to see and react to the big picture of health care may be a far more important skill set.[2] Because health care has become a complex business, it is no surprise that the selection of executives in all types of health-care settings has shifted from physicians and nurses to professional managers without patient care experience.

On the other hand, at the least, there needs to be some type of executive partnership with clinical professionals because of the nature and importance of the business. In some health-care settings, for example, executives relate to physicians as customers of the organization, whereas in others they are treated as equal partners in the business of health care. The reality is that regardless of the organizational relationship between executives and physicians, patients often think hospitals and the physicians treating them are the same entity. The melding and coordinating of the business and clinical prongs of health care may create the tension between executive clinical managers and executive business managers. They are very dependent on each other in order to provide the right care at the right place at the right time.

Regardless of the size or type of health-care setting, Ross argues that executive management boils down to three basic duties that do not change despite the challenges at any given time in health care, although the degree of responsibility may change from setting to setting. These duties are:[15]

✦ Increasing efficiency and financial stability through human resources, financial management, cost accounting, data collection and analysis, strategic planning, marketing, etc.

✦ Providing a basic social service—care of dependent people when they are most vulnerable.

✦ Maintaining the moral and social order of their organizations by advocating for patients, serving as arbitrator when there are competing values, and acting as the intermediary for the various professional groups.

These duties often conflict and contradict each other in a continually changing environment. Costs that increase as funding decreases, and patient demands that increase while the supply of health-care workers diminishes are part of the ongoing balancing act of health-care executives. However, the payoff for executives is that all of their hard, complicated work results in the satisfaction of helping individuals and their communities as a whole, albeit from an indirect, distanced, invisible, and often unappreciated position within health care.

Conclusion

Physical therapists and other health professionals may easily identify many opportunities for managerial opportunities in any type of health-care organization. Many of the communication and people skills that are required for patient care form a strong foundation for most of the responsibilities of managers. This realization may be the first step for many clinicians in determining their interest in shifting from patient care to broader managerial responsibilities for patient care.

REFERENCES

1. Lombardi DN. *Handbook for the New Health Care Manager: Practical Strategies for the Real World.* San Francisco, CA: Jossey-Bass/AHA Press Series; 2001.
2. Haddock CC, McLean RA, Chapman RC. *Careers in Healthcare Management: How to Find Your Path and Follow it.* Chicago, IL: Health Administration Press; 2002.
3. Morton-Cooper A, Palmer A. *Mentoring, Preceptorship, and Clinical Supervision.* 2nd ed. Malden, MA: Blackwell Science Ltd; 2000.
4. Kane-Urrabazo C. Management's role in shaping organizational culture. *Journal of Nursing Management.* 2006;14:188–194.
5. Magretta J, Stone N. *What Management Is: How It Works and Why It's Everyone's Business.* New York, NY: The Free Press; 2002.
6. Griffith JR, White K. *The Well-Managed Health Care Organization.* 5th ed. Chicago, IL: Health Administration Press; 2002.
7. Shortell SM. *Remaking Health Care in America: Building Organized Delivery Systems.* San Francisco, CA: Jossey-Bass; 2000.
8. Tongue JR, Epps HR, Forese LL. Communication skills for patient-centered care: Research-based, easily learned techniques for medical interviews that benefit orthopaedic surgeons and their patients. *Journal of Bone and Joint Surgery-American Volume.* 2005;87-A:652-658.
9. Aries NR. Managing diversity: The differing perceptions of managers, line workers, and patients. *Health Care Management Review.* 2004;29:172–180.
10. Zemke R, Raines C, Filipczak G. *Generations at Work: Managing the Clash of Veterans, Boomers, Xers, and Nexters in Your Workplace.* New York, NY: AMACOM; 2000.
11. Arsenault PM. Validating generational differences: A legitimate diversity and leadership issue. *The Leadership and Organization Development Journal.* 2004;25. Available at: http://www.emeraldinsight.com/0143-7739.htm. Accessed May 1, 2007.
12. Pechlivanidis P, Katsimpra A. Supervisory leadership and implementation phase. *The Leadership and Organization Development Journal.* 2004;25. Available at: http://www.emeraldinsight.com/0143-7739.htm. Accessed May 1, 2007.
13. Anderson JR. Managing employees in the service sector: A literature review and conceptual development. *Journal of Business and Psychology.* 2006;20:501–523.
14. Corrigan JM, Eden J, Smith BM. *Leadership by Example: Coordinating Government Roles in Improving Health Care Quality (Quality Chasm Series).* Washington, DC: National Academies Press; 2003.
15. Ross A, Wenzel FJ, Mitlyng JW. *Leadership for the Future: Core Competencies in Healthcare.* Chicago, IL: Health Administration Press; 2002.

Chapter 2

Health-Care Organizations and Physical Therapy

Learning Objectives

- Identify the artifacts of organizational culture.
- Determine the characteristics of the culture of health care.
- Determine the relationships among the levels of intercultural interactions and communication.
- Compare in-groups and out-groups and relate them to subcultures.
- Determine the culture of the physical therapy profession.
- Identify the interaction of professional and organizational cultures.
- Compare formal and informal socialization processes.
- Determine the importance of socialization in organizations.
- Determine managerial strategies for dealing with dramatic changes in an organization's culture.
- Discuss the key milestones in the development of organizational theory.
- Compare the types and structures of health-care organizations and physical therapy practices.
- Distinguish administration from management.
- Apply the Massachusetts Institute of Technology's (MIT) manifesto on the future of organizations to health-care organizations.
- Discuss salient issues in contemporary health-care organizations.
- Develop a worksheet for analysis of organizations.

Introduction

Many physical therapists accept managerial positions by investigating motivating factors, such as high starting salaries and good benefits, perfect location, and interesting job assignments. Not as many people spend time to understand how the organization that they are about to join works. This lack of understanding may result in an uncomfortable push and pull between the organization's need to socialize their employees to conform to the organization and the employees' need for the organization to conform to them.

Employees should not be surprised if potential employers ask for completion of a pre-employment assessment to increase their chances of a good match with potential applicants. At the same time, potential employees need to do their homework so that they are equally prepared for one of the most important decisions people make—where to work. This chapter provides a view of health organizations that may contribute to this understanding in a practical way. For instance, activities lead to the systematic development of a worksheet valuable for learning about organizations for job selection decisions or for improving job satisfaction.

Anyone who has worked for any type of organization, or has heard other people discuss their work, knows that dissonance between what one anticipates a job to be and what it actually is consumes a great deal of the attention of employers and employees. The better the pre-employment match, the less energy spent on the socialization required to reduce the conflict behind an employer explaining, "this is just how we do it here," and an employee's asking, "why on earth are we doing this?" More energy will then be available for the important matters of an organization—accomplishment of its common goal or purpose.

Organizational Culture

A good starting point for the investigation of an organization is culture. Culture is defined for this purpose as the shared attitudes, experiences, beliefs, and values of a group (an organization for instance). Culture also may be expressed as "the way we do it here" or "the rules of the game." It is best to think of an organization *as* a culture rather than to ask, what is the culture of the organization? From this perspective, becoming socialized into a new job is like moving to a new country and similarly, a major shift in an organization's goals or business is like living in country that experiences a major political or social upheaval.

The culture drives all aspects of a health-care organization's decisions about its operations and its relationships to its external stakeholders. Priorities that are set and problem-solving approaches employed depend on culture. The subtlety and power of culture as it unifies and controls the behavior of a group or sub-group should not be underestimated.[1] Activity 2.1 is the first step in developing a strategy for collecting information about a culture—particularly an organization's culture. The exercise may be useful in going beyond the usual interview questions that are developed in preparation for important career decisions, particularly for health professionals as they transition to new management roles.

Intercultural Communication in Organizations

Gudykunst's approach to the study of intercultural communication presents a useful model for understanding another aspect of culture—interactions with others. The three levels of interactions in this model may be applied to an understanding of organizational culture. Level 1 interactions in this model are based on the broad foundation of information collected about a culture—values, beliefs, norms, etc. Level 2 interactions are influenced by information about social groups or roles within the culture. This includes the categorizing of people by job title, gender, or age. Level 3 interactions are based on personal information about individuals in the Level 2 social sub-groups. This information determines how much an individual meets the stereotypes of a social sub-group within the expectations of the whole organization culture that they are part of.[2] Figure 2.1 shows the three levels applied to health-care organizations and the patients they care for.

Level 1 interactions are about health-care culture with its common values and norms that generally are related to helping people who are sick or injured. Level 2 interactions may reveal stereotypes that can be found regarding sub-groups such as physicians, nurses' aides, physical therapists, or patients from particular communities or ethnic groups. People in health-care organizations rely on this culture and subculture information in most of their interactions as they cope with a great deal of complex information—particularly when interactions with others are short-term—so that they can predict behavior and their responses to those behaviors. However, when relationships are long term, knowledge about an individual person, at Level 3 interactions, becomes more important in establishing strong patient-provider relationships in health-care organizations.

Health-care managers may need to provide opportunities to ensure that the norms and values of the organization are accepted by staff and that they understand the norms and values of the communities they serve. They also must encourage their staffs toward behaviors that reflect an understanding of the groups of people they commonly care for while identifying the differences and specific needs of individuals in those groups. Gathering information about

ACTIVITY 2.1
A STRATEGY FOR UNDERSTANDING ORGANIZATIONS

Developing a strategy to learn about organizations begins here. As a trial run of the process, look around (or visualize) the room you are in. Create a list (individually or in a group) of all of the "things" in the room and then identify the shared attitudes, experiences, beliefs, and values that you think these things reflect. For instance:

- In a classroom:
  - Are student chairs arranged in rows or do students sit together at tables? What does this chair arrangement suggest? What experiences are being shared?
  - Is there sophisticated audio/visual (A/V) equipment? What does the A/V equipment suggest about the culture that is the school of physical therapy?
  - Is there a flag hanging in the room? Trash strewn about? How is the lighting? Is the room used by students when classes are not in session?
- In a private room or home:
  - How is the furniture arranged? Is the room formal or casual? What does this furniture arrangement suggest? What experiences are being shared?
  - What is the color or decorating scheme? Is there sophisticated technology? What does the content and appearance of the room suggest about the culture of the people who occupy the space?
  - Is there trash strewn about? How is the lighting? How often is the room used? By whom?
- What else do you notice *or experience* when you are in the room? What are your assumptions about this culture because of these observations? In other words, what do the members of this culture value and believe? What are their shared attitudes and experiences? What norms of behavior are suggested by what you see?
- Asking "why" questions helps in this process. For example, why is there no one in the classroom unless there is a class? Why does everyone seem to congregate in the kitchen of a home? If the room is locked between classes, what does it suggest about the culture? Why are the chairs arranged the way they are?

- Next, move on to a health-care organization with which you are familiar. Begin to compile a list of the things you would look for—call it your health-care organization worksheet. Some suggestions are:
  - What do employees wear?
  - Are employees addressed by their first names? All of them?
  - How are patients addressed?
  - Are there oil paintings hanging on the walls?
  - Is there a wall of fame? Who is on it?
  - Do you see the organization's mission statement? Where?
  - What values and beliefs are reflected in the mission statement?
  - Are employees or volunteers at the information desk?
  - Is parking free?
  - Do they have a Web page? What is included?
  - What magazines are in the waiting rooms?
  - What jargon do the patients hear?
  - Is there a warm, homey feeling or does it feel cold and businesslike?
  - Where is the physical therapy department? How is it set up?
  - What else tells you something about the organization?
  - What else do you intend to notice *or want to experience* to gather information on the culture that is health care?
- Compare your list with those of others to develop a robust, thorough tool to investigate health-care organizations. What are the differences among lists? Why?
- Summarize your assumptions about health-care culture.
- How would you confirm your assumptions about the culture at this point?

an individual avoids misunderstandings that may result from assumptions drawn about the importance of cultural and social influences on a particular person.[2] For instance, managers who assume that all physical therapists value evidence-based practice or that all patients with a particular religious belief feel the same way about their rehabilitation may result in difficult interactions with staff members and patients. Health-care workers who treat all patients of a particular social or ethnic group the same may not be able to establish an effective ongoing relationship to accomplish therapeutic goals.

Managers also must be aware that the same three levels of interaction occur among health professionals. Level 1 interactions may arise when some coworkers do not value maintaining schedules or

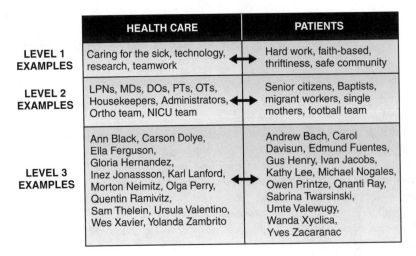

	HEALTH CARE	PATIENTS
LEVEL 1 EXAMPLES	Caring for the sick, technology, research, teamwork ⟷	Hard work, faith-based, thriftiness, safe community
LEVEL 2 EXAMPLES	LPNs, MDs, DOs, PTs, OTs, Housekeepers, Administrators, ⟷ Ortho team, NICU team	Senior citizens, Baptists, migrant workers, single mothers, football team
LEVEL 3 EXAMPLES	Ann Black, Carson Dolye, Ella Ferguson, Gloria Hernandez, Inez Jonassson, Karl Lanford, Morton Neimitz, Olga Perry, Quentin Ramivitz, Sam Thelein, Ursula Valentino, Wes Xavier, Yolanda Zambrito ⟷	Andrew Bach, Carol Davisun, Edmund Fuentes, Gus Henry, Ivan Jacobs, Kathy Lee, Michael Nogales, Owen Printze, Qnanti Ray, Sabrina Twarsinski, Umte Valewugy, Wanda Xyclica, Yves Zacaranac

Figure 2.1 ✦ Levels of interaction in health care.

others fail to follow the expected norm of offering unsolicited assistance. Level 2 interactions may be an issue if nurses rely only on their social stereotypes about physical or occupational therapists. The over- or underutilizing of the expertise of therapists in team decision making may result. Identifying opportunities for Level 3 interactions among work teams in order for them to get to know each other may be critical to increasing the effectiveness of patient care and job satisfaction. Managers in organizations that rely heavily on temporary workers, need to pay particular attention to the interactions of this subgroup at all three levels because of the potential influence they have on the work of organizations.

In-Groups and Out-Groups

In larger organizations, there may be several subgroups (subcultures) that are influenced by the unique nature of their work and the roles of the members in it. For example, in a large hospital, its business office subculture is different from the nursing subculture, which is different from the marketing department's subculture, which is different from the medical staff's subculture. These in-groups in health care are like all in-groups. Their members are expected to behave and think alike, and to cooperate with no expectation of equitable return on effort. They find comfort in the group because of their united view of out-groups—which are all other groups who present no emotional concern to the in-group, and from whom an equitable return for cooperating *is* expected by the in-group. Dividing

into in-groups and out-groups is universal to human nature, and individuals belong to many in-groups based on religion, social status, and job roles, for instance. The influence of an in-group is so powerful that separation or alienation from an in-group may be anxiety producing.[2]

In some cases, physical therapists as a whole may be an in-group. In other cases, there may be in-groups and out-groups of physical therapists in one organization's subculture of physical therapy. Physical therapists who work in the outpatient center of a hospital may consider the therapists who work in the inpatient units as an out-group. They may be reluctant to work in the other setting and minimally interact with each other. The outpatient team may be very willing to assist each other with patient loads demands because of their commitment to each other and patient outcomes. They are likely to agree on many aspects of care and how they do their work. The very same physical therapists, however, may be less willing to assist physical therapists working in the inpatient units unless there was some form of additional reward for doing so. They are less likely to agree on approaches to patient care and patient outcomes. The reverse scenario is also true.

In both cases a manager who disrupts the in-group/out-group dynamics may provoke a great deal of animosity among the staff. Creating opportunity for all of the physical therapists in an organization to be of one in-group may become important for accomplishing the goals of physical therapy practice within a large health-care organization. Managers need to delve into these components of organization culture to determine if the expected behaviors and attitudes of the organization are compatible with their personal and professional views of the world. See Activity 2.2.

ACTIVITY 2.2
PHYSICAL THERAPY CULTURE

Discuss the following:

- Is there a "universal" physical therapy professional culture that spans all practice settings? Describe that culture. For example: What are the expected behaviors of physical therapists (PTs)? What do PTs celebrate? How do they communicate? What jargon do they share? What are the symbols of physical therapy? What are the core values of physical therapy? What are the norms of physical therapy work? How is professional culture learned? How is it reinforced?
- Discuss how organizational culture impacts professional culture and vice versa.
- What are the physical therapy subcultures? How are they different? For instance, is physical therapy independent practice subculture the same as the subculture of a physical therapy department in a large teaching hospital?
- Are there physical therapy in-groups and out-groups? To what in-groups do physical therapists belong?
- How is physical therapy professional culture different from, and how is it the same as, the culture of other rehab professionals, such as speech language pathologist and occupational therapist?
- What will you add to your health-care organization worksheet from Activity 2.1 about subcultures and in-groups? About physical therapy culture?

Organizational Socialization

Although all newcomers to a culture experience reality (culture) shock, they have a strong basic need to belong and three things can happen when the shock wears off. They learn the rules of the game to fit in, they never fit in, or they may accept some of the culture and reject other parts as they attempt to change the organization. The attempts to change it are not necessarily a bad thing for an organization.[3] However, if the organization they want to change is their only potential source of income, some people may face difficult decisions about bucking the system. They may face what seems to be overwhelming odds to change the culture, and if there are no other job opportunities to turn to, failed attempts to change may create a very negative work experience.

The culture shock and fitting in is referred to organizational socialization—a dynamic, ongoing process through which people learn an organization's norms, values, attitudes, beliefs, and their expected role behaviors—the culture. This process is like culture itself—subtle, difficult to understand, yet powerful and important. It is helpful to consider this socialization process as a continuum with *totally socialized* anchoring one end and *no socialization at all* found at the other end.[3] The degree of socialization at any point in time may be anywhere along this continuum. Even when promoted within an organization, to a management position for instance, people must be resocialized as their roles in, and consequently their views of, the organization change.

Socialization is like a spiral that continues to twist and expand as people change, their social roles change, and the culture of the organization changes. Employees, therefore, may have ongoing phases of reality shock, reorientation, and resettling as their organizations change, or as they change jobs. Employees also bring their own personal and professional values and norms to a job that concurrently influence the organizational culture. Reciprocal balancing of these major influences is at the heart of managerial work.

For example, even as a physical therapist moves from one outpatient physical therapy position to another, socialization to the new, although similar, practice setting still occurs. Within the same organization, a physical therapist who moves from a staff position to a position of coordinator or manager is resocialized after being released from his or her patient-provider role to assume a new supervisory role. As another example, an outpatient center is restructured by some corporate mandate and people are resocialized to the cultural changes. This resocialization forces a reality shock that is unavoidable. It takes time to settle into these new situations in every instance, even under the best of circumstances. Likewise, organizations, although not as obvious, also experience a need for resettling as new people join and new in-groups are formed.

It is not surprising that actually doing one's job is typically complicated by the difficulty a person has grasping these nontangibles of organization culture that underlie all work. Connecting the implementation of concrete policies and procedures with the underlying reason or value—the why—that drives that work, may be difficult or confusing. Guiding the process of socialization is the responsibility of middle managers in most organizations. It may be very structured and formalized, or it may be a casual afterthought.

Formal Socialization

The larger the organization, the more formal the process for socialization becomes. New employees take part in individual and group orientation sessions, as well as ongoing employee development programs. The orientation sessions typically include presentation of the mission, policies and procedures, and safety regulations. The development courses are typically conducted to address some particular customer service or program issue. Mentors may be assigned to guide new employees formally as well. In either case, the underlying "whys" of the way work is done may be presented simply as the mission of the organization, and the opportunity to discuss potential conflicts of values and norms is rare. This type of socialization through orientation sessions is more about learning the formal rules of the organization, and the responsibility for their implementation lies with managers guiding people to behave accordingly.

Informal Socialization

The other component of socialization is informal. In larger organizations, informal socialization is sporadic and hit or miss. Responsibility for this socialization process lies more with coworkers as they take initiative to learn how to fit in with each other. This informal process more often occurs among peer employees, rather than between a boss and an employee, as the need for information arises, or when seasoned employees feel the need to set the new person straight (regardless of what they heard from the boss or during orientation sessions).

This informal socialization may be inconsistent with, if not counter to, the information gained in the formal sessions when a particular subculture emerges or loyalty to an in-group overwhelms loyalty to the organization. It may be a truer reflection of the norms and values of the organization than are presented as the written mission and goals.[3] Managers

who understand the importance of informal socialization, and encourage it, are at an advantage in both large and smaller organizations.

Socialization in Small Organizations

In small organizations, formal socialization methods may be minimal. Employees may find themselves just thrown into the work as they learn the ropes on their own, or they may find the informal socialization intermingled in their day-to-day work. Here are two examples of possible scenarios in small organizations. In the first scenario, a physical therapist who has never worked in a skilled nursing facility before, accepts a position as the only physical therapist there. Challenges may result because the formal socialization mechanisms may be nonexistent, or directed toward nurses and nursing care rather than the needs of physical therapists. Informal socialization will be through other health-care providers in the nursing home who may not or may not relate to the norms and values the physical therapist brings to the organization. In the second scenario, a physical therapist accepts a position in a small private physical therapy practice, and has a very different experience. Socialization to the practice—and to the profession—is likely to be more intense and more integrated into the day-to-day work because the entire organization is the in-group.

Effects of Socialization

These formal and informal socialization processes are vital to the organization as it attempts to meet its goals. For instance, the following aspects of work are impacted by the socialization of employees:[3]

- ◆ Cooperation and cohesion of employees needed by employers to get the job done
- ◆ Job satisfaction and job turnover
- ◆ Morale and productivity of individual employees
- ◆ Interactions among employees and with their supervisors

These socialization processes often are expressed as clichés, such as get onboard, join the club, fit in, get with it, in the groove, tow the line, or go along to get along. Although it may be hard to define how this happens, employees know that it does happen with varying degrees of comfort and ease. One of the major factors in the comfort level that health-care professionals experience as they join organizations is their concurrent professional socialization, which may either facilitate or impede organizational socialization. Novice physical therapists who are still defining their professional roles may find they are more heavily influenced by the culture of an organization than experienced physical therapists who are more likely to have strongly developed professional roles.

Although there is power in in-groups that influence organizations, managers cannot overestimate the power of individuals to do their own thing, and their reluctance to change. Understanding the success or failure of an organization and the success or failure of a person in the organization often boils down to the ability to align the values, personal as well as professional, of individuals with the organization's way of doing business. A reciprocal willingness to compromise becomes necessary. See Activity 2.3.

Organizations

Although every organization is a culture into which a person is socialized, not all organizations are the same nor have organizations always been the same. Many theories and models for organizations have evolved, yet understanding organizations continues to present challenges to scholars in a variety of disciplines including sociology, psychology, and business. A brief historical perspective of these theories is found in Table 2.1. Although efforts across the years have encouraged the move away from a controlled, structured approach to running a business, the influence of the bureaucratic, hierarchical model persists. Contemporary models of management and leadership that tend to align with organizational theories are discussed in the next chapter. This section explores three broad categories of organizations with a focus on health-care organizations.

ACTIVITY 2.3
PLEASANT GROVE PHYSICAL THERAPY

Read the following scenario and discuss the answers to the questions.

Pleasant Grove Physical Therapy has been the only physical therapy practice in the small town of Pleasant Grove for 15 years. The owner, Judy Jiminez, PT and her staff (Susan Solomon, PT and Andrew Bilirakis, PTA) have prided themselves on their commitment to serving the community, and especially in their flexibility in scheduling and office hours to meet the transportation needs of their rural patients who travel great distances to Pleasant Grove for their health care.

Judy decides to retire and sells her practice to National Physical Therapy Corporation (NPTC). It is an offer she cannot refuse and she is relieved to be told by NPTC that all of her good, hard work will continue. She has agreed to stay on until a physical therapist from another NPTC office relocates and takes over the practice. Susan and Andrew will become employees of NPTC and are pleased to learn that their salaries and benefits will increase as a result, although they will miss Judy.

Six months later, Susan and Andrew invite Judy to lunch to "catch up" because she has been traveling since her retirement. They report the new "outsider" boss is very difficult in his demands on their hours and imposed productivity goals. They report that many people are going to the hospital in the next town for their physical therapy although it is farther away. They feel like nothing is the same.

If you were Judy, what would you say to Susan and Andrew? Are their reactions to the changes in Pleasant Grove Physical therapy typical? What values and norms may have changed? What are policy and procedure issues? What do you expect the outcome for Susan and Andrew to be? What formal and informal socialization processes may have occurred?

What other questions, observations, etc. do you want to add to your health-care organization worksheet from Activity 2.1?

Public, For-Profit, and Nonprofit Health-Care Organizations

Regardless of their public (governmental) or private status, organizations share this common historical view of theories and models. Academically, however, private and public organizations are parallel studies in schools of business (think master of business Administration [MBA] degrees) and public administration (think master of public administration [MPA] degrees). Health-care administration (management) may be academic specialties in these

TABLE 2.1   A brief history of organizational theory

YEAR	THEORIST	CONTRIBUTION TO ORGANIZATIONAL THEORY
1900s	Max Weber	Bureaucratic, mechanical, logical approach. Absolute authority and division of labor. Laborers controlled by rules to reduce their potential threat to efficiency. Tight interdependency among subunits—cogs in a wheel that must mesh.
	Henri Fayol	Strategic planning, controlling, coordinating, etc. Motivating and guiding rather than controlling employees.
	Frederick Taylor	Standardization of work and role of training in factories. One best way determined by experts.
	Mary Parker Follett	Rejected Taylor's ideas. Organizations constantly changing. Focus on relationship of the parts to the bigger whole.
1920s	Elton Mayo	Hawthorne studies. Innate human behavior as important as external motivation. Importance of interactions and relationships in the workplace.
1930s–1940s	Abraham Maslow	Hierarchy of human needs. People have different needs and need different incentives. Need to go beyond monetary rewards to improve job satisfaction.
1940s–1970s	Douglas McGregor Peter Drucker	Theory X (people want direction and security and not responsibility) versus Theory Y (people want and accept responsibility, are self-directed, and seek self-actualization). Each perspective drives an organization differently. Management by objectives. Set goals, establish standards, and determine how well they are met.
	Foundation laid during Multidisciplinary Macy Conferences held in the 1940s and 1950s John Pfiffner & Frank Sherwood	Open and closed systems. Each organization unique because of interaction with external environment and unique problems to be solved that require interacting internal subsystems of processes rather than departments. No hierarchy. Lead to contingency theory.
1980s	William Ouchi (W. Edwards Deming)	Theory Z. Employee loyalty through high morale and satisfaction, which leads to low turnover and high productivity. On- and off-job responsibilities and needs met.
1990s	Peter Senge	Learning organizations. Constantly renewing themselves as extension of systems theory—not widely accepted.

schools or in schools of public health. Private organizations are further divided into for-profit and nonprofit organizations. The study of and the academic preparation for careers in nonprofit organizations may be an area of concentration for people with MBA, MPA, or master of public health (MPH) degrees. See Sidebar 2.1.

Health-care organizations are unique because of particular dynamics that set them apart, such as:

   ✦ their mission of service to alleviate pain and suffering and restore patients to health;
   ✦ the complex, highly regulated environment—internal and external—under which they operate;
   ✦ professional cultures (physicians, nurses, health-care managers);
   ✦ the rapidly changing health-care market.[4]

The distinctions among the three types of health-care organizations (public, for-profit, and non-profit) are less obvious to outsiders because of these common organizational qualities. Their source of funding (legislatures for public hospitals) may be the only factor that truly sets one hospital apart from other hospitals. Funding and profits may be of little interest to patients who are focused on access, quality, and costs when they need health care. For example, most people are not aware of the type of hospital they are in, nor may they have

Administrators and Managers

Although the terms often are used interchangeably, it may be helpful to make a distinction between administration and management. Management is a subcomponent of administration when administration is taken as the broader, general process of organizing people and resources to achieve common goals. Administration lies with executives of organizations responsible for setting strategy that guides decisions about the big picture of an organization. Administration also suggests bureaucracy. Management is about the day-to-day implementation of processes to accomplish the big picture goals. More important than making the distinction is acknowledging that organizations need people to conduct both levels of decision making, regardless of what their job titles may be. In smaller organizations, one person is often both the administrator and the manager. Looking at the verbs instead of the nouns also may be useful. Administer means to impose or formally apply. Manage means to direct, control, conduct, and to bring about.

a choice even if they did know. Except for the obvious governmental, bureaucratic control they may experience in public hospitals, all hospitals seem to be more or less the same to most people.

Both for-profit and nonprofit hospitals (and broader health-care systems) may be present in any community. About 70% of all hospitals are nonprofit organizations, however.[5] The reason for this leaning to nonprofit is related, at least partially, to the history of hospitals, which began as charitable institutions, often with religious affiliations. They were granted special corporate exemptions from taxes in return for their contributions to the community. As health-care needs increased over the years, other nonprofit corporations were created.

The other reason for formation of nonprofit health-care corporations is that they are exempt by law from paying any income or property taxes. In return for this favorable tax treatment, the nonprofit hospitals are expected to provide certain benefits to their communities. This contribution to the community ranges from nonpayment for services provided to the uninsured, loss because of bad debts, the provision of specialized services that lose money

(e.g., programs for people with severe burns), and patient education. Although nonprofit hospitals have received tax advantages that obligate them to meet the community needs, the level of charity care varies, and often the amount of the tax exemption received may exceed the value of the charity care provided.[5]

Conversely, for-profit hospitals are corporations that distribute their profits to individual investors (shareholders) who may be physicians or anyone, including their employees who may be offered stock options as an employment benefit. For-profit hospitals also contribute indirectly to the good of the community through the payment of taxes like any other corporation. See Sidebar 2.2.

In the private sector, efforts to meet these complex organizational challenges have led to two types of large organizational models. The first type includes networks (also called alliances) that may be comprised of independently owned multiple hospitals and other health-care providers (for-profit and/or nonprofit combinations) that join to centralize functions to improve their effectiveness and profits. Member organizations may drift in and out of these networks as their needs demand or members may be included only for selected functions. Health-care systems, on the other hand, are single ownership organizations with multiple units. Systems tend to be more solid than health-care networks because they are the result of the creation of new organizations through mergers and acquisitions. Only about 30% of all hospitals _are not_ affiliated with some type of system or network.[6]

Shareholders and Stakeholders

A _shareholder_ (stockholder) is a person or organization that owns shares of a for-profit corporation through the purchase of stock holdings in that company. Shareholders may be able to vote for the members of the board, take part in other decisions of the company, and share the profits.

Stakeholders are a much broader group because the term includes _anyone_ who has a legitimate interest (stake) in any type of organization. A stakeholder is anyone who may influence an organization or be affected by it. All shareholders are stakeholders but not all stakeholders are shareholders.

One successful type of health-care system has a small geographic focus, a large market share of the health-care business in that limited area, and, typically, nonprofit status. Other successful health-care models include religious-based, nonprofit hospital systems and for-profit chains of hospitals. The approach to the business of health care in these models is to direct their attention to smaller market shares in different markets spread over broad geographic areas.[6]

Contrary to popular opinion, nonprofit status does not mean that those organizations do not make profits. Some actually generate enormous profits. The creation of systems that include both for-profit and nonprofit organizations often arouse suspicion that, particularly at higher administrative levels of employees and among physicians, organizations may not truly "qualify" as nonprofit. At the least, a review of nonprofit status in health care requires some investigation. For instance, executives and physicians may be paid large salaries by a nonprofit hospital in a health-care network or system, although they spend most of their time generating revenue and thereby higher profits for stockholders in the for-profit hospital in the same system. The physicians and executives also may be stockholders in the for-profit hospital.

In the public sector, similar movement to a system or network model has also evolved. For instance, the Veterans' Administration's VISN (Veterans' Integrated Service Network) regionally integrates all health-care services for veterans.[7] They face the same challenges in a more bureaucratic and more poorly funded system. See Activity 2.4.

ACTIVITY 2.4
CURRENT EVENTS

Jennifer Atkinson is a physical therapist who is interested in taking the next step in her career. She wants to investigate management opportunities with potential for future executive positions within an organization. Where would she find information about what is currently happening with health-care systems and hospitals in her area? Nationally? How often does she need to check for changes in this information? Where does this type of information get included in your health organization worksheet? Share sources of information with others in a group discussion.

The Work in Different Organizations

Henry offers some perspectives that may be valuable in comparing work in private and public institutions that may apply to health-care organizations as well.[8] For instance:

- ✦ Is status more important than income?
- ✦ Is the need for income more important than the need to serve?
- ✦ Is it important to make a difference?
- ✦ Is a secure, long-term position important?

Although conducted in the 1970s, the results of a study of business school graduates to determine if there were predictors for their choice of employment in for-profit or nonprofit organizations may hold answers to these questions. The results of the study were that the two groups differed in some personality and value dimensions on several standardized instruments used to collect data. People with positions in nonprofit organizations were more dominant, flexible, and status-seeking than people in for-profit organizations who valued economic wealth more than their counterparts in the nonprofits. The authors suggest that it is indeed important to recognize that employees in different types of organizations may have different needs.[9]

The Future of Organizations

MIT's Sloan School of Management made a major effort to take a serious look at the future of organizations as we enter a period of global change that they believe is comparable to the changes that occurred during the Industrial Revolution at the beginning of the last century. In their manifesto, they present recommendations for action in today's organizations so that they may take a leadership role in averting major, potential global problems in this new millennium. Their recommendations include:[10]

- ✦ Creating new forms of production and new organizations to preserve the world's physical environment.
- ✦ Inventing organizations in new social systems that decrease the gap between the have's and have-not's.
- ✦ Developing processes that integrate rather than balance the work and personal lives of employees

so that success in work and satisfaction with home life are not exclusive.

✦ Identifying and making the goals of organizations explicit.

✦ Broadening the criteria for organizational success to include qualitative measures that address the triple bottom line of organizations— economic, social, and environmental.

✦ Rating organizations publicly so that comparisons can be made for employment and investment decisions.

✦ Promoting the development of guilds from existing professional associations, alumni groups, and other community-based organizations to meet the needs of independent contractors who will increasingly find that they are working in project-based virtual organizations rather than traditional companies.

See Activity 2.5.

ACTIVITY 2.5
WHERE TO WORK

What other considerations should potential managers include in a health organization worksheet? What components of private and public health-care cultures are important to consider? What is nonnegotiable in your personal career decisions? What can you live with that may not be the optimal circumstance? What role does the future play in the development of a worksheet? Do you think the MIT manifesto applies to health-care organizations?

The Structure of Health-Care Systems

Griffith and White suggest that all hospital systems are essentially open systems that transform resources into services to meet the demands of their communities while earning income. Change is a constant, so continuous attention to improvement is the only way to meet the ongoing, increasing demands of stakeholders (shareholders are major stakeholders in for-profit hospitals).[6]

The more clearly a health system is able to articulate its purpose, the better are its chances of meeting these demands. The ongoing effectiveness of an organization may be enhanced with a deliberate, formal plan to answer three basic questions: Why are we here (or what is our purpose)? Why did we select this purpose? What strategy is the best to achieve our purpose?[6] These also may be important questions to include in the health organization worksheet in Activity 2.1.

As health systems have evolved, strategies to achieve their purposes appear to lead to increased industrialization of all types of health-care organizations. Management professionals now direct most of the work of health professionals as physician control of hospitals continues to diminish.[4] Managers in health care, like any good business managers, want to control costs and increase profits. The bigger and more complicated hospital systems become, the greater their need for standardized processes based on scientific evidence to accomplish quality outcomes efficiently and effectively—sounds like a bureaucracy.

In addition to their industrialization, another characteristic of hospitals and health systems is that their organizational structures incorporate parallel hierarchical models—typically, there is one for physicians, one for other clinical service providers, and one for the provision of support nonclinical services. This organizational structure, more than anything else, makes health-care organizations unique and complex. Application of traditional organizational theories and models to these special places is often confusing and unsuccessful as a result.

Boards of Directors

Both for-profit and nonprofit corporations are required to have boards of directors that represent either the stockholders (for-profit) or the public (nonprofit) as they govern an organization. This *governance* role makes it easier to see how boards are comparable with the role of the legislature in public (governmental) institutions. Boards are responsible, in varying degrees of formality and direct responsibility, for defining an organization's purpose and all aspects of ensuring that its purpose is accomplished. How a board is appointed, how it is organized, and how it conducts its work are reflected in a variety of models that are just as complex as the organizations themselves. They are all legal entities with fiduciary responsibilities, but there are differences.[11]

For instance, board members of for-profit corporations are more likely to be paid for their services.

They direct their efforts to dispersing the organization's profits to stockholders, and may rely on lobbying efforts to advance their business agendas. Nonprofit board members are less likely to be paid, represent the public stakeholders in the organization, and direct their efforts to fundraising through charitable donations, grants, etc. The other differences among the boards of directors of organizations are how much responsibility they really have and their relationships to the chief executive officers (CEOs) and managers. Some boards may be intimately involved in the day-to-day management of an organization while others may be widely separated from management as they devote their energy to broader, long-term strategic planning and developing relationships with external stakeholders—a more administrative function. Some may serve to rubber-stamp decisions of managers while others are relied heavily upon for management decisions.[11] See Activity 2.6.

ACTIVITY 2.6
BOARDS OF DIRECTORS

1. The organizational chart of an organization may be very revealing. Select an organizational chart of any health-care system and analyze its components and their relationship. Share what surprises you and what you expected in a group discussion.
2. Select a nonprofit health-care organization that you would like to become more familiar with. Who are the members of the board? Are there any physical therapists? How can you become a member of a board of a health-care organization? Why would you want to be a member? What would you include in your health-care organization worksheet about boards of directors? What questions would you want answered about them?

Other Health-Care Organizations

Specialty hospitals like rehabilitation, cancer care, academic health centers, pediatric, and long-term, acute care hospitals appear organizationally as other hospitals, except their special missions (education, particular populations) set them apart. Although about one-third of health-care dollars are spent on

hospital care,[12] other health-care organizations, such as nursing homes, home care agencies, and community-based pediatric service agencies also are of interest to physical therapists who are interested in management positions. Some of these other health-care organizations may be included in broader health systems. For instance, a designated wing of a large hospital may be a certified skilled nursing facility. Nursing homes and home health agencies may be included in health networks or systems. Integrating multiple levels and types of services vertically and horizontally assists in meeting the needs of the community and increasing their efficiency, effectiveness, and profits. These other health organizations may be nonprofit, for-profit, or public organizations. They may be units in large national corporations, or independently owned corporations.

Comparative investigation of these other organizational cultures in health care is important to managerial career decisions because no opportunity should be overlooked or underestimated. For instance, the roles of nursing staff and the director of nursing, as one would expect in a *nursing* home have a major impact on those organizational cultures. Physician presence may be very different from the central role that physicians play in hospitals. This dynamic alone may be very appealing to managers who seek more autonomy and control in their work, and enjoy the "family" atmosphere of nursing homes. They tend to be less complex organizations although many of them may have more occupied beds than hospitals, and lengths of stays of patients are extended compared to hospitals. Typically, they are divided into residential and skilled rehabilitation units.

The culture of home care is very different from any health-care organization. Nursing again is the profession that historically drives these organizations from the days of the visiting *nurse* associations. They are unique because no setting is more patient-centered than a patient's home. The one-on-one interaction makes this culture compelling for health professionals who like the challenge of relying on their own instincts and patient care skills in the home, as well as the increased responsibility for independent decision making because interaction with other physical therapists is often minimal. This dynamic presents unique challenges for managers in these settings.

Pediatric health-care forms another set of unusual organizations. In addition to specialized hospitals that may have associated outpatient centers, and specialized home care agencies, many charitable organizations support pediatric rehabilitation services along with governmental agencies. Within these organizations, further clinical specializations may occur. For example, United Cerebral Palsy focuses on children with that diagnosis. Some of the Shriners Hospitals for Children may admit children with orthopedic conditions, while others focus on the needs of children who have suffered serious burn injuries. Physical therapy managers should be cautious in making assumptions that "peds" is "peds," when in reality a wide range of subcultures are included in this category of health care, particularly as applied to rehabilitation.

Education Organizations

An extended type of pediatric practice leads many health professionals (particularly in nursing and rehabilitation) to manage health services in public schools. As education rather than health-care organizations, managers must pay particular attention to the organizational culture of schools and socialization as part of an educational team rather than a health-care team.

Physical therapists may find themselves entrenched in several subcultures as school-based managers. First, pediatric physical therapy is a subculture in the profession that becomes an even smaller subgroup when confined to those therapists who work in school systems. Second, each school district is a subculture in a statewide education system. Each district may include a wide range of subcultures that rehabilitation professionals may identify as they travel among several schools at various levels of education in different communities. Delving into this complexity, which is compounded by intimate interaction with the subculture of each child's family, makes positions in this setting among the most challenging in terms of professional and organizational socialization.

Physical therapists who choose positions in higher education to teach in professional programs face similar challenges as they become socialized as teachers and researchers. They are at risk for inadequate socialization in their new culture as they identify the similar complex interactions of members of new subcultures that are found in health-care organizations. Regardless of the type of institution or unit that it is part of—public or private, religious-affiliated, a school of allied health, a medical school, or some hybrid unit—within each school of physical therapy a further melding of subcultures occurs as faculty with different scholarly and clinical experiences work to reach their organization's purpose and goals. Some faculty may hold degrees in some component of education such as curriculum design whereas program directors may hold degrees in higher education administration, and others hold degrees in the biomedical sciences. The levels of management in education organizations present the same complexity and opportunities as those in health-care organizations.

Other Physical Therapy Organizations

In addition to these organizations, physical therapy and other health-care managers have other private, typically for-profit, employer options such as rehabilitation corporations and physical therapy independent practices. The common factor among these organizations is the general focus of purpose—either interdisciplinary rehabilitation or physical therapy exclusively. Yet they may range from general practices that meet the needs of a broad community to highly specialized services that serve small niche markets. Their cultures may be very different. Physical therapists need to spend just as much energy on learning about these organizational cultures in their career decisions as they do investigating any other employer.

Of course, physical therapists have the option of not belonging to any organization as they directly seek contract work opportunities in a variety of health-care organizations. These therapists are least likely to be concerned about organizations, but they should consider the same issues as potential employees when accepting assignments. Providing contract services exclusively in one organization makes the line between an employee and a contractor a little fuzzier. Unlike the physical therapist who changes positions at the end of each contract period, staying in one organization is more likely to result in increased engagement in all levels of the culture of that one organization, regardless of employment status. However, the contract physical therapist may still belong to the out-group because they are contract therapists.

Physical therapists may also accept short-term assignments through one or more temporary placement agencies. These typically for-profit organizations present the same challenges to physical therapists who must gather data about an agency's culture, structure, and contractual arrangements with health-care organizations for placement of physical therapists and other health-care professionals. See Activities 2.7 and 2.8.

ACTIVITY 2.7
HEALTH ORGANIZATION WORKSHEET

Take the opportunity to update your worksheet from Activity 2.1 to include specific information you should gather on physical therapy services and practices. Identify all of the subcultures and/or in-groups that physical therapists may be part of in health care.

ACTIVITY 2.8
AMERICAN PHYSICAL THERAPY ASSOCIATION—APTA

Professional organizations are also a unique type of organization. Analyze the organizational components of the APTA. How would you describe it? How is it funded? Does the Board of Directors of the APTA serve the same purpose as the boards of directors in hospitals? What recommendations do you have for changing its organizational structure? What do you think about the APTA functioning as a guild as suggested in the MIT manifesto?

Contemporary Issues in Health-Care Organizations

The following issues are important to all health-care organizations, including those that are exclusively devoted to physical therapy services. Methods for addressing quality and safety processes will be specifically addressed in Section 2 of this text, but an overview of the salient problems to be addressed by managers are presented here.

Safety and Quality

The National Coalition on Health Care (NCHC)[13] is a watchdog group of more than 100 organizations that seeks to improve health care in the United States. They are provoked to action by facts such as health-care spending is currently 16% of the gross domestic product (GDP)—equivalent to $1.9 trillion, which is expected to continue to increase at accelerated rates to reach $4 trillion in 2015. In spite of all of these resources, the NCHC argues that our health care continues to be inefficient, poorly managed, and unequally distributed. The economic impact of health-care spending on individuals, employers, and society might not appear quite so outrageous if the impression were that the country—the people—were getting their money's worth.

Another watchdog group—the Institute of Medicine (IOM) of the National Academies agrees. IOM was created to ensure scientifically based, nongovernmental-generated advice to policy makers and the nation at large to improve health.[14] It recently conducted two very important studies suggesting that not only is the quality of health care highly questionable, but it also is dangerous to many people. For instance, in their report, *To Err is Human: Building a Safer Health System*[15] they report that more people die in a given year from preventable adverse events in hospitals alone than die from motor vehicle accidents, or breast cancer, or AIDS. Many of these errors are related to health-care culture and how health-care organizations are organized and managed rather than incompetence or carelessness of individuals. For instance, these terrible outcomes are linked to:

- ✦ A fragmented system in which rigid specialization and powerful influences make it difficult to hold people accountable.
- ✦ Resistance to the movement toward the implementation of information systems that are coordinated for patient-centered care.
- ✦ Limited financial incentives for health-care organizations to improve quality and safety.
- ✦ A medical liability system that is a serious impediment to efforts to uncover and learn from errors.

In the Committee on Quality of Health Care in America's *Crossing the Quality Chasm*,[16] the concern expressed is that the health care provided is not the health that could and should be provided because of outmoded *systems* of the work of health care that set employees up to fail. The only solution requires a total restructuring of health care to address both quality and cost concerns through improved administrative and clinical processes. The Committee recommends that all stakeholders need to support an environment for improvement through:

* Creation of infrastructures to support evidence-based practice
* Facilitation of the use of information technology
* Alignment of payment incentives
* Preparation of the workforce to better serve patients in a world of expanding knowledge and rapid change

The Committee encourages all health-care organizations to adopt six simple aims for improvement of the quality of care. Care should be:

* Safe—avoiding injuries to patients from the care that is intended to help them.
* Effective—providing services based on scientific knowledge to all who could benefit and refraining from providing services to those not likely to benefit (avoiding underuse and overuse, respectively).
* Patient-centered—providing care that is respectful of and responsive to individual patient preferences, needs, and values and ensuring that patient values guide all clinical decisions.
* Timely—reducing waits and sometimes-harmful delays for both those who receive and those who give care.
* Efficient—avoiding waste, including waste of equipment, supplies, ideas, and energy.
* Equitable—providing care that does not vary in quality because of personal characteristics such as gender, ethnicity, geographic location, and socioeconomic status.

Health-Care Organizational Ethics

Another contemporary issue is ethics in health care, particularly as health care moves toward domination by managerial rather than health professionals. Boyle has identified ethical challenges faced by all stakeholders in health care, which have become increasingly complex. Generally, these challenges arise when organizations do not apply their values consistently in decision making. These important organizational values include integrity, honesty, fairness, respect for others, promise keeping, and prudence. If employees feel that they are unsupported, undermined, or discouraged from pursing

good works that are based on these values, then cynicism, poor morale, and even shame may result.[4]

Boyle lists some examples of potential breaches of organizational ethics that may result if the eye of the organization is on tangible, monetary goals rather than goals related to care of the health of the community. For example, behaviors that suggest organizations may be unethical include misleading advertising, cover-up of errors, acceptance of poor quality, favoritism, suppression of rights, nondisclosure, corruption, etc.[4]

Health-care organizations must strike a balance between their social responsibility to increase profits (which is good) and their moral responsibility to meet the needs of the community (which is good). How best to pursue these often conflicting, yet equally noble objectives is the difficulty. What is the organization's moral compass and who is responsible for charting its course become critical questions. To be successful—ethically—organizations must first deeply value the importance of caring for the sick and injured, and live by these values at all costs. Second, they also must have processes in place to deal with the inevitable conflicts that arise from the good versus good decisions that arise from living those values.[17] Some may argue if an organization is successful in this process to address their moral obligations, all other successes, including financial growth, will follow without much difficulty.

Ending this chapter with questions about values as it began with questions about culture – the foundation of which is values—emphasizes the importance of values in organizations, and in the work of health professionals. The activities suggested in this chapter should have led to the beginning of a worksheet for analysis of these important aspects of health-care organizations that profoundly influence one's professional development. Take this final opportunity to add items about these issues and refine the worksheet from Activity 2.1. Engage in a group discussion for further development of this important tool.

Conclusion

Developing a strategy for understanding an organization is important for potential managers as well as people who have already been socialized in an organization. For many professionals, reconciling conflicts that may arise when professional socialization clashes with the socialization process of the organizations they join is a disturbing and difficult experience. Having tools available to identify these potential conflicts to decide where compromises can be comfortably made is important for all health professionals, but particularly important for those who transition to management positions.

REFERENCES

1. Ott JS. *The Organizational Culture Perspective*. Chicago, IL: Dorsey Press; 1989.
2. Gudykunst WB. *Bridging Differences: Effective Intergroup Communication*. 3rd ed. Thousand Oaks, CA: Sage Publications; 1998.
3. Klausner M, Groves MA. Organizational socialization. In Farazmand A, ed. Modern Organization: Theory and Practice, 2nd ed. Westport, CT: Praeger; 2002, p 207.
4. Boyle P, DuBose ER, Ellingson SJ, et al. *Organizational Ethics in Health Care: Principles, Cases, and Practical Solutions*. San Francisco, CA: Jossey-Bass; 2001.
5. Feldstein PJ. *Health Policy Issues: An Economic Perspective*. Washington, DC: Health Administration Press; 2003.
6. Griffith JR, White K. *The Well-Managed Health Care Organization*. 5th ed. Chicago, IL: Health Administration Press; 2002.
7. United States Department of Veterans Affairs. Facilities directory and locator. Available at: http://www1.va.gov/directory/guide/division_flsh.asp?dnum=1. Accessed March 3, 2007.
8. Henry N. Public, nonprofit, and private organizations: Similarities and differences. In: Farazmand A, ed. *Modern Organizations: Theory and Practice*. 2nd ed. Westport, CT: Praeger Publications; 2002, p 3.
9. Rawls JR, Ullrich RA, Nelson OT. A comparison of managers entering or reentering the profit and nonprofit sectors. *Academy of Management Journal*.18:616–623, 1975. Available at: http://www/jstpr.org. Accessed February 21, 2007.
10. Malone T, Ancona D, Bailyn L, et al. *What Do We Really Want? A Manifesto for the Organizations of the 21st Century*. Cambridge, MA: Massachusetts Institute of Technology; 1999.
11. McNamara C. Free complete toolkit for boards. Available at: http://www.managementhelp.org/boards/boards.htm. Accessed February 25, 2007.
12. Center for Medicare & Medicaid Services. National health expenditures—highlights. Available at: http://www.cms.hhs.gov/NationalHealthExpendData/downloads/highlights.pdf. Accessed February 25, 2007.
13. National Coalition on Health Care. Health insurance costs. Available at: http://www.nchc.org/facts/cost.shtml. Accessed March 4, 2007.
14. Institute of Medicine. About the Institute of Medicine. Available at: http://www.iom.edu/CMS/3239.aspx. Accessed March 4, 2007.
15. Kohn LT, Corrigan JM, Donaldson MS, eds. *To Err is Human: Building a Safer Health System*. Washington, DC: National Academy Press; 2000.
16. Committee on Quality of Health Care in America, ed. *Crossing the Quality Chasm: A New Health System for the 21st Century*. Washington, DC: National Academy Press; 2001.
17. Pearson SD, Sabin JE, Emanuel EJ. *No Margin, no Mission: Health-Care Organizations and the Quest for Ethical Excellence*. New York, NY: Oxford University Press; 2003.

Chapter 3

Leadership, Management, and Physical Therapy

Learning Objectives

+ Identify major milestones in the development of leadership theories.
+ Discuss the leadership-management continuum in the context of organizational characteristics.
+ Evaluate a leadership or management source of information.
+ Apply the four perspectives of leadership to selected identified leaders.
+ Discuss the value of leadership dimensions to analyze selected leaders.
+ Determine the link between leadership and influence.
+ Discuss leadership along the hierarchy–heterarchy continuum.
+ Discuss lateral leadership.
+ Discuss women in leadership roles.
+ Discuss leadership in the physical therapy profession.
+ Determine levels of management.
+ Discuss innate managerial ability.
+ Compare the three types of managers.
+ Reflect on the professional development of management skills.
+ Identify the contemporary roles of managers using the competing values framework.
+ Apply Drucker's management concepts to physical therapy practices.
+ Determine the factors to consider when deciding to pursue a management position.

Introduction

Although many serious scholars and a few short-lived gurus have written much, we continue to be fascinated and confused about how leaders and managers really accomplish the goals of organizations. The development of leadership and management theories and models has paralleled the development of organizational theories in the 20th century, which is not surprising because leaders and managers have had to change in order to accomplish the goals of changing organizations. Table 3.1 shows the historical relationship between leadership theories and the organizational theories that were presented in Table 2.1. Notice that management theory does not have a column of its own. Typically, management studies are intertwined with the study of organizations.

Like the study of organizations, the study of leadership and management is multidisciplinary, and formal studies are often specific to a particular type of organization—educational leadership is a good example. This fragmented approach during the last 100 years has lead to various, wider-ranging perspectives. Questions about leadership lack the more solid, common foundation for understanding found in organizational theory.

The lack of agreement about the interaction of leaders and managers in an organization complicates this understanding. Debates continue. For instance, can a leader and a manager be the same person? Is everyone, at some level, a manager? Is everyone a potential leader? Are leaders born or made? Clarification may begin by looking at the Latin origins of the words. Lead is derived from the Latin for

TABLE 3.1 Timetable of the development of organization, management, and leadership theories[1,2]

ORGANIZATION/ MANAGEMENT THEORIES	PERIOD	SCHOOLS OF LEADERSHIP AND THEIR RESEARCHERS	KEY POINTS
Bureaucratic, mechanical, logical approach. Absolute authority and division of labor and laborers controlled by rules to reduce their potential threat to efficiency. Strategic planning, controlling, coordinating, etc. Motivating and guiding rather than controlling employees. One best way determined by experts. Organizations constantly changing. Focus on relationship of the parts to the bigger whole. Hawthorne studies. Innate human behavior as important as external motivation. Importance of interactions and relationships in the workplace.	Early 20th century	Trait (generally accepted concept)	Great Man Theory. Characteristics of leaders that make them different from nonleaders. Leaders are born not made.
Hierarchy of human needs. People have different needs and need different incentives. Need to go beyond monetary rewards to improve job satisfaction. Theory X (people want direction and security and not responsibility) versus Theory Y (people want and accept responsibility, are self-directed, and seek self-actualization). Management by objectives.	1950s	Behavioral Lewin & Lippitt Katz, Maccoby, Gurin, Floor Stogdill and Coons Blake and Mouton	Focus on behaviors of leaders and how they treated followers. For example: democratic versus autocratic, and employee-oriented versus production-oriented. Basis of future models.
Open and closed systems. Each organization unique because of interaction with external environment and unique problems to be solved that require interacting internal subsystems of processes rather than departments. No hierarchy. Led to contingency theory.	1960s and 1970s	Contingency Fiedler House Kerr and Jermier Vroom and associates Relational School Dansereau, Graen, Haga Graen, Uhl-Bien, Scandura	Leadership effectiveness is dependent on factors, such as leader–member relations, task structure, and the position of power of the leader. Leadership is situational and style needs to match the situation. Includes path–goal theory, which creates barrier-free paths to get followers to the goals of the organization. Led to substitute-for-leadership theory, which identifies conditions under which leadership is unnecessary such as follower capabilities and clear organizational systems and procedures. Based on Vertical Dyad Linkage Theory, which is now Leader–Member Exchange (LMX) theory. In LMX, high-quality relationships (based on trust and mutual respect) generate more positive outcomes than low-quality relationships (based on satisfying contractual relations).
Theory Z. Employee loyalty through high morale and satisfaction, which leads to low turnover and	1970s and 1980s	Skeptics of Leadership Eden and Leviatan Rush, Thomas, Lord	Whether leaders made any difference was the question. Concluded that what leaders do is largely irrelevant. Evaluations of leaders really reflect attributions that followers make to

TABLE 3.1   Timetable of the development of organization, management, and leadership theories—cont'd

high productivity. On- and off-job responsibilities and needs met.		Calder, Meindl, Ehrlich Information-Processing Lord, Foti, De Vader Wofford, Goodwin, Whittington	understand outcomes. Leads to leap in research on leadership. Leader is legitimized when his or her characteristics match the expectation that followers have of the leader. Led to theory that cognition is related to behavior that in 2000s.
		The New Leadership (neocharismatic/ transformational/ visionary) Bass and associates Bennis and Nanus	Renewed interest in trait school and charisma. Transformational leaders are idealized (charismatic), visionary, inspiring leaders who get followers to transcend their interests for the greater good. As opposed to transactional leaders in which there is mutual exchange of costs and benefits between leaders and followers through rules, procedures, and bureaucratic authority.
Learning organizations. Constantly renewing them as extension of systems theory—not widely accepted.	1990s	Contemporary Kouzes and Posner Ekvall Nanus Sternberg Greenleaf Collins Argyris and Schon Senge Block	Leaders seek challenges, take risks, seek change, anticipate the future, and deal with uncertainty. Servant leaders who help others. Humility and will needed for organizations to transition to greatness. Big-picture flexibility. Learning imperative. Stewardship: the orderly distribution of power through service rather than control.

Source: Adapted from Antonakis J, Cianciolo AT, Sternberg RJ. Leadership: Past, present, and future. In Antonakis J, Cianciolo AT, Sternberg RJ, eds. *The Nature of Leadership.* Thousand Oaks, CA: Sage Publications; 2004, p 3 except section on 1990s, which is adapted from Isaksen S, Tidd J. *Meeting the Innovation Challenge: Leadership for Transformation and Growth.* Hoboken, NJ: John Wiley & Sons; 2006.

legislate and legitimate, and manager is from Latin for hand. Hence, a leader lays down the law and a manager uses a hands-on approach. However, the general public as well as scholars, have used these nouns interchangeably or inconsistently throughout the years to describe people in organizations. See Sidebar 3.1.

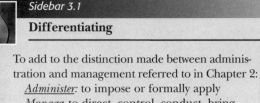

Sidebar 3.1

Differentiating

To add to the distinction made between administration and management referred to in Chapter 2:

Administer: to impose or formally apply

Manage: to direct, control, conduct, bring about

Lead: to guide, direct on a course, bring to some conclusion

A Leader-Manager Continuum

In the face of the confusion and interchangeability surrounding these terms, efforts to differentiate leaders and managers have become the norm. These differences between leaders and managers are found in Figure 3.1 in which leader and manager characteristics or roles are presented as anchors on continual dimensions rather than as "either-or" qualities. For example, the more a person's responsibilities are controlling and executing to reach specific objectives in a bureaucratic organization, the more the person manages rather than leads. Although people may have the management job title, in a more open system, they may be considered leaders rather than managers. Particularly when the attention of the person is directed to fulfilling the mission of the organization, identifying opportunities for new approaches, and pursuing opportunities through greater interaction with outside stakeholders, they may consider themselves, or be considered leaders by others. This continuum may help to understand the grayness and fluidity of these roles.

It follows from this model that whether a person is identified as a leader or manager also depends on the context of the organization. Regardless of the abilities of people to be effective in management or leadership roles, the context (organizational culture) is critical to determining where they fall along the leader-manager continuum and their success in either role. The hierarchical level of the position, the national culture, and leader–follower generational gaps may give rise to, or may inhibit, the behaviors and skills of leaders and managers.[1] Followers really determine whether a person is a leader or manager by assigning that person the designation regardless of actual job title or job description. Leaders are effective only when other people recognize them as leaders, and people expect their managers to be in charge, know what is best, and tell them the right thing to do. They become disappointed and confused when these expectations are not true.[3] See Activity 3.1.

ACTIVITY 3.1
LEADER OR MANAGER?

At this point in your professional development as a physical therapist, consider your skills and interests. Do you lean more toward being a leader or a manager on the leader–manager continuum? Why? If there were a magic wand to make you either the best possible leader or the best possible manager and you were able to select only one, which you would you choose? Why?

The Literature

Information overload in leadership and management literature is a concern. Determining the value of the latest studies and trendy approaches makes it difficult to decide who or what to believe. It sometimes appears that everyone who has managed or been managed or who is declared a leader writes a book about it. Readers must be cautious about books that focus on only one piece of the leadership-management puzzle.

Pfeffer urges people who aspire to leadership and management responsibilities to commit to the same level of expectations for evidence in business decisions that health professionals are expected to value in health care. Reliance on facts rather than conventional wisdom (e.g., to-do lists or rules of thumb) to determine what is true rather than what is new is no less important in leadership and management than it is in the care of patients.[4]

Because physical therapists are professionally prepared for evidence-based practice, they are at an advantage in assuming leadership and managerial roles. The demand for people in both clinical and managerial roles who can find and analyze information is vital for the success of health-care organizations. Facts are more valuable than opinions in the important decision making expected of health-care organizations. The ability to present and support facts may often be a key to success for new managers. Thinking and analyzing take precedence over how-to strategies and slogans. The following criteria are suggested as guidelines for evaluating business materials and courses:[4]

✦ Treat old ideas like the old ideas they are.
✦ Be suspicious of breakthrough ideas and studies—they usually are not.

LEADER ◆——————▶ MANAGER	
Purpose Driven	Objectives Drive
Emotional	Rational
Fulfill Mission	Fulfill Contracts
Do Differently	Do Better
Inspire Risk	Avoid Risk
Seek New Systems	Tweak Existing System
Look Outward	Look Inward
The Big Picture	Day-to-Day Routine
Take Initiative	Seek Control
Confront Order	Maintain Order
Set Organizational Context	Plan and Execute
Transformational	Transactional
Innovative	Stable
Flexible, Supportive	Well-Ordered
Open Systems	Bureaucracies
Do the Right Thing	Do Things Right
Change Things	Keep Things Running
Coordinate and Cultivate	Command and Control
The Future	The Present

Figure 3.1 ✦ The leadership–management continuum.

✦ Celebrate collective ideas and communities not gurus and individuals.

✦ Look at pros and cons of each idea, approach, etc.

✦ Use success and failure stories as a source of evidence but not valid evidence.

✦ Be neutral.

✦ Base decisions and actions on evidence rather than ideas that are in vogue.

See Activity 3.2.

ACTIVITY 3.2
CRITIQUING THE LEADERSHIP/MANAGEMENT LITERATURE

Step 1. Select any contemporary, popular text on leadership or management (leaders or managers). Using the suggested guidelines in the text, determine the value of the text to potential or current leaders and managers who seek to improve their effectiveness. Discuss your findings.

Step 2: In groups, identify sources of _peer-reviewed_ studies of leadership, management, and administration in health-care organizations. Select contemporary studies in these journals for critique. Discuss the findings of each study. How does this research differ from physical therapy research?

Step 3. Compare your findings in Steps 1 and 2.

Leadership

Although leadership is not easily defined, there have been leaders as long as there have been groups of followers who need one to accomplish a common goal. Leadership in society appears to be vital, yet the contributions of individual leaders to the outcomes of particular organizations are nebulous. Getting a handle on leadership is a little more difficult than grasping the roles of managers because _leader_ really is not a job title with a clear job description. Announcements for managerial or administrative positions typically do not say, "Leader Wanted," although what the employer really wants is someone who can lead. Defining those leader responsibilities and measuring the effectiveness of the ability to lead when hiring and evaluating performance is critical. Developing in-house programs to "grow their own" leaders is a strategy used by some organizations, while

others continue to rely on an "I-know-it-when-I-see-it" approach to identifying potential leaders for organizations. Another catchphrase that may be useful is "Take me to your leader." If someone said, "Take me to your leader," to whom would you go to? What position does this person hold? Does the position held automatically make them a leader?

Depending on the circumstances, leaders may come and go, or they may assume varying levels of leadership over a given span. Consider political or military leaders. They may function effectively and without much fanfare, performing many managerial duties until an occasion arises that moves them along the continuum to a leadership role—they rise to the occasion. Winston Churchill during World War II may be such an example. His political career had been relatively mediocre until the war in which he is credited as a major contributor to the victory of the Allies. After the war, his leadership ended rather abruptly. President Jimmy Carter is a reverse example. He was a strong leader while in the military and Georgia politics, yet while President of the United States, he was considered a relatively weak leader. He went on to became an influential statesman who received the Nobel Peace Prize for his efforts in human rights and social development after he left office. Another catchphrase, "timing is everything" appears to be very true for leadership, or perhaps it is time to start a new phrase, "context is everything in leadership."

These two examples of leadership are a good test for the four perspectives of leadership identified by Grint.[5] Activity 3.3 asks which perspectives of leadership explain the achievements of different leaders.

ACTIVITY 3.3
LEADERSHIP PERSPECTIVES

Identify contemporary, well-known leaders. Which of the following perspectives best explains their abilities to lead? Which of the following perspectives is best for explaining the success of leaders in health-care organizations?

Person Perspective. Is it who leaders are that makes them leaders?

Results Perspective. Is it what leaders achieve that makes them leaders?

Position Perspective: Is it where they operate that makes them leaders?

Process Perspective: Is it how they get things done that makes them leaders?

Defining Leadership

We know that leadership is an influencing process (see Sidebar 3.2), which reflects the characteristics and behaviors of leaders as they are perceived by their followers, to accomplish organizational outcomes in a particular context.[1] This definition is similar to the one proposed by the Global Leadership and Organizational Behavior Effectiveness (GLOBE) research project. GLOBE defines leadership as the ability of an individual to influence, motivate, and enable others to contribute to the effectiveness and success of the organizations of which they are members. Based on a study conducted in 1996 of leaders in 62 countries, they developed an instrument to measure the degree to which selected leaders held the values of the leadership dimensions (like continua) they identified in their analysis. The identified leadership dimensions are:[6]

- ✦ charismatic/value-based (visionary, inspirational, integrity, decisive)
- ✦ team-oriented (collaborative, integrative, diplomatic)
- ✦ participative (non-autocratic, allow participation in decision making)
- ✦ autonomous (individualistic, independent, unique)
- ✦ humane (modest, tolerant, sensitive)
- ✦ self-protective (self-centered, status-conscious, face-saver)

Whether it is the GLOBE model or not, it is important to have a framework for determining what it is that makes leaders successful, and how much leaders are really contributing to the overall expected outcomes of an organization. For instance, it is impossible to determine how much and what kind of development leaders may need to become more successful if the organization does not define and measure the roles and efforts of leaders.

Subcultures and out-groups may also have leaders. These leaders also may have a large impact, albeit potentially more negative than positive, on the accomplishment of the organization's goals. Although a direct link between organizational culture (and its subcultures) and leadership is uncertain, if what a leader proposes works, it continues to work because it becomes a shared assumption (a major factor of culture) among followers. Leaders are highly symbolic of the beliefs about the goals of

---

Sidebar 3.2

Understanding Influence[8]

- ✦ Influence is the mechanism for using power to change behaviors or attitudes. Influence produces an effect without direct command or force.
- ✦ Influence is more powerful than direct power because it is a process of acceptance and mutual agreement that results in commitment and good work.
- ✦ When influenced, people feel that decisions made are their choices.
- ✦ Direct commands typically result in discontent and take more effort because employees need to be constantly supervised to ensure their compliance.
- ✦ People would rather not be told what to do unless it is a dire circumstance when they welcome the fact that someone takes control.
- ✦ Influence is a two way rather than top-down process.
- ✦ To exert influence, a person must be willing to be influenced by others, and be open to new information. Of course, to be influential a person has to "walk the talk."
- ✦ People need to be taken seriously by the influencer, or the influencer will be quickly discredited.

---

an organization and they create the culture that drives management.[7] See Sidebar 3.2.

The Leadership Paradox

Another interesting view of leadership is consideration of all of the apparent paradoxes associated with it. This paradox view further contributes to the complexity and the confusion about leadership. For instance, Pfeffer suggests that leaders must:[4]

- ✦ Be in control and project confidence yet realize their limitations because of organizational realities.
- ✦ Be wise yet modest to avoid self-enhancement.
- ✦ Lead, yet get out of the way – no leadership may be the best leadership.
- ✦ Build systems and teams yet take little direct credit for their successes.

It is suggested, of course, that the secret to leadership success is to balance the contradictions rather than choosing one or the other.[9] This balance becomes particularly important as organizations move from vertical to horizontal structures and from hierarchy to heterarchy models (see Sidebar 3.3). A paradox also exists in distributing leadership throughout an organization at all levels when this progressive approach to organizations depends on strong leaders to effect the change.[4] The reality is that organizations are some hybrid along a continuum of hierarchy—heterarchy. Some unit has to have global responsibility for an organization, and even the most rigid bureaucracy devotes some effort to seeking input from others.[10]

Lateral Leadership

The idea of distributing leadership throughout an organization is perhaps best expressed as lateral leadership—leading from alongside people rather than leading them from above. Lateral leaders function as mentors and consultants to teams of workers who are typically enmeshed with several outside vendors or contractors to achieve the goals of an organization. Members of these teams may be reassigned as the needs of the organization demand, which means that people have different leaders for different projects. Lateral leaders rely more on teaching and persuasion than directing and controlling. These are leaders who are neither controlled nor controlling, and, in fact, may have no formal authority over others.[11]

Advances in communication technology have played a major role in facilitating lateral leadership. With technology, more people have more information more quickly. The freedom created by access to information enables people to work harder and more creatively in reaching decisions. The more creative, flexible, and self-motivated people need to be, the more decentralized—lateral—leadership needs to be.[12] The idea that no leadership is the best leadership is derived from these concepts. However, larger, more complex organizations need more than lateral leaders to reach their full potential. They also need a leader or leaders whose roles are to innovate, to communicate the vision, and to rock the boat (while staying in it).[11] The juggling of all of these contradictory responsibilities and multifaceted roles is the reason leadership is such tricky, exciting business. See Activity 3.4.

Sidebar 3.3

Heterarcy and Hierarchy

Heterarchy is a system model characterized by an *equal* sharing of power and responsibilities at the same horizontal level of a hierarchy, or a heterarchy can be a stand-alone organization. This model facilitates cooperation, dialogue, participation; and allows different criteria for performance for different elements of the organization. Multiple skills, styles, and types of knowledge are all valued without any particular group or individual having privileges over another. Each unit has a great deal of autonomy, which allows for flexibility and innovation.

Hierarchy is a model composed of layers of heterarchies with power and privilege assigned only to the highest level of the system. In hierarchies, each unit is connected directly or indirectly to the highest level heterarchy. Division of labor and consistency of organizational structures are important in order to be as efficient as possible.

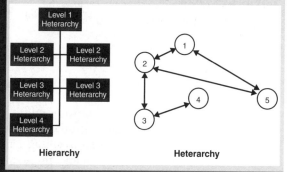

ACTIVITY 3.4
PHYSICAL THERAPISTS AS LATERAL LEADERSHIP

Discuss how the professional education and clinical roles of physical therapists prepare them as lateral leaders.

Female Leaders

From 2002 to 2004, the percentage of women in the executive, administrative, and managerial occupations in the United States increased to 46% from 18%. Some of this growth is the result of the creation of new positions in those 2 years. However, in health care, human resources, and educational organizations, women dominate leadership roles with increased representation in big business as well.[13] The increased presence of women in political positions at all levels of government has been striking, although not overwhelming.

Eagly attributes this recent upsurge to several social changes. First, between the sexes there is a greater equality in the division and amount of labor in housework, whether women are working or not, because the number of children per family has declined. Those women who choose to work, have decreased levels of family/work conflict. Secondly, the educational level of women has increased. Women hold more than one-half of all Bachelor of Science (BS) degrees earned in the United States, and the gap between men and women on science and math scores has diminished. The proportion of women in medical and law schools continues to increase. Third, working women value the same things that working men do such as freedom, challenges, prestige, and power. Like men, they are willing to pursue these rewards by taking risks and being assertive.[13]

Meanwhile, the expectations for leadership have become more feminine. For instance, democratic principles, work teams, participatory decision making, delegation, growth, and more diversity in the workforce demand sharing information, fairness, and enhancing self-worth. All of these demands and strategies are considered softer, more feminine skills. However, acceptance of women in leadership roles appears to remain culture dependent, and women still have a long way to go for acceptance in many organizations.[13] Women see themselves as the hub of a circle with spokes out rather than in a command and control hierarchy. They are expected to become the future leader of leaders because of this softer approach that is based on openness, transparency, consensus, and relationships. They tend to be more successful at leading themselves, leading within organizations, and partnering with other organizations.[14] See Activities 3.5 and 3.6.

Management

This part of the chapter shifts focus on the other end of the leader-manager continuum. The descriptors in Figure 3.1 suggest that managerial roles and skills are a better fit in more traditional, bureaucratic organizations that require more structure and control to meet their goals. Bureaucracies continue to dominate the world of work despite contemporary trends and new organizational models. Because of their hierarchical structures, there are layers of management, which means there are many managers with different roles in the same

---

ACTIVITY 3.5
FEMALE LEADERS

Think about a famous female leader. Which of the following perspectives best explains that woman as a successful leader? How does this differ from your answers to Activity 3.3?

Person Perspective. Is it who leaders are that makes them leaders?

Results Perspective. Is it what leaders achieve that makes them leaders?

Position Perspective: Is it where they operate that makes them leaders?

Process Perspective: Is it how they get things done that makes them leaders?

Which of the GLOBE leadership dimensions do you perceive as feminine?

Charismatic/value-based (visionary, inspirational, honest, decisive)

Team-oriented (collaborative, integrative, diplomatic)

Participative (non-autocratic, encourages participation in decision making)

Autonomous (individualistic, independent, unique)

Humane (modest, tolerant, sensitive)

Self-protective (self-centered, status-conscious, face-saver)

ACTIVITY 3.6
LEADERSHIP IN THE PHYSICAL THERAPY PROFESSION

Identify the past and current leaders in the physical therapy profession. Discussion questions:

Go back to Activity 3.3. Is there a predominate perspective of leadership in physical therapy?

The number of female physical therapists continues to be consistently greater than the number of males. Is this true of its leadership? Why do you suppose?

Are the leaders of the profession the same as the leadership of the American Physical Therapy Association? Why?

organization. Typically the levels are senior (top or upper) management, middle management, and low-level management (supervisors or team leaders).

More recently, middle management levels have become compressed or eliminated in many organizations that have been downsized or re-engineered to meet cost-saving goals. Their major function, as a go-between for lower and upper management became redundant, as computers allowed direct transfer of much more information from workers to decision makers in many organizations. The need for a layer of people to supervise the work of subordinates and generate reports for superiors appears to diminish in organizations with a heterarchical viewpoint. It is important, therefore, in reading management literature to ascertain which level, or levels, of management is being addressed as well as to consider where along the leader-manager continuum the expectations of an organization under consideration lie.

Management itself is a misunderstood concept. In everyday life, we all have more direct contact with managers of businesses and organizations than we do with leaders. Our experiences may be less than pleasant because managers are the "people in charge" to whom we go when things go wrong in the grocery store, a bank, or at a restaurant; so we are already emotionally charged in lodging our complaints. When things are going well, we do not really pay much attention to how a business is managed. We just know it is well-managed when we have no problems with it.

Experiences at work with bosses also lean toward the difficult. In any organization, 60% to 75% of people report that the worst (or most stressful) part of their jobs are their immediate supervisors.[3] On the other hand, the great managers who take care of our complaints and the great bosses who make us better than we thought we could ever be, are those who make great organizations, often without much notice.

It is not surprising that contemporary management naysayers predict that management is dead, and they say good riddance. This eagerness to eliminate managers is compelling if the role of management is limited to the supervision of others—middle management. From that perspective, in contemporary high-tech and virtual organizations driven by self-organizing teams with lateral leaders, the traditional middle manager may be obsolete.[15]

Magretta suggests, however, that all organizations need management because it is not just about supervising others or rungs in the corporate ladder. It is the process for turning complexity and specialization into performance. In this broader definition, the more complex an organization becomes and the more specialized work becomes, the larger the role management plays to effect an integrated outcome. Although there is an expectation that individuals will take more initiative and assume more responsibility at work and that more and more of us will become independent contractors, organizations are still needed to get things done.[15]

Innate Ability to Manage

Management is really one of the most transforming innovations of civilization[15] and it will continue to play a major role in our lives because there is very little that one person may accomplish independently. Management in the broadest sense will endure because it is so fundamental to human nature for people to "organize" to achieve some common goal. Any time the needs exceed the resources available, things need to be managed—whether it is prehistoric hunters and gatherers, family budgets, or generating profits for shareholders. Because humans have always had needs that exceeded their resources, management is really a generic, innate ability rather than the specialized know-how that it has become through the successful efforts of publishers, consultants, and speakers on the circuit.

All people have the basic skills it takes to be managers. All people manage many things at their work without the job title of manager, and most people manage their nonwork lives effectively. Physical therapists manage patient care all the time but patients and others do not call them or consider them to be managers. The skills of managing patient care are basically the same as those needed to manage a staff or special project. Just as they developed their clinical skills to accomplish patient outcomes through actual practice, physical therapists must have hands-on practice to transfer their innate, managerial skills to positions that focus on the outcomes of the organization.

There is a model of management types that suggests that there are three types of managers—affiliative, personal, and institutional:[8]

✦ *Affiliative Power Managers:* Want to be liked more than they want to get the job (patient care) done so they make decisions based on what makes people (staff) happy.

- *Personal Power Managers:* Strong bosses who make employees feel strong. Democratic but turf building and self-aggrandizing so friction between units of an organization (Physical Therapy, Occupational Therapy, Speech Language Pathology) results. They are competitive, and not team players because decisions are based on "me" first.
- *Institutional Managers:* Of service to the organization. Mature and eager to reward performance. They put the organization before themselves in decision making.

It is possible to suggest that these perspectives may be found in patient/client management as well. Relationships with patients also can be affected by the management type of the therapist. Some physical therapists may become powerful in their clinical positions as they seek to be liked and to please their patients, while others may compete with other members of the team to be powerful or successful in patient care, and others may find power by putting the needs of patients before their own. See Activities 3.7 and 3.8.

ACTIVITY 3.7
MANAGEMENT SKILLS

Identify the specific behaviors of physical therapists and managers that reflect the power perspectives of managers.

ACTIVITY 3.8
PROFESSIONAL DEVELOPMENT REFLECTION

Take time to reflect on your current patient/client management skills. What management opportunities have you had in positions you have held? How did they go? Think about managing your day-to-day life. How does it go from a management perspective? Where do leadership and management beyond patient care fit in your professional development plans based on what you know so far?

Competing Values Framework of Management

Regardless of the configurations of organizations—from flat heterarchies to complex hierarchies, certain things need to be accomplished through some processes to reach an organization's goals. Management is this process of affecting groups of people and manipulating resources towards the accomplishment of goals that are beyond the scope of individual effort.

Quinn and his associates developed a competing values framework of management that reflects the snowballing effect of the development of management theories. They have combined the four major historical stages of management (organizational) theories to form the foundation of their framework, which is presented in Figure 3.2.[16] To put the framework in context, Table 3.2 compares Fayol's traditional view of how managers reach organizational goals with the contemporary view of managerial roles defined by Quinn and his associates in the competing values model.

This framework of competing values has received a great deal of attention from researchers and consultants. Managers and others find it compelling because it incorporates the four major schools of thought on management (organizations) into one all-encompassing framework, which links the interrelationships of the models rather than showing them as competing views. The premise is that not one of the four models alone is adequate because each one was developed as one perspective of a very complex construct—managing organizations. Therefore, not one model should be rejected because all four perspectives are critical to organizational effectiveness. The competing values framework is synergistic, dynamic, and logical. Figure 3.2 also reflects the paradoxes of managing through the relationship of the arrows through the center. Managers need to contend with internal processes while in an open system, and balance human relations (people) responsibilities with their fiduciary responsibilities.[16]

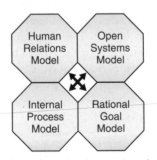

Figure 3.2 ✦ Quinn and associates' competing values framework of management. (Adapted from Quinn RE, Faerman SR, Thompson MP, McGrath MR. *Becoming a Master Manager: A Competency Framework.* 2nd ed. New York, NY: John Wiley and Sons; 1996.)

TABLE 3.2 Traditional and contemporary views of managerial roles in the competing values model

TRADITIONAL FUNCTIONS[17]	CONTEMPORARY ROLES[16]	RELATED COMPETING VALUES MODELS[16]
Organizing ──────────→	Producer: task-oriented, driven, time management	Rational Goal Model
Leading ──────────→	Director: clarifies goals and visions, plans, delegates	Rational Goal Model
Planning ──────────→	Coordinator: scheduling, logistics, designing work, projects	Internal Process Model
Controlling ──────────→	Monitor: checks on compliance of individuals and groups, facts and figures, details	Internal Process Model
*Coordinating**	Facilitator: builds teams, manages conflict	Human Relations Model
	Mentor: helpful, open, fair development of others	Human Relations Model
	Innovator: adaptation, creates change, trend analysis	Open Systems Model
	Broker: external resources, image, reputation, negotiator, liaison, presents ideas to others for acceptance	Open Systems Model

*Coordinating has been deleted in revisions of Fayol's work.

Understanding the competition among the four models for the attention of a manager is the strength of this all-inclusive framework. From large complex bureaucracies to small businesses, such as solo practitioners in physical therapy practices, managers must be prepared for all of these contemporary roles and have the ability to shift emphasis from one role to another as the goals of an organization demand.

It is not hard to understand why many people are reluctant to assume managerial positions. These positions seem daunting and overwhelming to outsiders, and often confusing and unclear to insiders. Hopefully, the competing values framework is helpful in demystifying management so that the rewards and advantages of these important responsibilities are realized by more people. Transitioning from a clinician to a manager is not as unrealistic or unattractive as many people think. Many clinicians find themselves pushed (coerced by higher management or driven by a sense of responsibility to step up when no one else is available) to move from patient care to management positions because they are good at what they are currently doing. Why do so many physical therapists take to it once they are in a management position despite their reluctance? As suggested before, one reason is that management skills are innate, and physical therapists have already developed the softer management skills that are currently desirable through their patient care experiences.

All managers assume all eight management roles defined in this framework. Consider how a physical therapist serves as producer, director, coordinator, monitor, facilitator, mentor, innovator, and broker in patient/client management. The actual day-to-day duties associated with these roles may differ from one level of management to another, and the emphasis on particular roles may shift within the same managerial position. Effectiveness as a manager at any level lies with the ability to integrate these competing roles—to deal with the paradoxes that are the result of four different models of management. New managers need to realize that the cultural shock that occurs in a move from one level of management to another demands some reorientation because of revised duties rather than new roles. See Activities 3.9, 3.10, and 3.11.

ACTIVITY 3.9
PULLING IT TOGETHER

Create a table with four columns and nine rows.

Label the four columns: Contemporary Role of Managers, Staff Physical Therapist, Mid-Level Manager of any organization, Upper Level Manager or CEO of any organization.

Enter the eight contemporary roles of managers along the left side.

Complete the table by identifying duties and responsibilities performed by each level of manager in each of the eight roles.

Place an asterisk next to the _one_ role that you think receives the most attention in each position.

Compare and discuss your table with others to clarify your understanding of managers.

ACTIVITY 3.10
CAN THEY BE PULLED TOGETHER?

What do you think?

Can a leader and a manager be the same person?

Are leaders born or made?

Are managers born or made?

What does it take to be a leader? A manager?

How do organizations determine who is a leader and
who is a manager?

How does a manager become a leader? Vice versa?

manage themselves according, will build successful, productive, achieving organizations all across the world by establishing standards, setting examples, and leaving a legacy of a greater capacity to produce wealth and a greater human vision:[19]

1. Management's task is to make people capable of joint performance so that their strengths are effective and their weaknesses are irrelevant. We depend on management for our ability to contribute to society and achieve our personal goals.

ACTIVITY 3.11
CASE STUDY

Jordan Janko has been a physical therapist for 4 years. She has been focused on her patient care responsibilities, and she is in the final stages of preparing to sit for the board certification examination in neurology. She has worked in the same large medical center since graduation. Her performance evaluations have been outstanding and she has enjoyed her role as clinical instructor for the last 2 years. Her patients love her. She is very satisfied with her position and the organization as a whole, although there have been several periods of major organizational changes. For instance, she has reported to four different people in 4 years because of changes in the organization or changes in the people in those positions. From her perspective, some of these changes have been good while others have not.

Jordan is flattered when the Vice President of Clinical Services (VPCS) approaches her with a new opportunity. She has heard the rumors about yet another impending reorganization so she is not surprised that four new management positions are being created in the rehabilitation services department. The VPCS is offering her one of the new positions—Coordinator of Adult Neurorehabilitation. The position involves the management of a new interdisciplinary team that will include approximately 20 people who will report to her. Many of her coworkers with whom she has enjoyed working will be on the team and there will be some new hires. The VPCS tells Jordan that management wants rehab to become an exemplary model for patient outcomes and satisfaction and it is agreed that she is the only one who can lead the neuro unit to excellence. Should Jordan take the job? What pros and cons should she consider?

Where on the leader–manager continuum would you place this new position?

The Final Word on Management

It is difficult to say "management" without saying Peter Drucker. A seven-time winner of the prestigious McKinsey Award that is presented to author of the best article in the *Harvard Business Review* each year, he is credited with breaking the ground for management's body of knowledge, which includes 25 books. Both practical and theoretical his contributions have endured for more than 60 years.[18] It seems appropriate to end this chapter with a summary of his thoughts on management. According to Drucker, managers who understand the following seven principles and

2. Management is deeply embedded in culture. What managers everywhere do is the same, but how they do it is very, very different.

3. Management's job is to think through and exemplify an organization's objectives, values, and goals so that people are committed to them. Without this commitment, there is no enterprise (organization), there is a mob.

4. Training and development that never stops must be built into every aspect of an organization.

5. Every organization is built on communication and individual responsibility because people

have many different skills and knowledge to do many different types of work that must be pulled together.

6. Just as we need a diversity of measures to determine human performance, we need a diversity of measures to determine the performance of an organization and its continuous improvement.

7. The results of organizations are not within its walls. Results only exist on the outside in the satisfied customer, the healed patient, and the student who learned something and puts it to work 10 years later.

REFERENCES

1. Antonakis J, Cianciolo AT, Sternberg RJ. Leadership: Past, present, and future. In: Antonakis J, Cianciolo AT, Sternberg RJ, eds. *The Nature of Leadership.* Thousand Oaks, CA: Sage Publications; 2004, p 3.

2. Isaksen S, Tidd J. *Meeting the Innovation Challenge: Leadership for Transformation and Growth.* Hoboken, NJ: John Wiley & Sons; 2006.

3. Bellman GM. *Getting Things Done When You Are Not in Charge.* 2nd ed. San Francisco, CA: Berrett-Koehler Publishers; 2001.

4. Pfeffer J, Sutton RI. *Hard Facts Dangerous Half-Truths & Total Nonsense: Profiting from Evidence-Based Management.* Boston, MA: Harvard Business School Publishing; 2006.

5. Grint K. *Leadership: Limits and Possibilities.* New York, NY: Palgrave Macmillan; 2005.

6. The GLOBE Foundation. *Syntax for GLOBE National Culture, Organizational Culture, and Leadership Scales.* Glendale, AZ: Thunderbird School of Global Management; 2006.

7. Den Hartog DN, Dickson MW. Leadership and culture. In: Antonakis J, Cianciolo AT, Sternberg RJ, eds. *The Nature of Leadership.* Thousand Oaks, CA: Sage Publications; 2004:249.

8. Harvard Business School. *Harvard Business Essentials: Power, Influence, and Persuasion: Sell Your Ideas and Make Things Happen.* Boston, MA: Harvard Business School Press; 2005.

9. Lucas JR. *Broaden the Vision and Narrow the Focus.* Westport, CT: Praeger; 2006.

10. Schwaninger M. *Intelligent Organizations: Powerful Models for Systemic Management.* New York, NY: Springer; 2006.

11. Harvard Business School. *The Results Driven Manager: Getting People on Board.* Boston, MA: Harvard Business School Press; 2005.

12. Malone TW. *The Future of Work: How the New Order of Business Will Shape Your Organization, Your Management Style, and Your Life.* Boston, MA: Harvard Business School Publishing; 2004.

13. Eagly AH, Carli LL. Women and men as leaders. In: Antonakis J, Cianciolo AT, Sternberg RJ, eds. *The Nature of Leadership.* Thousand Oaks, CA: Sage Publications; 2004, p 279.

14. Gergen D. Women leading in the twenty-first century. In: Coughlin L, Wingard E, Hollihan K, eds. *Enlightened Power: How Women are Transforming the Practice of Leadership.* San Francisco, CA: Jossey-Bass; 2005, p 1.

15. Magretta J, Stone N. *What Management Is: How it Works and Why it's Everyone's Business.* New York, NY: The Free Press; 2002.

16. Quinn RE, Faerman SR, Thompson MP, McGrath MR. *Becoming a Master Manager: A Competency Framework.* 2nd ed. New York, NY: John Wiley and Sons; 1996.

17. Fayol H. *General and Industrial Management.* London, England: Pitman Publishing Co.; 1949.

18. Harvard Business School. *Classic Drucker.* Boston, MA: Harvard Business School; 2006.

19. Drucker P. Management and the world's work. *Harvard Business Review.* 1988;66:65.

Chapter 4

Introduction to Health Care as a Unique Insurance-Based Business

Learning Objectives

+ Discuss the unique needs and characteristics of patients as customers.
+ Link population statistics to a community's health-care needs.
+ Determine the role of employment and employers in health-care insurance.
+ Identify all components of the provision of health care in a given community.
+ Discuss the regulation of health-care insurance.
+ Compare and contrast types of private and public health-care insurance.
+ Explore online health-care insurance resources.
+ Identify the challenges presented to physical therapy managers by the underinsured and the uninsured.
+ Analyze the health-care insurance issues presented in a case study.
+ Identify contemporary challenges in the payment for health-care services.

The Unit of Business in Health Care

Health care is a business and, in many ways, its management parallels the management of all businesses. Finances, human resources, capital equipment needs, the control of costs, and the generation of profits are just as much a part of the business of health care as they are the substance of other businesses. On the other hand, the business of health care is unique because of its purpose—preventing, managing and curing diseases, and healing injuries—and the complex manner in which health care is conducted and paid for. A patient (and an employer if applicable), a health-care provider, and an insurer comprise the basic unit of health-care business that is influenced by health-care policy. Refer to Figure S1.1 in the introduction to this section to recall these interrelationships and the complexity of health care that health-care managers face. Types of private and public health insurance are introduced in this chapter with activities to enhance the basic understanding of the exchange of goods and services in health care from a manager's or a provider's perspective.

Patients

The business of health care places all of its customers with special needs—patients—in an unusual consumer position. When receiving health-care services in any setting, or when purchasing medications, durable medical equipment, or other supplies; patients must contend with several intervening influences. The simple exchange of money for goods and services in other businesses becomes complicated in health care as patients deal with what their health insurance pays for, preauthorizations, meeting deductibles, and making co-payments, etc. Patients also must determine how and if the rules of conducting business in health care have changed as their needs move them from one type of health-care setting to another, as their insurance coverage for health services and goods changes from year to year or employer to employer, and as they move from private to public insurance.

These special business circumstances are often confounded because people who require health care are often seeking it when they are most vulnerable and anxious—at times of sickness or injury. It is understandable that this emotional state often leads to a feeling of helplessness and frustration with "the system" on one hand and relief when, on the other hand, their health problems are alleviated. For many people, the only major choice involved when they are sick or injured is whether to use health care or not. Once they have decided that they need health care, most decisions about that care are out of their hands. A health-care consumer relies on payers and providers to determine what they need, how much they need, and where to get it. For instance, a typical scenario may be:

1. A person becomes very ill and suspects a virus.
2. That person sees a doctor who has been assigned by the person's health maintenance organization (HMO) or selects a doctor from a list of approved doctors provided by the person's preferred provider organization (PPO).
3. The doctor orders tests, prescribes medications, or makes a referral to a another health-care provider. All of these decisions about what and how much health care to provide are determined in a large part by the preauthorization policies and drug formularies of the HMO or PPO.
4. The person trusts that the health-care decisions made on his or her behalf are the best choices. (Although more recently, a person may "Google" for information.)
5. More often than not, people recover from illnesses and injuries and they are satisfied with the process of health care and its positive outcome—a return to health—without much question.

How the average person deals with health care and insurance depends more on socio-economic and employment status than other factors. See Activities 4.1, 4.2, and 4.3.

Patients Who Are Employees

Maintaining employment status to be eligible for health insurance benefits has been an important decision for many people. This strategy may be less of an option as employers reduce their health-care benefit expenses by reducing the number of employees who are eligible for health insurance benefits. Reductions in force or converting employees to part-time or contract (per diem) status are two such employer

---

ACTIVITY 4.1
FACTS AND FIGURES EXERCISE

Go to the U.S. Census Bureau Fact Sheet found at http://factfinder.census.gov/home/saff/main.html?_lang =en. Make your way to the Fact Sheet for the latest population estimates for the United States.

Create a table with five columns and about 20 rows. Label column one census data and label the rows: Population of the United States; Males; Under age 5; Population 25 years and over; Over 65; Bachelor's degree or higher; In the labor force (population 16 years and over); One race; Two or more races; White; Black or African American; Asian American; Native Hawaiian and Other Pacific Islander; Some other race; Foreign born; Hispanic or Latino (of any race); Disability status (population 5 years and over); In labor force (population 16 years and over); Per capita income (in 2005 inflation-adjusted dollars); Families below poverty level; Individuals below poverty level. Add other categories of interest if you like. Label the columns: Latest Year National Figures; Percents National; Latest Year Local Figures; Percents Local.

Select your hometown city, county, or zip code and complete the table. Are the data consistent with your personal experiences with people in your community? Where are you in the table? Compare the chart for your selected community with that of other communities that have been investigated by others in your group. Did you include other rows? Explain why.

ACTIVITY 4.2
WHAT DO THESE FIGURES MEAN?

Consider each datum in the table in terms of the impact on health-care delivery in the selected community. What is the impact of each of these factors on health-care services in the selected community? How does this information influence the responsibilities of health-care managers?

ACTIVITY 4.3
YOUR OWN HEALTH-CARE EXPERIENCE

What has been your personal experience, or that of your loved ones, with the health-care system? Think about who made decisions and how they made them about your care. Were you satisfied? Share your impression in a small group discussion. Based on these personal experiences, develop a list of factors for managers to consider in the experiences patients have in their organizations.

---

their families. Rather than providing a more expensive broad-brush of benefits for everyone, alternative models allow employees to select less expensive plans with fewer benefits to meet their specific needs. These cost-control efforts often result in frequent changes in the contracts that employers have with health insurance companies. Each year employees must sort through much new information to select the health-care benefits most appropriate for their needs because employers negotiate annually with insurance companies for policies and plans to reduce their costs of offering these benefits to their employees.

The challenge for employees during open enrollment is that the selection of a plan has become very complex. Should they pick a PPO or a HMO? A health savings account (HSA)? Should they have a plan with a high deductible and high co-payments? What is an acceptable maximum annual total insurance payment? Should they switch plans although their current physicians are not on the panel of doctors in the less expensive insurance plan they may enroll in for next year?

People feel differently about this decision process. For young, healthy, single people whose health status is good and who have had very little need for health-care services, these may be casual decisions. Even accepting a position without health insurance benefits may seem of little consequence especially when the salaries may be more without this benefit. On the other hand, a single mother with a complex medical history including a chronic condition requiring ongoing medication, with two children who need immunizations and frequent doctor's visits for ear infections faces a big decision. She may feel overwhelmed by the complexity of options she faces as she attempts to calculate the financial implications of each health plan choice when weighed against the odds of sickness or injury occurring in her family.

strategies. More recently, in efforts to control the rapidly increasing costs of health-care benefits, employers have developed some new strategies. Large employers have begun to offer several different health-care plans (similar to the Medicare Part C approach) for their employees to choose from that are geared to more specific needs and resources of individuals and

Another concern for those employees eligible for health insurance benefits is the ability to afford the payroll deduction contributions for premium payments. Employees may choose to refuse health insurance benefits to increase the amount of their take-home pay to meet other household and family expenses. Even if the payroll deduction is only 20% of the total cost of the health insurance premium, many people cannot afford it. They also may choose individual rather than family coverage to reduce their payroll deductions. Activity 4.4 presents the challenges employees face and the implications for physical therapists.

ACTIVITY 4.4
TYPES OF HEALTH INSURANCE PLANS

There are several types of health insurance plans—HMO, PPO, POS, PSO, HSA etc. Select a large business (maybe an affiliated hospital, a university, or an employer you are familiar with) and identify all of the types of health insurance plans that are offered to their employees. Define the characteristics of each. Rank them according to quality of benefits. Rank them according to cost of premiums and other out-of-pocket expenses. Determine the coverage of physical therapy services in each policy. Which type of plan do you think health-care managers prefer patients to have? Why?

Employers of Patients

Legally, employers are not required to offer health insurance benefits. Historically, the whole health insurance industry ballooned when employers decided that they could not continue to raise wages if they wanted to control costs and taxes on wages, but could offer benefit packages to attract employees instead. Employers also perceived advantages to keeping workers healthy and ready for work, so health insurance was considered a wise investment for reducing sick day benefits. Fueled by collective bargaining units (unions) and competition for workers, benefits packages, however, have become a major expense of doing business.

In addition to these insurance expenses, local governments also may tax private health businesses for their contributions to the care of poor people in the community. For example, a private hospital that does not admit patients with Medicaid, may pay state and county taxes that are used to support the funding of either a public county hospital, or to support the Medicaid payments to other private hospitals who do provide services to people insured under the Medicaid program.

The other related cost of doing business is workers' compensation. Employers may reduce their costs by locating the businesses in states or other countries where workers' compensation laws are more employer-friendly. The cost of workers' compensation insurance is high although states tightly regulate this system. Workers' compensation benefits paid to injured workers also are high so many insurance companies are reluctant to enter the market. This lack of competition among insurance companies creates problems for employers who must meet state regulations for obtaining it. Organized businesses and organized labor are in a push-pull influence on state political processes to reduce the costs to businesses and to increase the benefits to workers. Go to Activity 4.5.

ACTIVITY 4.5
WHAT IF. . .

Discuss the following question from the perspectives of both the employer and the employee. What would change if, effective the first of the year, all employers, except the government (federal, state, local), just stopped paying for health insurance as an employee benefit? Would this action be a good thing for employers? For employees? For managers of physical therapy services? Why or why not?

Providers

Health care is provided in a wide range of different settings that are all some form of health care. For comparison, a grocery store is a grocery store. Although they may vary in size and they may offer different brands of products, grocery stores are all the same with the same basic rules of marketing, conducting business, serving customers, achieving profits, and competing for a market share of the grocery business. Small, freestanding, individually operated "mom-and-pop" grocery stores may be a thing of the past as large corporations with stockholders that control chains of grocery or convenience stores prevail, but they are all basically providing the same goods and services.

On the other hand, the term health-care provider covers a wide range of services. Health care may happen in a physician's office, a large teaching hospital, a pharmaceutical company, a drugstore, or a home care agency, etc. It also may be a private physical therapy office with a solo owner, a chain of corporate-owned outpatient physical therapy centers, or a specialized rehabilitation hospital. Each of these components of our health-care "system" is regulated differently, provides services differently, and measures success differently. These different health-care organizations, whether private or government supported, are all competing for the same limited, ever-decreasing number of health-care dollars through their negotiations with public and private health insurance companies.

The current trend toward health-care alliances and mergers that are developed to capture a larger share of the health-care market, just as grocery-store chains do, should be no surprise. Independent health-care providers may find it more difficult to flourish in health care as a result. These mega health-care business deals often confound the legal status of health-care organizations from for-profit (in which shareholders receive stock and are paid dividends from the profits) to nonprofit (there are no shareholders, they are tax-exempt in return for providing needed services to the community, and their profits are reinvested in the corporation).

These large organizations are typically named something such as Overall Regional Health Care System as they become a major, if not the only, provider of health care in a community. They seek to vertically and horizontally integrate health care so that one large health-care system offers one-stop shopping for people across their life spans, and across their needs for services. They strive to provide for any particular episode of care from the emergency room to home care services and hospice care, while encompassing all outpatient care, diagnostic services, and physician visits in between. Shifting this care from expensive inpatient care to the less expensive outpatient care, as much as, and as soon as, possible has become a rule of doing health-care business. See Activity 4.6.

Individual health-care professionals and the professional organizations that represent them are faced with numerous challenges as the result of the tension created by providing professional services in a business environment. These tensions, which influence the decisions of managers in health care, are presented more in depth in other chapters of this text.

ACTIVITY 4.6
HEALTH CARE IN A SELECTED COMMUNITY

Identify <u>EVERY</u> organization that provides health-care goods and services in the community you selected in Activity 4.1 or some smaller component of it that is a manageable size. Analyze their relationships to each other. Determine if each one is a private or a governmental (public) organization. How much does the total economy of the community rely on these health-care organizations? Where does physical therapy practice fit into this health care? How do the number of health-care providers relate to the number of people identified in each category in Activity 4.1?

Insurers

The means for receiving payment is unique for health-care businesses with unusual customers—patients. Payment for specialized health-care goods (e.g., drugs and durable medical equipment) and the services of health-care providers rarely is made totally out of the pockets of patients. Rather, the providers of both the goods and services in health care are paid, typically, through their contracts with health insurance companies that insure the patients and the collection of co-payments and deductible fees from those patients.

Unlike the restaurant owner who receives the same payment for a meal regardless of who buys it, the doctor, or other health-care provider may receive different payments for providing the same service depending on which health insurer is buying it and the terms of the contract with that insurer. Likewise, patients may pay a different amount for the same health-care goods and services as their health-care insurance policies change from year to year. Because employers are seeking the most cost-effective insurance as an employee benefit, employees are faced with fluctuations in their contributions to the payment of insurance premiums made by their employers, and the amount of their deductible payments, and co-payments.

Health-care providers may have contracts with several different health insurance companies and may need to "adjust" their decisions about each patient with the same condition according to the contract terms and guidelines for the treatment of specific diseases. Because these guidelines seem to be established or adopted by insurance companies inconsistently and arbitrarily, changes require the constant vigilance of managers.

One source of insight into health insurance companies is through their lobbying organization, the America's Health Insurance Plans (AHIP). It represents 1,300 companies that provide health insurance to more than 200 million Americans through private and public employers and directly to consumers.[1] This group seeks, of course, to expand access to health care through insurance by affecting health-care financing and delivery policies, which will help to control their costs (including the payment of benefits) and increase their profits.

For instance, they have supported the continuation of health-care insurance of adult students and increased access of small businesses to affordable health-care coverage. They made improvements in state-managed insurance pools for those unable to afford to purchase insurance in other ways. Health-delivery issues that affect the costs of insurance companies include the wide variations in health care across the country because of the lack of evidence to support best practices in health care, and the number of medical errors that increase the costs of health care.

The call for insurance reform places insurance companies at odds with the National Association of Insurance Commissioners (NAIC), which is composed of the 50 state insurance regulators.[2] The job of state insurance commissioners is to protect the public who are consumers of health (and other types of) insurance by regulating insurance companies so that they are competitive and financially solvent. The NAIC seeks to coordinate the regulations among states. This consistency across states is obviously important to a large, national insurance company, such as Blue Cross/Blue Shield, that must comply with different rules in every state where they do business. See Activity 4.7.

Find the Web page for any state's commissioner or office of insurance regulation. What are the state's views on health insurance? Is the public protected?

Types of Health-Care Insurance

Some additional groundwork on the health insurance business is indicated because, like health care,

health insurance, which is the major source of payment for health care, is also different from any other insurance business.

Car insurance is an example for comparison. Although most people are required to produce evidence of automobile insurance to receive a driver's license, choosing which policy and paying the premiums is the decision of the car owner. The car owner decides how much risk he or she is willing to take, which determines the cost of the insurance premiums. The risk taken is often influenced by the value of the car. For instance, a higher deductible reduces the car insurance premium and may be desirable if the car has been previously owned and is of limited value. Minor repairs to a car may be covered out of pocket, or ignored entirely, thus an insurance policy with a high deductible may make sense. However, if the car is a new luxury car, a higher maximum coverage for damages may be desirable, although the insurance premiums will increase as a result. Few people are willing to risk a high out-of-pocket payment for expensive major repairs to maintain the pristine condition of an expensive car.

In either case, the expectation is that filing an insurance claim is highly unlikely, but the coverage provided by car insurance is necessary "just in case" and for many people, they ***must*** have insurance to drive it. Auto insurance companies' decisions are driven by competition to sell policies to as many policyholders as possible to widely distribute the risks of paying claims. Of course, this competition for the business of car owners is important to controlling costs of car insurance and increasing profits of insurance companies in a market-driven economy.

Private and public health-care insurance companies both have the same business objectives as companies insuring drivers, but how health insurance is purchased and administered is different. To complicate matters, private and public health-care organizations accept payment from both private and public health insurers.

Private Health Insurance

Most people who are employed receive a health insurance policy as an employment benefit—the employer assumes all, or a large percentage, of the burden of the cost of health insurance policies for employees. Until recently, this meant that an employer negotiated with a health insurance company, such as Blue Cross/Blue Shield, without input from employees (unless they were part of collective bargaining units). Employers simply presented the insurance policy to the employees who accepted it without much question, except perhaps to ask the amount of their monthly contributions to pay the premiums on the selected policy. Employees assumed that their employers had negotiated a good contract for good health-care coverage, and considered it a benefit to be taken for granted. Because of the need to control their health insurance costs, employers now negotiate with several insurers and offer a wide range of policies and plans for employees to select from to encourage greater cost sharing on the part of employees.

Other Private Insurance

Employer-provided is only one source of health insurance in the broader category of private health insurance. Some employees may receive a health insurance policy through a union that contracts with an insurance company. Others may purchase an individual policy directly from a private company if they are employed and health insurance is not a benefit, or if they are unemployed. The availability of health insurance policies that are individually purchased like this may vary from one part of the country to another, and there may be more restrictions related to pre-existing medical conditions a person may have and the allowable expenses included in the policy. Of course, finally, a person may choose to be uninsured and risk paying for all medical expenses "out of pocket."

Personal Injury Protection (PIP)

Also of interest to physical therapists, PIP is yet another type of no-fault insurance that is the primary insurance for medical expenses related to motor vehicle accidents. Although private insurance companies provide PIP, states legislate the insurance requirements that apply to everyone who operates a motor vehicle. Activity 4.8 presents the opportunity to review personal health insurance policies.

Government-Supported Health-Care Insurance

The U.S. government is heavily involved in the health-care insurance business. This section includes

---

ACTIVITY 4.8
PERSONAL HEALTH INSURANCE

Look at your own (or another person's) health insurance card and/or health-care policy and answer these questions:

How did you get it?
Who pays for it?
What kind of plan is it?
What does it cover?
What is the deductible?
What are the co-payments?
Does it pay for physical therapy?
Does it pay for a rehabilitation hospital stay?
How much does the policy cost?
How much of the cost is yours to pay?
Who decided what services the policy covers?
Do you have any other health insurance?
Does everyone in your family have the same insurance?
If not, answer the same questions about their other health insurance policies.
In your family or discussion group, who has the best health insurance? Why?

---

the programs available to government and military employees. Entitlement programs are addressed in the following section.

Civilian Government Employees

The government (federal, state, and local) is the largest employer in the United States, employing an estimated 15% of the workers in the country.[3, 4] Civilian employees of the federal government receive health-care insurance through the Federal Employees Health Benefits Program, which includes current employees, retirees, and survivors.[5]

The people who work for state and local governments also are insured through programs in each state, county, or city. As expected, controlling health-care costs is as important to public employers as they are to private employers. Public employees face the same issues in terms of contributions to premiums and choices of plans, etc., which private employees face.

Military Employees

The federal government also insures the health of military employees through the U.S. Department of Defense's Military Health System, which is managed by Tricare.[6]

Tricare was the HMO system that replaced the Civilian Health and Medical Program of the Uniformed Services (CHAMPUS) for its armed forces, their dependents, and retirees. Health-care services may be provided through the system of military hospitals at home and overseas, and through contracts with private health-care providers that are willing to participate in the program.

Veterans

Although they are not employees of the government, military veterans are included in this section because as former military employees, they also receive federally supported health care through the Veterans' Administration system of hospitals and clinics. Eligibility is determined by the need for health care, which is based on the level of service-connected disabilities and the veteran's level of income and assets.[7]

Federal Entitlement Programs

The government also collects taxes through employers to offer health-care insurance in two entitlement programs that were created in the 1960s for special populations—Title XVIII of the Social Security Act established Medicare for the aged and disabled, and Title XIX created Medicaid for the poor, which has traditionally been linked to Aid to Families with Dependent Children (AFDC) in each state.

CMMS

These programs are managed by the Centers for Medicare and Medicaid Services (CMMS or CMS) within the Department of Health and Human Services through contracts with private insurance companies called intermediaries (for Part A) and carriers (for Part B). Moving from the original system in which the government ran Medicare itself, private insurers now are the primary insurers of Medicare through their contracts with the government. The intent was that, like private sector insurance, this would open Medicare to market forces and competition to reduce costs. This potential promise has not materialized.

Medicare Beneficiaries

Medicare beneficiaries include people ages 65 or older who are eligible for social security, people under the age 65 with certain disabilities, and people of all ages with end-stage renal disease. Medicare has four parts. People are automatically enrolled in Part A of Medicare at no cost when they turn 65 or meet the eligibility requirements for the other categories of beneficiaries. It provides health insurance for hospital services, nursing homes, and home health care. Part B of Medicare is voluntary. People may choose to have deductions made from their social security benefits each month to pay for Part B coverage, which provides insurance for outpatient health services including physical therapy and visits to the doctor. Both Parts A and B may have deductibles and co-payments.

Recently, Congress enacted legislation as part of its Medicare reforms to add Medicare + Choice (commonly called Part C and now known as Medicare Advantage), which offers beneficiaries who are already enrolled in Medicare A and B a wide range of alternative coordinated care plans in Part C such as HMOs, PPOs, HSAs, POSs, (points of service), provider sponsored organizations (PSOs), etc. These plans may require additional premiums, but include expanded benefits. Medicare Part D (the Medicare Prescription Drug, Improvement, and Modernization Act of 2003) includes prescription drug benefits for Medicare enrollees for the first time.

Other Medicare Expenses

A popular misconception is that Medicare is free, but as with private insurance, Medicare recipients face a wide range of out-of-pocket expenses that are dependent on the Medicare plan and the level of coverage they select. The sicker a person is, the quicker they will reach the maximum limits of their insurance coverage, and the more they will pay out of pocket for deductibles and co-payments for the care they receive. It should be no surprise that insurance companies offer, and many people buy, Medigap insurance policies to cover those health-care expenses not covered by Medicare plans, and long-term care insurance policies for extended nursing home care. Another unique aspect of Medicare is that it often involves the coordination of benefits for beneficiaries who may have concurrent health insurance policy through an employer, a spouse who works, or through pension plan benefits.

Medical Necessity

A final important point—Medicare benefits are based on medical necessity, which means that Medicare only covers medical services and treatments that are considered necessary and reasonable according to evidence-based standards of care.

Carriers and intermediaries have complex mechanisms for determining what services are reasonable and necessary. These determinations are often open to interpretation to the chagrin of providers and patients. This lack of consistent interpretation, preauthorization requirements, and limits of coverage affects billing and payment rules and decisions from one insurance company to another. Because these insurance companies also have divisions for insuring nonMedicare recipients, they often apply Medicare rules for coverage of these services. For example, a Medicare recipient who has Part B Medicare through ABC Insurance Company may be preauthorized for outpatient physical therapy services three times a week for 3 weeks. A nonMedicare patient with an ABC policy may be limited to the same level of physical therapy services as ABC seeks to standardize their payments for a given condition.

Medicaid—A Federal/State Entitlement Program

Unlike the use of age as the reason for entitlement in the Medicare program, Medicaid is a means-test entitlement, in which enrollment is limited to people below certain limited income and asset levels. Each state creates and manages its own Medicaid program following federal guidelines to qualify for matching federal money. The amount that each state receives varies and is dependent on each state's ability and willingness to provide medical care to this needy population.

Medicaid is much more complex than Medicare because eligibility for which health-care services, how they are paid for, and who delivers them are highly variable from state to state. New waiver programs add to the confusion about who is eligible for Medicaid. Also, within any state, the way the Medicaid program is administered for children and families may be different from the way it is administered for the elderly. One group's health insurance may be managed as an HMO and another group's as a PPO, for instance. It is best to think of them as two systems within Medicaid. Within those two groups, many subgroups are eligible for Medicaid. Some of them are mandatory beneficiary groups that each state must include in its Medicaid program to receive federal funds, and others are optional.

Other Medicaid Beneficiaries

Over the years the people who may be included in a Medicaid program has expanded beyond the initial groups of beneficiaries—the very poor, families with dependent children, and the disabled. For instance, certain pregnant women and children from higher income families have been added. Recently, demonstration waiver projects for special groups like uninsured women with breast cancer, people with tuberculosis, and legal immigrants have been approved by Congress. Each Medicaid group may receive different benefits, and people within the same group may receive different benefits from one state to another.

States also must provide Medicaid insurance to anyone who receives Supplemental Security Income (SSI). This program was Title XVI of the Social Security Act, and it provides cash assistance to the aged, blind, and disabled below certain income levels. States may decide to offer Medicaid coverage to others. For instance, people who are not eligible for SSI but require nursing home care, or people with disabilities who work but are not eligible for other health insurance may have Medicaid benefits.

Finally, some Medicare beneficiaries have such low incomes that they also are eligible for Medicaid. A complicated cost-sharing arrangement is implemented that may include, for instance, Medicaid payment of Medicare premiums, deductibles, and co-payments. Medicaid is further complicated by the fact that not all people below the poverty level are eligible for Medicaid, and neither do all people who are eligible for Medicaid receive its benefits. People may not know they are eligible or they may not feel a need for health insurance.[8]

State Children's Health Insurance Program (SCHIP)

SCHIP is another federal/state program (Title XXI of the Social Security Act) to provide health-care insurance to children whose family's income and assets were too much to qualify for Medicaid, yet not enough for a obtaining a private insurance policy. Each state receives a given amount for SCHIP based on population and other factors. In some states, SCHIP is part of the Medicaid program, in other states it is freestanding, while hybrid models are used in others. As a block grant program, the money for this 10-year program is limited. Unless Congress renews funds for the program, it ends after the 10-year period, or some states may spend their allotted funds in less than the 10 years.

Individuals with Disabilities Education Act (IDEA) and Individuals with Disabilities Education Improvement Act (IDEIA)

Other federal legislation that has a peripheral healthcare component of particular interest to physical therapists is the IDEA) which was revised as IDEIA in 2005. This civil rights legislation creates a federal/state program to aid children with disabilities through support of special education in school systems and related services, which include physical therapy and medical equipment. This aid also reaches infants and toddlers through early intervention programs.[8]

Workers' Compensation

Another public program that lies on the fringes of health care, legislatively, is workers' compensation (workers' comp). It is driven by state statutes to provide no-fault insurance programs to protect workers who are temporarily or permanently injured or sick because of their work, while protecting employers from legal action from injured or sick employees. This is a system in which employees have some guarantee of benefits regardless of fault for the injury or sickness, and employers are able to anticipate payments of mandated benefits rather than risk huge, unpredictable losses from lawsuits arising from injuries and illness. Because of this legislation, employees cannot sue their employers when injured or when they become sick because of their work.

There is no standardization to workers' compensation from state to state. Employers may pay their premiums to any insurance company, they may be self-insured, or they may contribute to state-operated funds for workers' compensation as their only option. In some states, all three options are available. Which employers must carry workers' compensation insurance and how much they carry is variable.

Two Components of Workers' Compensation

In any case, workers' comp is a two-prong program. First, workers are compensated for lost wages and loss of future, potential wages because of injury or illness. Although the benefits are variable, injured workers typically receive about two-thirds of their salaries while they are disabled or more if the disability is permanent. Survivors of people killed on a job also are compensated. Compensation also includes payment for pain and suffering, and the cost of retraining, if necessary, so that each worker who is able returns to work. The second prong is medical benefits for the treatment and care of these injured or sick employees, which includes physical therapy for rehabilitation of injuries and disease to improve the ability to return to work. The cash benefits and medical care are established by state formulas and provider payment schedules that are typically administered in the states' departments of labor.[9]

It should be no surprise that there is a parallel workers' compensation program for federal employees and other special categories of workers, such as longshoremen, the merchant marines, miners with black lung, and employees of the U.S. Energy Commission—typically these programs address employees of interstate commerce types of businesses because they work in more than one state.[10]

Workers' Comp Issues

Although this sounds fine, there are issues. The compensation schemes are based on types of injuries and proportional loss of the use of body parts. For instance, the benefits for a worker who loses an arm is different from those of a worker who is paralyzed from the waist down. The idea is a "partial" person should be able to return to "partial" work. An example of this is a worker with a back injury who is assigned to light duty work. Whether that person can find such work is not part of the formula. Another issue is that the system does not keep up well with new injuries and illnesses that arise from new types of or trends in contemporary work. Physical therapists are often challenged by patients enmeshed in the tug of war between rehabilitation to return to work and the promise of compensation for loss of potential wages resulting from their work injuries.

Litigation

It is not unusual for physical therapists to hear patients who are receiving workers' comp talk as much about their attorneys as they do their physicians. Although the system was established to avoid work-related litigation, injured workers are often embroiled in lawsuits to address new injuries, or to increase the values established for particular injuries, which may not be adequate to support a person for the rest of his or her life. This amount of compensation is often dependent on the work the person does. The classic example is the loss of a finger. The change in potential earning capacity is different for a renowned concert violinist than it is for a bank teller.

The other legal dimension of workers' compensation is that false claims by employees may result in litigation if employers contest these claims, typically through administrative judges within the state agencies or state appellate courts. On the other hand, in some states, employees may bring discrimination suits against employers because of action based on previous workers' comp claims, or if they were fired because they filed a claim. Other legal claims are the result of injured workers who think that the insurance company acted illegally or unfairly, or employers who feel that insurance premiums are unfair or inflated. See Activity 4.9 and Sidebars 4.1 and 4.2.

ACTIVITY 4.9
FIND OUT MORE

1. Go to the Web pages for Military Health and Veterans' Administration. Find the health-care facilities nearest you in each system. What benefits do beneficiaries have?
2. Go to the Centers for Medicare and Medicaid Services (CMMS or CMS) Web page. Link to the Medicare, Medicaid, and SCHIP Web pages. What can you find out about payment for physical therapy?
3. Find Medicaid information on your state's Web page. What does it say about physical therapy?
4. How is IDEA/IDEIA managed in your state? In your local school district?
5. Go to the Workers' Compensation Web page for your state. What are the rules for employers? What are the benefits for employees?
6. As a citizen, are you happy (comfortable, satisfied) with these public government programs?
7. As a physical therapist, are you happy (comfortable, satisfied) with these public government programs?

Sidebar 4.1

Federal Resources

The best sources of information on federal government programs are the Congressional Research Service (CRS) Reports to Congress that are prepared through the Library of Congress. The reports of their Domestic Social Policy Division are most relevant to this section. However, these reports are not meant to be accessible to the public. If you do a Web search beginning with CRS followed by health or Medicare for example, you may find these reports. The Thurgood Marshall Law Library at the University o f Maryland catalogs these reports related to health-care policy and they can be found at http://www.law.umaryland.edu/Marshall/crsreports/index.asp.

Sidebar 4.2

Vocabulary

At the CMS Web page, http://www.cms.hhs.gov/, notice the tab for acronyms. Not only is the alphabet soup of abbreviations explained, but there also is a link to a glossary.

The Uninsured and Underinsured

The uninsured have no health insurance,[11] and the underinsured have insurance that is inadequate to meet their health-care expenses. Although insured, the underinsured face responsibility for a share of the high premiums and out-of-pocket expenses for co-payments and deductibles that place them at the same risks for debt and bankruptcy that the uninsured must face. Ongoing dealings with collection agencies or the need to significantly change one's life style to pay medical bills may become necessary. Health-care debt is one of the major reasons for bankruptcy in this country.

Both groups are less likely not to seek needed medical care in the first place, or they may fail to adhere to instructions because they cannot afford them. For example, they may not fill a prescription, or they may be a "no-show" for their physical therapy appointments because they are unable to make the co-payment "due at the time the service is rendered." This failure, or inability, to adhere to instructions may progress what would be a minor, manageable health problem to a more serious and expensive chronic problem.

The poorer and sicker people are, the more likely they have no or too little insurance. Of course, the frightening thing is that any one of us can become uninsured or underinsured at any time. Any worker can be suddenly unemployed, even temporarily, and become temporarily uninsured. Anyone can develop a major catastrophic illness or injury that leads to the maximum amount of a health insurance policy very quickly. They become immediately underinsured, and that inadequate policy may not be renewed. If people are lucky enough to recover from these major catastrophes, they are then likely to be left with some preexisting condition that is uninsurable, or that will limit any new policy to new conditions only. We may all be lucky enough to become old and unlucky enough for the benefits in Medicare to be cut back, and thereby become uninsured. See Activities 4.10 and 4.11.

ACTIVITY 4.10
NO INSURANCE COVERAGE

Yvonne Mendoza is the manager of an outpatient clinic with the following policy and procedure.

POLICY: Physical therapy services may not be provided to patients who are uninsured or unable to make co-payments at the time of service.

PROCEDURE: The office manager is to advise each patient of this policy. Visits for physical therapy may not be initiated unless there is documented evidence of insurance coverage and the patient signs an agreement to make co-payments and/or meet deductibles at the time of each visit. Patients with no insurance coverage for physical therapy must pay the total fee for each visit at the time of visit. All due fees must be paid before another visit may be scheduled.

Here are three patients who require physical therapy services that have been referred to the clinic:

- Abigail is a young woman who was recently laid off from her job as a waitress so she is temporarily unemployed and uninsured. She fell while running across the street and fractured her right distal tibia and fibula. A cast was applied in the emergency room at the time of the accident. It was removed today, 6 weeks later. In addition to the expected limited range of motion (ROM) and atrophy, she appears to have complex regional pain syndrome. The nurse in the emergency room told her she needs physical therapy and arranged for a prescription for physical therapy, which she brings to your clinic. She is very eager to return to work.
- Barry is employed as a waiter. He has health insurance and is pleased that it covered so much of the cost of his recent hospitalization when he needed an appendectomy a few months ago. A few weeks ago, he hurt his back as he was moving furniture to his new apartment. He has been off from work and his sick days have run out. He is able to move well enough to begin outpatient physical therapy and has a prescription from the doctor for "evaluate and treat 3X/week for 3 weeks for severe lumbar strain." He is surprised when the business manager tells him his insurance does not cover outpatient physical therapy. He wants to get back to work.
- Carl is a former headwaiter in your city's most exclusive restaurant. However, major reversals in his life have resulted in very negative circumstances. He has been living on the streets and in various homeless shelters for more than 6 months and contracted a Community-associated Methicillin-resistant *Staphylococcus aureus* (CA-MRSA) infection that went untreated, resulting in major surgery to debride his left foot and lower leg. He is also diabetic and relies on services at a clinic for the homeless. The nurse there has called you to ask if you might provide physical therapy services to improve his ability to walk and promote healing of the surgical incision. The clinic is willing to pay a small stipend for each visit.

Go to the Web pages of the American Physical Therapy Association (APTA) and find the *APTA Guide for Professional Conduct*. Review the applicable principles of the *APTA Guide for Professional Conduct*. Then discuss the answers to these questions:

- These three patients should receive physical therapy services as soon as possible. What should Yvonne do? What are her alternatives?
- What should Yvonne do about the policy and procedure?
- Rewrite the policy and procedure to be consistent with the *APTA Guide for Professional Conduct*.
- What are the financial implications of the decisions Yvonne makes?

ACTIVITY 4.11
A HEALTH-CARE CASE STUDY

Read about the Rosen family and discuss their health care through the questions at the end of the case.

John Rosen is a 19-year-old student at a university. He is the son of Susan Rosen who has worked for a large manufacturing company, ABC Widgets for 25 years and Sam Rosen who is a self-employed electrical contractor. John, his father and his two sisters have been insured by the family coverage plan of the health insurance policy that his mother holds through her employer all of those years. ABC Widgits has always contributed 80% of the monthly premium for a health insurance policy for its employees and Mrs. Rosen has paid the remaining 20% through deductions from her pay. Although her payroll deductions have been increasing, she is satisfied with the policy and her health care so she has not taken the opportunities presented by her employer every year to change the type of health insurance plan she has or her insurance company.

Although Mr. Rosen has eight employees, he does not have a health insurance program for them. As required by law, he does contribute to the Workers' Compensation program in his state.

The Rosen's have been very fortunate. Except for the usual childhood immunizations and minor injuries, short-term illnesses from viruses and other infections, the birth of her children, and Mr. Rosen's short hospitalization because of a gastrointestinal (GI) problem, they have not required health-care services and have not given their health care much thought.

However, Mrs. Rosen just received a notice from the health insurance company that when John turns 20 in 60 days, their family coverage policy will no longer include him. She calls John, tells him to enroll in the university's student health insurance program temporarily, and that she will investigate the alternative health plans that will be available to her for next year during the annual open-enrollment period at work in October, 9 months from now.

Mr. and Mrs. Waterson, John's grandparents, are both 78 years old. They both became eligible for and enrolled in Medicare when they were 65 and opted for inclusion in Medicare Part B. In addition, Mr. and Mrs. Waterson continue to receive other health insurance benefits because Mr. Waterson is a retiree of ABC Widgits. Their health-care providers must pay attention to their coordination of benefits. He also is a veteran who was wounded in the Korean War, so he is triply insured. Mr. Waterson takes medication to control his hypertension and diabetes. He sees his doctor monthly. Mrs. Waterson was recently hospitalized for a mild stroke and is receiving outpatient physical and speech therapy services. They are confused by the numerous ads they hear on TV or receive in the mail almost daily about different Medicare plans and options. Explanation of benefits reports they receive from Medicare and their other insurers are a mystery to them. They pay every bill they receive promptly and without question. They spend winters in Florida and summers in North Carolina.

John's aunt and uncle, James and Jane Waterson, live about 600 miles away. They have two preschool aged children. James is the sole wage earner for the family. As an independent construction worker, he opts to take higher hourly wages rather than a wages and benefits package because he likes the freedom of selecting jobs that pay the most while selecting only to take the types of work he prefers. They have been uninsured since they have been married, but able to afford health-care expenses, like the birth of their children without difficulty because of their ability to maintain a large pool of savings.

Unfortunately, work opportunities are slim this year, and although his income is very limited, it is not low enough for the family to qualify for Medicaid to cover their potential health-care costs and they are dipping into their savings much more than they would like. The Waterson's have just learned that their oldest child who is ready to begin kindergarten is asthmatic, the baby has been diagnosed as developmentally delayed, and James has developed an unrelenting back problem, which also has contributed to his reduced work effort. They rarely go to a physician and treat the usual run of childhood problems on their own with over-the-counter medications and home remedies. Because he is a contractor and not an employee of any particular company, he is not eligible for workers' compensation benefits. Jane is considering taking a part-time job if she will be eligible for health insurance and can afford the payroll deductions for coverage. Her neighbor told her there is something called SCHIP that insures children and she is trying to find out more about that.

ACTIVITY 4.11
A HEALTH-CARE CASE STUDY—Cont'd

Discussion Questions:

• What are the health risks for each member of the Rosen family?

• What health insurance do they have? Should they have? How would you describe their health insurance coverage?

• If the Rosen's lived in your state, what would be Mr. Rosen's obligations to his employees for health insurance and workers' compensation?

• List the things that Mrs. Rosen must consider in selecting a health insurance policy for her family next year? What type of policy do you think is best for her?

• Each time that the elder Waterson's need health care, what, if any, are their insurance challenges? What are the challenges for their providers? Which of their three insurance policies do you think are the "best" for them?

• Are the younger Waterson's better off insuring just their children? Why?

Conclusion

The case study of the Rosen's extended family reflects the challenges of our health-care system from the perspective of the people who need it, or who may need it. Like many people, the Rosen's extended family does not quite have a handle on health-care costs and payments and the role of insurance in their care. Their other insurance policies on their home or their cars offer protection for unexpected catastrophes. They may never collect benefits on those policies in their lifetime and they may insure with the same company for these policies forever.

However, over that same lifetime, several different insurers may pay for the health care each person receives, or there may be periods of no insurance at all. The contributions for the premiums to pay for the insurance and the out-of-pocket expenses for deductibles and co-payments vary as people move between the private and public "branches" of the health-care system across their life spans. This movement in the health-care system may be provoked by changes in socioeconomic, employment, marital, or disability status.

On the other hand, the Rosen's family, like most people, feels that health care should be a right but are a little less clear about who should pay for it, or even how it gets paid for, and especially unclear about how much it really costs. Their health-care benefits reach far beyond catastrophic, unexpected events to include routine visits to the physician, prescriptions, and the management of chronic conditions. It would be similar to having an auto insurance policy that pays for tune-ups and the gasoline that keeps a car running.

Health-care managers and providers also face health-care system challenges. Dealing with the complexity and shifts in private and public insurance within the communities they serve, as costs continue to rise and payments are controlled by insurers, places managers in health care in unique, challenging positions. These issues are addressed further in Sections 2 and 3.

REFERENCES

1. America's Health Insurance Plans. America's health insurance plans. Available at: http://www.ahip.org/. Accessed March 7, 2007.
2. National Association of Insurance Commissioners. Our mission. Available at: http://www.naic.org/index_about.htm. Accessed March 9, 2007.
3. Federal Jobs Net. Government jobs overview. Available at: http://www.federaljobs.net/overview.htm#Introduction and http://www.bls.gov/oco/cg/cgs042.htm. Accessed March 7, 2007.
4. Bureau of Labor Statistics. State and local government; excluding education and hospitals. Available at: http://www.bls.gov/oco/cg/cgs042.htm. Accessed March 9, 2007.
5. U.S. Office of Personnel Management. Insurance programs. Available at: http://www.opm.gov/insure/health/. Accessed March 7, 2007.
6. Office of the Assistant Secretary of Defense (Health Affairs). Welcome to tricare.mil. Available at: http://www.tricare.mil/. Accessed March 7, 2007.
7. United States' Department of Veterans Affairs. Health care—veterans health administration. Available at: http://www1.va.gov/health/. Accessed March 7, 2007.
8. Herz E, Hearne J, Stone J, et al., eds. *How Medicaid Works: Program Basics.* Washington, DC: Library of Congress

Congressional Research Service Report for Congress received through the CRS Web; 2004 http://www.law.umaryland.edu/marshall/crsreports/crsdocuments/RL3227703162005.pdf. Accessed March 7, 2007.

9. House Committee on Ways and Means. *Green Book 2003: Workers' Compensation: Overview.* Available at: http://waysandmeans.house.gov/media/pdf/greenbook2003/WorkersComp.pdf. Accessed March 7, 2007.

10. U.S. Department of Labor. Federal Employees' Compensation Act. Available at: http://www.dol.gov/esa/regs/statutes/owcp/feca.htm. Accessed March 7, 2007.

11. DeNavas-Walt C, Proctor BD, Lee CH, eds. *Income, Poverty, and Health Insurance in the United States.* Washington, DC: U.S. Census Bureau Government Printing Office; 2006.

Responsibilities of the Physical Therapy Manager

Each chapter in this section addresses one of the major responsibilities of physical therapy managers, which are listed below. Those in bold are the core responsibilities of managers, that lie under the umbrella of its vision, mission, and goals. These core responsibilities are based on a foundation composed of legal and ethical, risk management, and communication responsibilities. The last chapter guides readers in the development of a feasibility study.

- ✦ Vision, mission, goals (Chapter 5)
- ✦ **Policies and procedures (Chapter 6)**
- ✦ **Marketing (Chapter 7)**
- ✦ **Staffing (Chapter 8)**
- ✦ **Patient care (Chapter 9)**
- ✦ **Fiscal (Chapter 10)**
- ✦ Risk management (Chapter 11)
- ✦ Legal and ethical (Chapter 12)
- ✦ Communication (Chapter 13)
- ✦ *The Feasibility Study (Chapter 14)*

The relationship of these responsibilities is represented in Figure S2.1. If not totally responsible for the development of the vision, mission, and goals, managers certainly are *always* responsible for ensuring that their decisions are aligned with these documents as they address issues that arise in the five major areas of responsibility—policies and procedures, marketing, staffing, patient care, and fiscal.

Underlying these decisions are the responsibility for the risks involved, compliance with the laws affecting the organization and health professionals, and the defense of ethical principles. Effective verbal and written communication with all stakeholders is the basic management responsibility for the accomplishment of an organization's goals that underlies all of the others.

Strategic Planning

Reaching an organization's goals requires that managers develop an ongoing, self-correcting process for defining and redefining these responsibilities to get from where

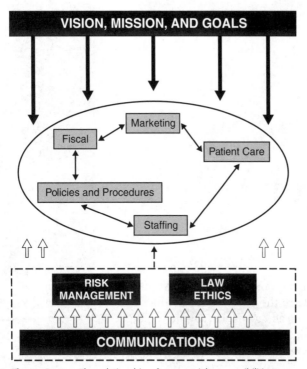

Figure S2.1 ✦ The relationship of managerial responsibilities.

the organization is now to where it wants to be in the future. Commonly called strategic planning, this process reflects the direction of an organization's goals, supplies the answers to the questions related to what the organization should do, and how it does it. Strategic planning applies to lofty, broad organizational issues as well as day-to-day problem-solving. Kaufman[1] suggests an approach to strategic planning, based on the ability to correctly assess the needs of an organization. A need is defined as the gap between the efforts of an organization and the results to which they aspire—their goals. Needs must be expressed in terms of measurable *results* rather than the processes or resources used by the organization.

In the next step in strategic planning, managers gather and analyze data on the gap between what is and what should be. They then decide whether the need is important enough for the organization to invest the resources required to meet it by answering important questions:[1]

✦ Can the need easily be eliminated or ignored?

✦ What will it cost to ignore the need?

✦ What is the impact of meeting the need on society? External stakeholders? Internal stakeholders?

✦ How much will meeting the need cost?

✦ How high a priority is the need?

According to Kaufman, selecting a need to be met (or gap to close or reduce) becomes a problem (challenge) for managers to solve. Considering which of their responsibilities are most likely to meet a need is helpful to managers as they tackle the challenge. Said another way, managers need to identify and use key concepts and ideas to achieve important results—they need a strategy. Figure S2.2 illustrates a simplified example of using this strategic planning model to address the need to reduce the number of patient no-shows and cancellations. This model will be presented for application to given challenges throughout this section.

Feasibility Studies

The formal writing process to present a feasibility study provides managers the means to clearly describe and analyze the business or project they intend to develop. It forces managers to project the future, consider the financial implications of their plans, and identify potential sources of funding—develop a strategic plan in other words. Having a written feasibility study keeps managers on track toward business success. This planning process also identifies barriers managers need to overcome, or it determines whether the intended project needs to be stopped before it begins because the barriers are insurmountable. Perhaps most importantly, a strong, complete, clear feasibility study serves as the foundation for a successful business plan that potential investors or lenders are more likely to support.

REFERENCE

1. Kaufman R. *Strategic Planning for Success: Aligning People, Performance, and Payoffs.* San Francisco: John Wiley; 2003.

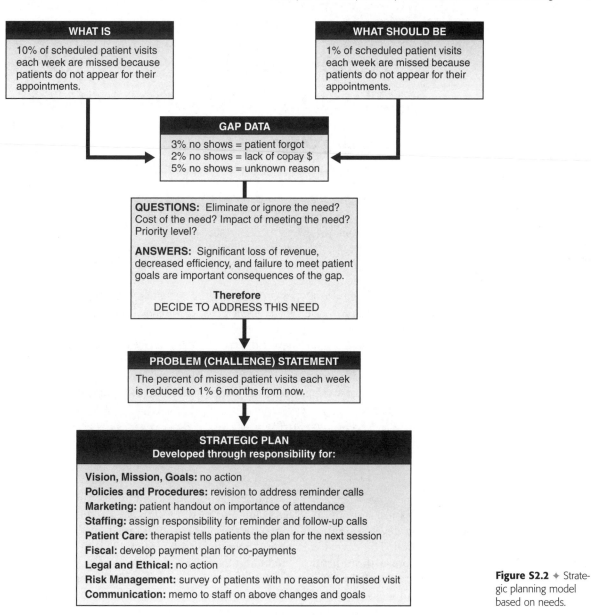

WHAT IS

10% of scheduled patient visits each week are missed because patients do not appear for their appointments.

WHAT SHOULD BE

1% of scheduled patient visits each week are missed because patients do not appear for their appointments.

GAP DATA

3% no shows = patient forgot
2% no shows = lack of copay $
5% no shows = unknown reason

QUESTIONS: Eliminate or ignore the need? Cost of the need? Impact of meeting the need? Priority level?

ANSWERS: Significant loss of revenue, decreased efficiency, and failure to meet patient goals are important consequences of the gap.

Therefore
DECIDE TO ADDRESS THIS NEED

PROBLEM (CHALLENGE) STATEMENT

The percent of missed patient visits each week is reduced to 1% 6 months from now.

STRATEGIC PLAN
Developed through responsibility for:

Vision, Mission, Goals: no action
Policies and Procedures: revision to address reminder calls
Marketing: patient handout on importance of attendance
Staffing: assign responsibility for reminder and follow-up calls
Patient Care: therapist tells patients the plan for the next session
Fiscal: develop payment plan for co-payments
Legal and Ethical: no action
Risk Management: survey of patients with no reason for missed visit
Communication: memo to staff on above changes and goals

Figure S2.2 ✦ Strategic planning model based on needs.

Responsibility for Vision, Mission, and Goal Setting

Learning Objectives

✦ Distinguish organizational visions, missions, values, and goals from each other.
✦ Determine the roles of the statement of a vision, a mission, the values, and the goals in the management of physical therapy practice.
✦ Critique vision and mission statements.
✦ Relate vision, mission, and values to organizational culture.
✦ Determine the potential influence of mission statements on individuals in organizations.
✦ Determine the appropriate relationship between vision, mission, values, and goals of the American Physical Therapy Association and those of physical therapy practices.
✦ Analyze various levels of goals for the management of physical therapy practices following given criteria for effective goals.
✦ Develop strategies for communicating and promoting acceptance of a physical therapy practice's vision, mission, values, and goals.

Overview

The importance of visions and mission statements in the initial start-up and ongoing development of businesses cannot be overestimated. The caveat is that they need to be derived from a thoughtful process that includes the input of all stakeholders on what the organization values and seeks to accomplish. Including key stakeholders in the preparation of visions and missions accomplishes two things. It increases the chance that they will truly reflect the organization at all levels, and it increases the chance of buy-in when it is time for everyone to "walk the talk."

After they are created, the power of visions and mission statements lies in the role they play in the culture of the organization as they guide the decision making and the expectations of all of its stakeholders. This power is dependent on managers effectively communicating and sharing the vision and mission statement of the organization to develop a sense of unity and security. A shared common purpose results if an organization and its members "walk the talk" of its vision and mission. If, however, the stakeholders perceive them as empty expressions that are forced upon them, the result is more likely to be disillusionment and low morale.

Because of their important role, establishing the vision and mission is a critical first step of strategic planning for new organizations. Clarifying the difference between mission and vision statements is important and the question of whether the vision or mission comes first in strategic planning probably boils down to a matter of choice. Typically, however, a new business looks to the future and establishes the premise for the business (its vision) and then focus on what it needs to be to get there—its mission. Simply put: A vision is what the business seeks to become and is a source of inspiration for stakeholders. A mission statement reflects what the business is about—its purpose—now. It reflects what the business values and believes as it defines customers, processes, and performance expectations.

Visions

Managers cannot dismiss determining the vision of an organization as unimportant, or approach its development casually. Identifying this broad, over-riding goal is critical to determining the direction of an organization through a realistic picture of the future. Stakeholders need to address important questions about the organization like what it should stand for, and what it should become. Visions should challenge the performance and ideas of stakeholders. A vision leads employees (and entrepreneurs) to:[1]

+ Commit to the organization because the vision energizes them.
+ Develop a sense of the meaning of their work as part of a bigger whole.
+ Strive to achieve a standard of excellence that stimulates improvement.

For instance, compare these vision statements:
McHale and Associates Physical Therapy
To be the physical therapy provider of choice in Jones City, Alabama
New Jersey Pediatric Rehabilitation Services
To serve all children with special needs in New Jersey
The McHale vision seems to suggest a small independent business whose future lies in being good at what it does. The implication is that this practice sees itself as a vital part of its community, and that it will grow as the community grows. The New Jersey Pediatric Rehabilitation Services vision projects an image of a large, growth organization whose strategic plan will focus on the expansion of a complex, interdisciplinary organization to meet the needs of a particular population throughout an entire state.

In either case, without a vision and overriding goals to strive for, it would be difficult for either organization to accomplish its business goals. Many entrepreneurs may have a vision but they may not write it down or share it. The problem with failing to share the vision is that it will be difficult to get others to follow without it—they do not know where they are headed. The managerial decisions made without a shared vision will have no context. Employees and other stakeholders may then erroneously interpret, or ignore, what appear to be empty decisions.

An unshared vision is problematic, but no vision at all may prove disastrous to an organization. Although a cliché, it is true that it is hard to get anywhere if you do not know where you want to go, and it is equally difficult for people to follow, or contribute, if they do not see the vision. For example, a person who is very good at making pies receives encouragement to sell them. Without a vision, the pie maker may approach the pie business in a hit-or-miss, casual manner by selling pies when someone asks for one or by participating in local bake sales.

With a vision, whether it be to supply pies to all restaurants and catering companies in her community, or to be the next Mrs. Smith's or Marie Callender's with worldwide distribution of specialty pies, the first step in strategically planning for a serious business is taken with a vision statement. As another example of the impact of a vision statement, the staffing to build a small enterprise may be very different from the staff chosen to create an international company. Developing and then sharing the vision helps in determining which potential employees will be the best match in an organization.

A vision may not include a target date for realizing the vision, but an estimated date is necessary during its formulation. Beginning the vision with a phrase like "by 2015" or "in ____ years," whether it appears in the final version or not, helps to make the vision more concrete (rather than a fanciful dream). A deadline also provokes discussion about whether or not the vision is realistic and achievable.

For example, how long should it take for McHale and Associates Physical Therapy to become the provider of choice in Jones City? How long would it take for New Jersey Pediatric Rehabilitation Services to realize its vision? The level of organizational complexity, resources already available, resources needed, and prior business experience are examples of factors that influence the target date for realizing a vision. For developing businesses, a good vision time line is 3 to 5 years. See Sidebar 5.1 and Activity 5.1.

> *Sidebar 5.1*
>
> ### The Vision Statement Checklist
>
> + Clear, vivid picture of the future of the organization
> + Challenging
> + Hopeful
> + Memorable
> + Realistic
> + Achievable
> + Guides the long-term action plan

1. Using the characteristics in Sidebar 5.1, improve upon the vision statements of McHale and Associates Physical Therapy and New Jersey Pediatric Rehabilitation Services:
   McHale: "To be the physical therapy provider of choice in Jones City, Alabama."
   New Jersey: "To serve all children with special needs in New Jersey."
2. Compare the organization cultures that might be expected in these two practices. What would it be like to be employed in each one?
3. Find the vision of a physical therapy practice or other health-care organization you would like to know more about. What does its vision statement tell you about the organization? Does it meet the characteristics expected of a vision? Does the vision meet your professional expectations for an employer?
4. In small groups, compare and contrast vision statements.

Mission Statements

A mission statement provides a current path to realize the future that is presented in the vision of an organization, and that is in line with its values. Mission statements may have a direct bearing on the bottom line and success of the organization because, like the organization's vision, they are dependent on the degree of buy-in by stakeholders. Like its vision, an organization's mission statement also becomes a source of power for an organization because it enables its sense of purpose. The mission statement clarifies its legal role, expectations of its stakeholders, and, perhaps most importantly, its moral duty—what it *ought* to be doing. Unless its mission is socially desirable and justifiable, an organization may fail to create the enthusiasm and excitement among its stakeholders to "walk the talk."[2]

A mission statement reflects the principles under which an organization acts and the standards by which it will be judged. It boosts morale and strengthens its reputation when the organization lives up to it. Conversely, it may damage morale and reputation if it is perceived to be weak, hypocritical, or not trustworthy.[3] If the vision for an organization has already been determined, a beginning point for establishing its mission is to ask why the vision exists. What is the purpose of the vision? Other questions to be addressed during development are:

- What does the organization wish to be remembered for?
- What are its unique strengths and weaknesses?
- How is it distinguished from its competitors?

The mission statement is an emotional call to action that is easily transferable to the actions of employees and other stakeholders. It helps an organization focus its energies and drives the organizational culture, if it is used consistently in decision making.[4]

For example, McHale and Associates Physical Therapy might ask *why* Jones City needs their practice to be the provider of choice as they develop their mission statement. The answers may lead to a mission statement like:

McHale and Associates' Mission Statement
McHale and Associates are board-certified physical therapists who provide the highest quality care to prevent and rehabilitate the movement disorders of people of all ages in Jones City. Our individualized, hands-on approach to improving the quality of life of our patients is available at times most convenient for them in our modern, state-of-the-art facility. We believe our patients are at the center of our efforts as we consult with other health-care professionals to coordinate a comprehensive plan for their health.

A mission statement written with input from its stakeholders assures the inclusion of the values and beliefs of all constituents. Without this input, using a mission statement to make decisions, identify and resolve differences, and clarify expectations of employees becomes more difficult for managers. For instance, when reading its vision and mission physical therapists considering employment with McHale and Associates may expect that they should hold a board-certified specialization, they will need to be flexible in their work hours, and comfortable with one-on-one contemporary patient care in Jones City. Patients who read this mission will have expectations about the qualifications of their therapists and they will be confident that their therapists collaborate with their physicians and other health-care providers. Should their experiences fall short of these expectations, the reputation of McHale and Associates may be at risk. See Sidebar 5.2 and Activity 5.2.

ACTIVITY 5.2
MISSION STATEMENTS

1. Using the characteristics in Sidebar 5.2, improve upon the mission of McHale and Associates:

   McHale and Associates are board-certified physical therapists who provide the highest quality care to prevent and rehabilitate the movement disorders of people of all ages in Jones City. Our individualized, hands-on approach to improving the quality of life of our patients is available at times most convenient for them in our modern, state-of-the-art facility. We believe our patients are at the center of our efforts as we consult with other health-care professionals to coordinate a comprehensive plan for their health.

2. Review the revised vision created for McHale and Associates in Activity 5.1. Is the new vision aligned with the final mission statement?

3. Given the vision of New Jersey Pediatric Rehabilitation Services from Activity 5.1, write a mission statement that meets all of the criteria in Sidebar 5.2:

   "To serve the needs of all children in New Jersey with special needs."

4. Find the mission statement of a physical therapy practice or other health-care organization you would like to know more about. What does its mission statement tell you about the organization? Does it meet the characteristics expected of a mission statement using the components in Sidebar 5.2? Does this mission statement meet your professional expectations of an employer? In small groups, compare and contrast your mission statements.

Broader Health-Care Mission Statements

Because of their importance in the management of health care, developing mission statements that capture the unique and enduring purpose, practices, and values of an organization is an urgent need. Economic pressures and the service mandate of health care often are in conflict, so managers must sustain a unified sense of purpose and values through a powerful mission statement that motivates individuals and the organization as a whole to reconcile these competing interests of health-care organizations.[5]

The results of a thematic analysis of hospital mission statements conducted by Williams and others are useful to health-care managers who are addressing this need regardless of their type of health-care setting. The consistent, outstanding theme among these hospitals was the importance of exemplary patient care. Other than this commitment to patients, they found wide variation in the mission statements they studied, although they expected otherwise because the Canada Health Act recommends specific health-care values. The mission statements were far from standard, boilerplate missions. They did find common themes among the mission statements that may be expected in the mission statements of physical therapy practice as well.[5] These identified themes included:

✦ Values
✦ Identity (image)
✦ Services provided (geographic area served)
✦ Employees and staff
✦ Resources

They concluded that the mission statements studied were laudable and if internalized by the employees, they provided moral guidance that could be translated into behavior. Their study reinforced the importance of understanding that behavior is a manifestation of what people truly value. Therefore, for mission statements to translate into action, they must address values.

They recommended the following management initiatives to improve commitment to the mission of health-care organizations:[5]

1. Consider the perspectives of all stakeholders to promote ownership and authenticity of the mission.

2. Make the mission and value statements the central pillars of ethics awareness programs.

3. Increase the relevancy of the mission and value statements by making them part of decision making and policy-development processes.

4. Provide incentives for mission/value adherence and explicit consequences for nonadherence.

5. Actively promote the mission/values in all relevant internal and external communication.

6. Express and reinforce management's commitment to the mission and values.

See Activity 5.3.

ACTIVITY 5.3
WALK THE TALK

Select the vision and mission statement from an organization in this chapter or from an actual health-care organization. Do they also have a value statement? Identify 10 actions or behaviors that might be expected of employees that would reinforce the intent and purpose of these statements. In other words, how would they "walk the talk" in the selected organization?

Value Statements

Recently, some organizations have chosen to separate the values component of the typical mission statement into a separate statement. Value statements often begin with "we believe. . .", or "we are committed to. . .", or simply "we value. . .". This approach results in mission statements that are more direct, typically shorter, and limited to a clear definition of what they do. An accompanying value statement supplies the why's of the mission and offers support for the vision.

All organizations have values that drive its culture. Although not always explicit, the values of an organization determine the qualities that command respect. They generate the principles that guide the actions of the employees and other stakeholders as they judge themselves and are judged by others.[3] The values statement typically identifies the four to six most important values, or things that are valued, which are presented in rank order with the most important value listed first. A physical therapy practice's value statement may address (in no alphabetical order):

- ✦ Access
- ✦ Accountability
- ✦ Diversity
- ✦ Education
- ✦ Financial success
- ✦ Honesty
- ✦ Innovation
- ✦ Productivity
- ✦ Quality care
- ✦ Respect
- ✦ Teamwork
- ✦ Work/home balance

For example, the values statement of New Jersey Pediatric Rehabilitation Services reads:

New Jersey Pediatric Rehabilitation Services values teamwork that includes family participation in its provision of innovative quality care to children with special needs in New Jersey.

See Activities 5.4 and 5.5.

ACTIVITY 5.4
VALUES STATEMENT

Take this opportunity to brainstorm 10 additional values that might support a physical therapy practice. Define these values.

ACTIVITY 5.5
RELATING TO THE AMERICAN PHYSICAL THERAPY ASSOCIATION

Discussion questions:

1. What are the vision and mission of the American Physical Therapy Association? Do they meet the criteria for a vision and a mission statement provided in Sidebars 5.1 and 5.2? How do you think they might be improved?

2. Why did the American Physical Therapy Association separate its core values from its vision and mission statement?

3. What should be the relationship between the vision, mission, and core values of the profession and those of individual physical therapy practices?

Goal Setting

The goals, or results desired, for the organization are equally powerful and important in planning and implementing a new practice or new component of an organization. Organizational goals are also a means for controlling, coordinating, and evaluating work performance. In large organizations, conflict commonly arises because the many goals established to carry out a mission and achieve a vision may seem to contradict each other. The focus of an organization's goals also may change at different times as factors influencing the business of health care force a change in the priority rank of goals.

Fry, Stoner, and Weinzimmer offer a model for understanding the levels and types of goals in organizations that are a helpful foundation for goal writing.[6] Their general rules for goals are in bold and applied using holiday shopping as an example:

1. Goals must be **phrased in terms of outcomes** (accomplishments) not processes. Example of an unacceptable goal as process: Go shopping. Example of an acceptable goal as outcome: Purchase all gifts for family members by end of the day on December 15th.

2. Goals must be **measurable:**
   Example: Purchase five stocking stuffers for under $10 each by the end of the day on December 10th.

3. Goals must **challenging but realistic:**
   Example: Make all gift purchases at the Midway Mall.

4. Goals must be **communicated:**
   Example: Use text messages, posted notes, memos, policies, and procedures, etc. to get the point across.

The following example of combines all of these goal criteria:

In a phone message to Sam from Susie:

"We will meet at Midway Mall at 9 a.m. on Saturday, December 15 to complete our entire holiday gift shopping by 5 p.m. The gift list includes five stocking stuffers for less than $10 each for the children and 10 total gifts for our parents, your three sisters, my brother, and our bosses limiting our spending to less than $50/person."

Another common approach to goal writing is SMART, an acronym for:

- ✦ **S**pecific
- ✦ **M**easurable
- ✦ **A**ction-oriented
- ✦ **R**ealistic
- ✦ **T**imebound

In the shopping example, SMART criteria are met as:

"We'll meet at Midway Mall at 9 a.m. on Saturday, December 15 to complete **(A)** all **(S** and **R)** of our holiday gift shopping by 5 p.m. **(T** and **R)**. The gift list includes five **(M)** stocking stuffers for less than $10 **(M)** each for the neighborhood children and 10 total **(M)** gifts for our parents, your three sisters, my brother, and our bosses limiting **(A)** our spending to no more than $50/person **(M)**."

In another approach, Fry and his associates have identified three types of goals that apply to any strategic planning. They all demand deadlines and evaluation feedback to determine if they have been met:[6]

- ✦ **Horizon goals**—broad and less specific goals that are to be met over the course of the overall planning time span of years.

- ✦ **Near-term goals**—also called short-term goals, with results or accomplishments expected in the next operating cycle, typically 1 year. They serve as progress points toward horizon goals.

- ✦ **Target goals**—very short-term and specific to time and measurement. They generate action that can be accomplished in days or weeks. Targets goals need to be checked regularly to determine if they remain consistent with near-term and horizon goals.

Target goals require action plans that include the identification of barriers to reaching the targets. Barriers can be insurmountable in which case the target is abandoned and an alternate goal is set. Other barriers are temporary if the target can be set aside for a short time so that the barrier can be overcome or resolved.[6] For example, a near-term goal may be that all staff earns transitional doctor of physical therapy (t-DPT) degrees by the end of the year. A barrier may be that one of the contracts with a third-party payer was not renewed and revenue did not meet projections. As a result, funds to support the tuition of staff in transitional programs were not available so their studies were postponed.

Because there is no practice too small for strategic planning, the following fictitious solo practitioner's practice will be used to demonstrate the target goal (results) setting component of strategic planning.

Michael Somski's vision and mission for his Chronic Pain Relief practice are:

VISION: To practice physical therapy exclusively to resolve complex chronic pain conditions of people who have previous failed attempts for relief of their pain.

MISSION: To provide focused, one-on-one care to people with chronic pain following an efficient, effective multifaceted approach provided by a board-certified physical therapist who is a fellow of the International Pain Society that results in the clients' ability to participate in meaningful work and leisure activities.

This vision and mission statement may lead to the following horizon goals for Chronic Pain Relief.

By 2015:

✦ 100% of patients receiving care at Chronic Pain Relief will be referred, or seek care on their own initiative, because of its reputation for success in resolving complex pain problems.

✦ Chronic Pain Relief's start-up debt will be paid in full.

✦ 100% of the patient load will be patients with chronic pain.

✦ Patient volume will be consistently six patient visits/day.

✦ 85% of patients who receive care at Chronic Pain Relief will report either a return to work or normal daily activities if not employed.

Near-term goals for Chronic Pain Relief may include the following.

In 1 year:

✦ 25 physicians will refer at least one patient/ month to Chronic Pain Relief.

✦ The practice's treatment area, reception room, and office will be completely furnished.

✦ The Chronic Pain Relief Web page will be recognized by ABC Website Review for excellence.

✦ Contracts with 20 health insurance companies will be fully negotiated and in place.

Typically target goals are presented in a chart like the one below for a given week in the Chronic Pain Relief practice.

See Activities 5.6 and 5.7 for more attention to goals.

A Manager's Responsibility

Health-care managers have responsibility for the development, implementation, and ongoing review of visions, mission statements, and goals as a major component of strategic planning for a new organization. Remaining true to them in an often unpredictable and confusing health-care system demands the attention

TARGET	BARRIERS	ACTION	DEADLINE
Hire receptionist/office manager.	Timely posting of ad for position. Time for interviews during patient care.	Have ad in Sunday paper. Select applicants and schedule three interviews after 5 p.m.	Wed. noon By the end of the next week. Start date for receptionist first of month.
Market-call three physicians.	Arranging appointments with physicians.	Call to confirm office appointment. Make reservations for lunch. Pick up muffin basket for office staff.	By end of week
Finalize and implement billing system.	Limited computer skills.	Arrange 8-hour session with computer consultant.	Saturday
Average three appointments/ day next week.	Limited referrals.	Follow-up calls to 10 physicians to ask for referrals.	In next 2 days

ACTIVITY 5.6
CRITIQUE OF GOALS

1. Critique the goals established for Chronic Pain Relief using SMART or the general rules for goals. Revise as necessary.
2. Determine how attainment of the goals will be evaluated.

ACTIVITY 5.7
ESTABLISHING GOALS

Write goals for McHale and Associates and New Jersey Pediatric Rehabilitation Services based on the final versions of their visions and mission statements.

of managers at all levels of an organization as well. Perhaps most importantly, managers must persuade and empower people to achieve the vision and live the mission to accomplish the goals of an organization. The following actions are examples of some of the managerial roles related to visions, missions, and goals:[1]

+ Determine whom to involve in their development.
+ Determine current status and possible directions for the organization.
+ Develop these documents.
+ Select strategies to communicate them and to receive feedback.
+ Assure management behavior that is consistent with them.
+ Allocate resources to make them happen.
+ Check periodically that the vision, mission, and goals remain appropriate.

Independent practitioners cannot afford any less investment in the establishment of a vision, mission, and goals for their organizations. Particularly in the early developmental stages of a new business, all decisions about a new practice depend on understanding where the organization is headed and how it intends to get there. These processes also assist new entrepreneurs in clarifying answers to the tough questions posed by investors or lenders as they determine how well thought through a business plan is. Managers in established organizations may devote more time to looking for gaps between a current vision, mission, and goals and one that will best prepare them for the future. See Activity 5.8.

REFERENCES

1. Lansdell S. *The Vision Thing (ExpressExec Strategy; 03.04) (eBook)*. Oxford, United Kingdom: Capstone Publishing Ltd; 2002.
2. Bryson J. *Strategic Planning for Public and Nonprofit Organizations: A Guide to Strengthening and Sustaining Organizational Achievement*. San Francisco, CA: Jossey-Bass; 1995.
3. Talbot M. *Make Your Mission Statement Work: Identify Your Organisation's Values and Live them Every Day*. Oxford, United Kingdom: How to Books Ltd; 2003.
4. Luke RD, Walston SL, Plummer PM. *Healthcare Strategy: In Pursuit of Competitive Advantage*. Chicago, IL: Health Administration Press; 2004.
5. Williams J, Smythe W, Hadjistravropoulos T, et al. A study of thematic content in hospital mission statements: A question of values. *Health Care Management Review, 2005,* 30:304–314; 2005.
6. Fry FL, Stoner CR, Weinzimmer LG. *Strategic Planning for New and Emerging Businesses: A Consulting Approach*. Chicago, IL: Dearborn, A Kaplan Professional Company; 1999.

ACTIVITY 5.8
STRATEGIES FOR COMMITMENT

Referring to the strategic planning section on pp. 61–62 and the worksheet below develop a strategic plan to address the need for staff commitment to the vision, mission, and goals of an organization. iscuss how to determine the effectiveness of these strategies.

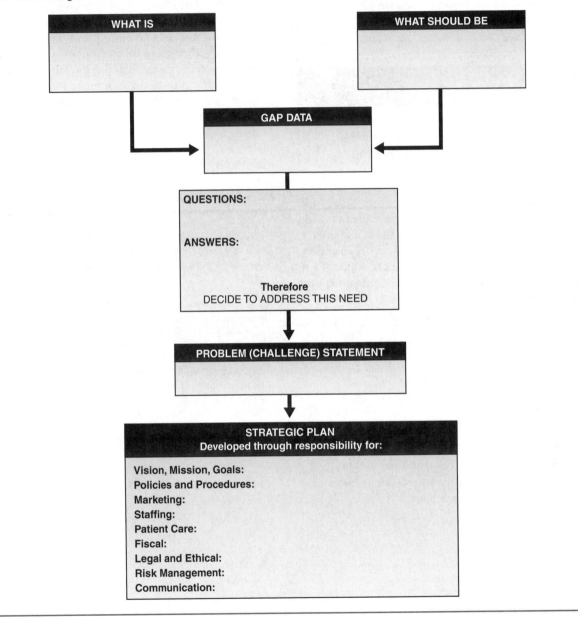

WHAT IS

WHAT SHOULD BE

GAP DATA

QUESTIONS:

ANSWERS:

Therefore
DECIDE TO ADDRESS THIS NEED

PROBLEM (CHALLENGE) STATEMENT

STRATEGIC PLAN
Developed through responsibility for:

Vision, Mission, Goals:
Policies and Procedures:
Marketing:
Staffing:
Patient Care:
Fiscal:
Legal and Ethical:
Risk Management:
Communication:

Chapter 6

Responsibility for Policies and Procedures

Learning Objectives

- Determine the purpose of policies and procedures.
- Distinguish between policies and procedures.
- Identify some expectations of The Joint Commission for policies and procedures.
- Identify managerial actions that increase the value of policies and procedures.
- Compare policies and procedures to other documents used by health-care organizations.
- Critique given policies.
- Prepare a policy and procedure using a given template.
- Discuss the responsibilities of managers for policies and procedures.

Overview

In large health-care organizations, the development, review, and implementation of policies and procedures are driven by The Joint Commission (formerly The Joint Commission on Accreditation of Health-care Organizations) and other accreditation and licensure requirements. One intent of these requirements is to ensure that policies and procedures are multidisciplinary. A multidisciplinary approach is expected to reduce confusion and inconsistencies about patient care that may occur among various units and disciplines.[1] Because of this requirement, and the complexity of large health-care organizations, responsibility for policies and procedures often falls to a system-wide standing committee devoted to the ongoing development and review of its policy and procedure manual. Software and packaged materials also are available to assist in the development and monitoring of policies and procedures. See Sidebar 6.1.

Although it will be less complex, a policy and procedure manual is equally important to even the simplest organization—a solo physical therapy practitioner. There are several good reasons to develop and implement policies and procedures:

- To meet the requirements of licensing or other agencies that may demand them.
- To avoid the potential trap of relying on memory to assure consistency in conducting business over time.
- To demonstrate thoughtful, thorough attention to the details of the business to stakeholders.
- To serve as evidence during legal proceedings. Note: wording that suggests absolutes like "always" should be avoided; use typically, usually, etc. instead.
- To reflect the compliance of an organization's commitment to state and federal laws.

A completed policies and procedures manual is typically not included in feasibility studies or business plans. However, the people who are making decisions about supporting the plan may welcome at least the proposed table of contents for policies and procedures in an appendix as evidence of the detail of thought given to the plan.

Sidebar 6.1

Selected Policies and Procedures Required by The Joint Commission

- Abuse: Recognition, Reporting, and Patient Care
- Age-Appropriate Care
- Confidentiality of Patient Information
- Consent
- Do Not Resuscitate Orders
- Human Resources Management Plan
- Infant and Child Security
- Restraint Use: Med-Surg and Behavioral Health
- Infection Control Surveillance
- Interpreter and Translation Services
- Medical Device Safety
- Medical Record Review

- Medication Administration
- Multidisciplinary Progress Notes
- Patient, Procedure, and Site Verification
- Patient Rights and Grievances
- Pain Management
- Patient Care Planning
- Patient and Family Education
- Plan for Provision of Patient Care
- Sentinel Events
- Universal/Standard Precautions
- Verbal and Telephone Orders

Basic Principles of Policies and Procedures

A policies and procedures manual only has value if it is used. Access to the manual is the first important criteria. A cumbersome manual that serves only as a space taker on a manager's bookshelf will be of no value if it is opened only when a compulsory review of it must be done. An online version of a manual in which employees may search for terms, increases its usability and implementation, and reinforces the use of standardized formats as they are developed. To be more usable, the policies and procedures manual for any health-care organization must:[1]

- Be current and relevant to contemporary work.
- Exclude clinical guidelines and protocols.
- Exclude entries that are simply information sharing.
- Be consistent in format (e.g., worded as do's rather than as do not's).
- Emphasize expectations rather than what is unacceptable.
- Be accessible and easily retrievable.
- Include a complete history of changes made to the document.
- Include guidelines for writing, revising, and reviewing the manual.

Deleting outdated policies and procedures is probably as important as writing new ones, particularly for health-care organizations that struggle to keep up with ongoing changes in technology, manpower, and organizational structures. Not only do managers want everyone to be on the *same* page, but it is critical that the page they are on is the *right* page. Developing a policy and procedure to manage policies and procedures is the critical first step. Fortunately, computer software programs and other resources have made the development, review, revision, and tracking of changes in policies and procedures manuals easier and timelier.

Policies Versus Procedures

Policies

A policy is a broad statement of an expectation that guides decisions about actions to be taken in an organization. Policies reflect the general rules that govern organizational procedures. A policy addresses who, what, when, and where about some component of an organization. Some examples of policies in a fictional health-care organization are:

- NONSMOKING FACILITY. All buildings, facilities, and public spaces (including covered walkways and covered parking lots) on the campuses of the Hillsdale Health System are nonsmoking areas. Each campus chief executive officer (CEO) may implement more restrictive policies, but none that are less restrictive.
- BUSINESS RULES. All employees will adhere to the business rules of the Hillsdale Health

System. The following activities will result in disciplinary action, up to and including termination of employment: commercial endorsements of products related to the employee's discipline, expression of private opinions or endorsement of political candidates, and acceptance of personal gifts or gratuities.

✦ NETWORK SECURITY. Nonclinical information is a principal asset of the Hillsdale Health System and must be protected from unauthorized modification, destruction, or disclosure, whether accidental or intentional. All network participants are responsible for the security of the Data Communications Network as a shared resource.

✦ KEYS AND LOCKS. The Chief of Physical Plant Services is responsible for responding to all requests for replacement or issuance of new keys or keycards, duplication of existing keys, keying changes, installation, or repair of locks (rooms, desks, file cabinets, deadbolts, etc.) throughout the Hillsdale Health System. Reproduction of keys is prohibited by anyone other than the locksmith designated by the Chief of Physical Plant Services. It is a misdemeanor crime to possess, use, duplicate, or cause to duplicate any keys to buildings or other secured spaces without proper authorization of the Assistant Vice President of Operations.

✦ INTERVIEW EXPENSES. Job applicants selected for interviews may be reimbursed for certain, limited traveling costs. However, reimbursement will not be granted if the applicant is offered a job with Hillsdale Health System but refuses it.

See Activity 6.1.

ACTIVITY 6.1
POLICIES REVIEW

Discuss your impressions of these policies. Are they good, or do they need to be improved? Are who, what, when, and where addressed? What do these policies tell you about the culture of these organizations?

Procedures

A procedure describes a particular way of accomplishing an action. It is a series of steps to provide details to reach an end or to describe how to carry

out a policy. Unlike policies, which tend to be more enduring, the wording of procedures generally allows some variation in actions that are acceptable as long the intent and outcome of the procedure is reached.

Procedures also tend to evolve more over time because of the impact of new technology and processes on tasks completed and responsibilities met. For example, the policy on reimbursement of interview expenses is not likely to change, but the procedures for an applicant to receive reimbursement may change. Despite this flexibility and modification, procedures are the established methods for conducting the business of an organization. See Activity 6.2 and Sidebar 6.2.

ACTIVITY 6.2
WRITING PROCEDURES

Prepare an accompanying procedure(s) for the policies listed in Activity 6.1. Include a *draft* of the steps necessary to carry out the policies. For example, for the Nonsmoking Policy, a procedure may be:

The Chief of Physical Plant Services:

1. Posts and maintains nonsmoking signs at all entrances and other appropriate locations.
2. Designates two outdoor smoking permitted areas and posts smoking permitted signs.
3. Places appropriate receptacles in each designated smoking permitted area.
4. Checks on the condition of the signs and smoking areas biweekly.
5. Replaces or repairs signage or areas as necessary within 24 hours.
6. Receives reports of incidents of smoking in violation of the policy from employees and guests.
7. Reports incidents of smoking violation to the Assistant Vice President of Operations within 24 hours.

Policy and Procedure Template

Policies and procedures are more likely to be effective if they accurately describe an activity using consistent terminology to ensure the consistency of the results. They must be logical, detailed, free of spelling and grammatical errors, and understandable. There should be no gaps in the steps to ensure adherence and the desired outcome. A template or standard format for policies and procedures is valuable for improving their

---

Sidebar 6.2

Other Organizational Documents

✦ Policies and procedures should be distinguished from the bylaws of a health-care organization, clinical guidelines, and protocols.

✦ *Bylaws* are the essential legal framework of a corporation that typically addresses procedures for holding meetings, electing officers, and defining the duties and powers of the corporation. Shareholders or boards of directors adopt *bylaws* to provide detailed implementation of the articles of incorporation of their organizations.

✦ *Clinical practice guidelines* (pathways) are systematically developed statements based on established standards to assist in the decision making of practitioners and patients about appropriate health care for specific clinical conditions.

✦ *Protocols* are specific, detailed plans for treatment regimens (or a scientific study). Protocols are about doing and clinical practice guidelines are about deciding.

---

effectiveness. Although the layout of a policy and procedure may vary, they typically include the following sections:

  ✦ Title and tracking number
  ✦ Effective date
  ✦ Review/revision date
  ✦ Policy
    ✦ Purpose
    ✦ Persons affected
    ✦ Scope
    ✦ Background
    ✦ Definitions
  ✦ Procedures
    ✦ Responsibilities
  ✦ Approval signatures

This format reflects a system that combines policies and procedures in one document. Some organizations may choose to separate policies and procedures into two manuals that are cross-referenced. There is a risk that people are less likely to look up the information they need in two sources because it is more difficult for readers, but because procedures are revised more

frequently than policies, some organizations find it easier to keep policies and procedures separate. Use Activities 6.3 and 6.4 for further consideration of these issues.

ACTIVITY 6.3
DEVELOPING A TEMPLATE

Select the policies and procedures of any organization by searching policies and procedures on the Web. Critique the template used against the list of sections provided. Improve upon the list or the template reviewed if necessary. Using a selected policy and procedure template as a model, refine the policy and procedures developed in Activity 6.2.

ACTIVITY 6.4
PACKAGED POLICIES AND PROCEDURE

Search for software or another commercial package available for health-care policies and procedures. Critique the product. Share your impressions with that of other members of a group. Are these products a good investment for managers?

A Manager's Responsibility

Policies and procedures are about accountability for decisions at all levels of an organization and the processes that are required to accomplish its goals. Managers are responsible for preparing them from the reader's viewpoint to assure their implementation. It is unreasonable to expect people simply to know what to do. They may bring assumptions from prior work experiences that are no longer applicable, or they may be expected to perform duties that are new to them. Even experienced employees may need to be reoriented to their work as changes in the organization or technology result in new ways of doing things or new responsibilities.

Managers need to be the experts on their organizations' policies and procedures. Questions often arise because of the difficulty in identifying every possible step and possibility in a procedure, or because the procedures themselves are added or changed faster than they can be written or revised. Mangers are expected to be the people to turn to resolve these questions. They must then revise the policies and procedures in question to so that they may be followed effectively.

Encouraging those affected by policies and procedures to participate in their review and to make recommendations for improving them is likely to be an important institutional policy that increases ownership (increased commitment to) of the manual. Managers who assign new employees to read and then sign off on a policy and procedure manual during the orientation process may discover this is a meaningless exercise. An alternative may be to introduce questions or problems during orientation sessions or meetings and ask employees to find the relevant policy and procedure to address them, either individually or in groups. This approach also presents the opportunity to update or revise policies. Particularly important are policies and procedures related to their legal rights and responsibilities that employees need to understand.

Managers must be vigilant to new actions or technologies that require revisions or new policies and procedures in a timely manner. In institutions with policy and procedures committees, managers must initiate these processes rather than wait to be reminded to update or add to them. Writing policies and procedures earlier than later saves time and diminishes the chances for potential errors or inconsistencies in performance.

Because a policy and procedure manual may be used when employees seek legal solutions to problems with their employers or when patients question the care they have received, managers also must consider the manual a potential risk management and quality assurance tool. Being confronted with a manual during legal proceedings, a manager would not want to be caught in the awkward position of reporting that it is outdated and not really the way things are done. When forced to choose, courts often will interpret actions by organizational personnel as representative of the organization's preferred course of action over related, documented policies that may not be consistent with those actions. See Activity 6.5.

REFERENCE

1. Paige JB. Solve the policy and procedure puzzle. *Nursing Management.* 2003; March 34(3) 45–48 Available at: http://www.nursingmanagement.com. Accessed on January 12, 2008.

ACTIVITY 6.5
POLICY AND PROCEDURE REVISIONS

Currently, staff at Greendale Hospital has not been involved in the review of policies and procedures. Now that they are more easily accessible online by all employees, Greg Ovinio, the CEO, has asked Marsha Morris, the rehabilitation manager to come up with a plan to assure that all of her staff review the policies and procedures and make their recommendations for changes and additions during the next 3 months. How would you suggest that Marsha tackle this problem? Refer to the strategic planning section on pp. 61–62 and the worksheet below.

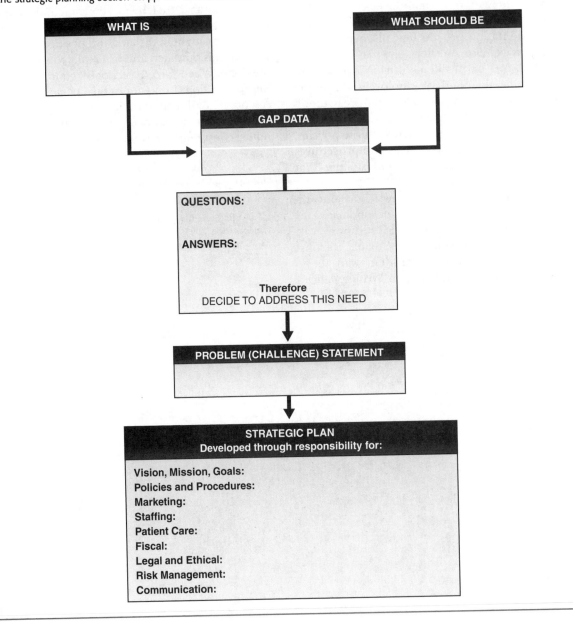

WHAT IS

WHAT SHOULD BE

GAP DATA

QUESTIONS:

ANSWERS:

Therefore
DECIDE TO ADDRESS THIS NEED

PROBLEM (CHALLENGE) STATEMENT

STRATEGIC PLAN
Developed through responsibility for:

Vision, Mission, Goals:
Policies and Procedures:
Marketing:
Staffing:
Patient Care:
Fiscal:
Legal and Ethical:
Risk Management:
Communication:

Chapter 7

Marketing Responsibilities

Learning Objectives

+ Discuss the reasons for modification of the traditional four Ps of marketing in health care.
+ Compare the characteristics and purposes of inbound and outbound marketing.
+ Distinguish among advertising, publicity, promotion, and public relations.
+ Compare traditional and social marketing strategies.
+ Compare the cost and effectiveness of branding and other marketing tools.
+ Discuss the need to consult with marketing professionals.

Overview

Despite its long history that has lead to a variety of models, as a management tool, marketing is relatively new to health care. Provoked by the dramatic changes in health-care reimbursement, hospitals and other components of the system were faced with consumers who had become more street smart about their health care and needed to be related to differently. The days of "the doctor is always right," and "hospitals know how to take care of you" were changed by patients who were finding their own information and asking more questions. At the same time, new hospital executives brought along trusted business tools that included marketing plans as they moved to health care from other industries. As a result, marketing is now enmeshed in the responsibilities of managers at all levels of all health-care organizations.

For the purposes of this chapter, marketing is a process that includes a wide range of activities to make sure that an organization meets its goals by meeting the needs of its customers. The focus of marketing is the exchange of something of value. For instance, a physical therapist treats a patient in exchange for money from the patient and/or from a third-party payer, a physician receives staff privileges at a hospital in exchange for admitting patients there, or an employer pays insurance premiums in exchange for health-care coverage for its employees. Marketing enhances all of these transactions and it is considered successful when the goals of both parties are met.[1]

Traditional marketing approaches have been modified in health care because of the uniqueness of its business. Customer satisfaction became patient satisfaction and new ways to measure satisfaction had to be developed. Unlike other customers, patients are rarely the ultimate decision maker about "buying" health-care services, and they usually do not have a choice when they need a service. They do not know the price of a health-care service so patients do not base selecting a service on price, even when they have a choice. Patients require the referral of professionals to services that they often know little about, making it difficult for them to judge their quality.[1] Consider the differences in the buying processes when a person needs a new television and when a person needs a total joint arthroplasty, for example. See Sidebar 7.1 for a classic marketing approach.

Sidebar 7.1

The Four Ps

The classic approach to marketing is control of the Four Ps. Although discounted by some marketing professionals as inappropriate for health-care organizations, they do clarify marketing issues:

✦ **PRODUCT:** the goods, services, and ideas offered by an organization. A lasting, loyal relationship is often considered the product of health care for marketing purposes.

✦ **PRICE:** the charge for the product including professional fees, insurance premiums, deductible and co-payments, etc. *Effort costs* are often included in health-care marketing. In addition to money, patients and clients must relate costs to long-term benefits of care, including lifestyle changes that demand a great deal of effort on their part.

✦ **PLACE:** the manner in which goods and services are distributed to consumers. Place often enhances the perceptions of quality in health care. Place includes communications that are not face to face like online information, 24-hour nursing consults, and the ability to share medical records electronically.

✦ **PROMOTION:** any means used to inform a market that an answer to their need is available to facilitate an exchange. It is often a mix of advertising, direct sales, sales promotions, publicity, etc.

Thomas[1] suggests that marketing should be viewed as processes that are both inbound to the organization and outbound from the organization. He describes these processes as follows:

✦ *Inbound marketing* includes marketing research to identify potential customers and their needs, the means to meet those needs, analysis of the competition, and positioning and pricing a new service (finding a niche).

✦ *Outbound marketing* is the promotion of a product or service through advertising, public relations, and sales strategies.

Marketing typically focuses on one particular service or product at a time because the activities used to be successful may be very different one from another. Success depends on attention to *both* inbound and outbound marketing processes. Until recently, health care focused primarily on outbound marketing, typically without much attention to or analysis of its effect. Physicians were often the only focus of hospital marketing efforts. Patients, employers, third-party payers, and many others also have become customers. Today, health-care systems often have vice presidents of marketing who guide plans that are implemented at all levels of an organization. Even solo practitioners must assume responsibility for marketing to reach the goals of their smaller organizations. This chapter identifies some major components of inbound and outbound marketing.

Inbound Marketing

Target Markets

According to Thomas[1] (and many others), the first inbound marketing responsibility is to identify the potential groups of patients or clients with specific needs to be met, or to survey a broad group of people in a community to identify opportunities for new programs that may need development. This development is particularly important in health care where increasing the patient base is very important to increasing revenue and profits when costs and reimbursement are so tightly controlled. Target markets can be identified or described by age, sex, income/educational levels, profession/career, type of residence, and zip code, etc. Marketing success is dependent on knowing customers likes, dislikes, goals, and expectations. In other words, answering the question—What will satisfy them?

Technology for data collection and analysis has made these processes easier and has lead to a boom in the data management. It has become easier to gather information about specific groups, often called *target markets* or *market segments*, and their needs. These techniques include: simply having employees report what customers ask for or complain about, directly asking customers in person about their needs, or having patients submit comment cards. Focus groups, case studies, and surveys (i.e., mail, phone, and Internet) also are commonly used. See Sidebars 7.2 and 7.3 and Activity 7.1.

Product Clarification

Because of this inbound process, managers should be able to describe clearly the product or service from the eyes of the target market group. Emphasizing special features that have been designed to anticipate their particular needs builds satisfaction and loyalty. Determining how a product or service is packaged and priced is the next step. Finally, the demand for a product or service in health care needs to be identified as much as is possible. Understanding the demand can be challenging because of the complexity of access to services, variable payment for those services, the unpredictable nature of injuries and diseases, and frequent changes in reimbursement policies.

Competition

Managers also need to direct their attention to the competition. If a product or service is new or unique, there may be no direct competition. More often, in health care, there may be a great deal of competition. Managers need to first decide their attitudes about their competition. Competitors may be ignored so that all energy is focused on other aspects of the business; or managers may obsessively track the strategies of competitors to outdo them, or they may imitate them. In any case, managers need to establish the uniqueness of their products and identify a name, or brand, to reflect that image to set them apart from the competition.

The starting point of this process is competitor analysis. This is another critical component of inbound marketing, which helps to determine the advantages an organization has over another. It helps in forecasting returns on possible future investments in the organization. One way to analyze the competition is for managers to ask some key questions:

✦ Who are the competition for meeting specific customer needs or preferences?

✦ What is the competition's profile? Location? Vision, mission, and goals? Organizational structure? Ownership? Growth? Other products and services? Market segments served? Customer loyalty? Facilities? Capacity? Number and types of employees?

✦ What strategies do they use to meet their objectives?

✦ What threats does the competition pose?

✦ How do competitors' products and services differ from each other and from the planned product or service?

- ✦ What are the strengths and weaknesses of the competitors' product or service?
- ✦ Are differences in prices important?
- ✦ How satisfied are the competition's customers?
- ✦ Who are the competition's partners and supporters?
- ✦ How is the competition doing overall?
- ✦ What are possible actions to beat the competition? Can they be done?
- ✦ How will the competition react to the projected changes if they are made?
- ✦ Who are potential new competitors?

Gathering data to answer these questions requires putting together information from a variety of sources which include published reports and brochures; and asking suppliers, customers, and former employees. Simple, disciplined, direct observation of advertising, press releases, trade-show presentations, and other social contacts also provide information. Tracking changes in the competition's advertising may reveal new directions, products, and services or a change in the focus of their strategies.

Benchmarking

A tool for comparing competitors is benchmarking. Using ideal standards that have been identified as best practices for a variety of key success factors, comparisons among organizations are made. Managers use benchmarks to identify necessary initiatives to improve their competitive position.

Managers must first identify which areas of an organization would benefit from benchmarking, and the costs and importance of changes that may result from a study. When an area (usually financial resources or products and services) has been selected for benchmarking, the variables to be measured are identified. The best in class companies are then selected because of their performance on the selected variables—lowest cost, or highest patient satisfaction, or lowest employee turnover are examples. These companies may be direct competitors or the best at a particular variable in another industry. Data may be gathered from a wide variety of sources, or an organization may contract with a company that gathers data for organizations. See Sidebars 7.4 and 7.5.

In the next step of the benchmarking process, managers analyze the collected results to identify gaps in the performance of their organizations when compared

with the best in class with the best estimates available. Then comes the hard part, developing and implementing a strategic plan to meet or exceed the competition that may range from doing the same things better or developing an entirely different approach. The final managerial responsibility in benchmarking is monitoring and analyzing the result of the new plan and using the results as the basis for future benchmarking. Of course, becoming best in class may be an important outcome of this process.

The SWOT Strategy

SWOT is another classic marketing analysis strategy. SWOT identifies the **S**trengths and **W**eaknesses of an organization (i.e., internal factors, such as resources and capabilities) and the possible **O**pportunities and **T**hreats (i.e., external factors, such as competition, reimbursement, and governmental policies). SWOT is generated through an environmental scan that is a systematic surveillance of the internal and external events and conditions that affect the organization.

SWOT allows managers to summarize and filter key points about their organizations. See Activity 7.2.

ACTIVITY 7.2
DETERMINING A MARKET

Sid Williams is a physical therapy manager of his own practice. He attends the World Confederation of Physical Therapy Convention and is impressed with a program using a new approach to increasing physical activity of elderly people who live independently in a community. He thinks he would like to develop a similar program in his practice. It might be good for business and the community. How should Sid decide if this would be a good business decision?

Outbound Marketing

Outbound marketing has shifted somewhat from image advertising to specific, targeted promotions that include more informational content for specific products and services. Advertising and promotions are supplemented with sales and public (or media) relations that focus on an organization as a whole. They are complemented by customer service and satisfaction efforts. If inbound marketing efforts have been effective, outbound marketing should easily fall into place. If inbound marketing was skipped or ineffective, no amount of outbound marketing may lead to the desired level of use of a product or service. The days of developing a product or service and then convincing people they want it seem to be over.

Branding

Health care faces the challenge of marketing intangible concepts like quality and professionalism to develop a perception of the organization. This requires establishing a mindset of the image of the organization and its services. Services are often difficult to quantify and evaluate because they are personal, subjective experiences that are not open to the same type of quality controls that goods are. They reflect the persons who are providing them, and really cannot be owned or transferred. The solution to this dilemma is a brand—some name, symbol, or other feature that distinguishes an organization from other similar organizations or services. Branding is less common in health

care but because brands incorporate intangible values, images, and benefits into some visual feature that stimulates demand, it may become a more important health-care marketing tool. See Activity 7.3.

ACTIVITY 7.3
BRANDING

Using printed and online resources identify branding efforts of health-care organizations or physical therapy practices. Describe your impressions of the organization because of its branding.

Selecting Marketing Tools

Managers have to decide the comparative value of efforts expended, funds available, and costs associated with a wide range of outbound marketing possibilities. Particular attention must be given to which target market(s) to appeal to and what message is to be communicated. The most preferred and effective means for delivering the message is balanced against what is affordable and practical. Some selected tools are:

- Sponsorships of sport teams, charities, and the arts
- Memberships in community and civic organizations
- Memberships in professional associations
- Community outreach, such as participation in health fairs and other educational programs
- Logos on stationary supplies, apparel, and signage
- Publication of newsletters and brochures
- Hard copy advertising in newspapers, community directories, entertainment programs, billboards, and banners
- Media advertising
- Publicity and promotions
- Web-page development, including message boards and links for more information
- Networking

Determining which of these possibilities may bring the biggest bang for the dollar depends on understanding the target market that is the focus of advertising and other possible interventions. The direct impact of general advertising on the desired results of an organization may be difficult to assess, although important, particularly in the early stages of the development of a new practice. Establishing guidelines for supporting and participating in community activities may be wise. Without them, there is a risk of insulting someone while trying to please everyone.

For instance, considering how many people in a target market actually attend high school football games may help a manager decide whether or not sponsoring a small billboard on the athletic field is a wise investment. Participating in a fraternal organization or an association of business owners may be time better spent than preparing and mailing a newsletter to every household in a selected zip code. Networking activities that develop and nurture relationships among businesses may be very comfortable for health professionals. Arranging social activities that bring people together for this purpose are often viewed positively, particularly when little time is available for face-to-face interactions.

Web sites provide an opportunity to be discovered by people conducting searches for physical therapy services, and may include many educational resources attractive to more than one target market segment. Again, the time, efforts, and costs of Web pages may seem exciting and cutting edge, but may not be effective marketing. If the number of people in the community with Internet access is limited, word of mouth may be a much more powerful marketing tool. It goes a long way with little costs except the efforts necessary to develop good will. Sidebar 7.6 clarifies some marketing terminology.

Marketing Physicians and Others

A target market of particular concern to all independent practitioners are the physicians and other health professionals who may refer to a physical therapist practice. Not only must managers establish referral relationships, and identify and meet the needs of the people who refer, but they must be able to sustain a consistent commitment from the physicians and others for referrals. Establishing and sustaining relationships with case managers, vocational rehabilitation counselors, employers, and attorneys to increase referrals is equally important in many practices. As physical therapy practices compete with each other for a limited number of contracts with third-party payers, strategies to meet the needs of decision makers in insurance companies also becomes critical. See Activities 7.4 and 7.5.

Sidebar 7.6

Advertising, Publicity, Promotion, and Public Relations

<u>Advertising</u> is publicity and nonmedia efforts that is paid for and controlled by an organization.

<u>Publicity</u> is appearing in the media. Organizations do not control the message that is developed by media reporters and writers.

<u>Promotion</u> is ongoing advertising and publicity that keeps the product or service in the minds of the customer and helps stimulate demand.

<u>Public relations</u> is the process to ensure that an organization has a strong public image and to help the public understand the organization. Advertising and publicity contribute to this image either negatively or positively, so the message conveyed is very important.

EXAMPLE

<u>Advertising:</u> Flyer on bulletin boards in local restaurants reads—Fourth St. Physical Therapy Center. Hours 7 a.m. to 7 p.m. Mon.–Sat.

<u>Publicity:</u> An expert on peripheral vascular disease gives a 1-hour presentation on Open House Night at Fourth St. Physical Therapy and is interviewed by a reporter for the health section of the newspaper.

<u>Promotion:</u> 1-hour presentation on a different diagnosis the first Friday of every month during Fourth Street Physical Therapy Open House Night.

<u>Public Relations:</u> Fourth Street Physical Therapy receives an award for outstanding physical therapy practice in the state.

ACTIVITY 7.4
REFERRAL RELATIONSHIPS

1. Laura Phillips has decided that physicians in her community are her most important target market. What should she learn about these physicians?
2. Compose a cover letter introducing her practice that she will send to almost 300 physicians.
3. Develop an outline for Laura to follow when she visits personally with key physicians.
4. What should Laura do to sustain and consolidate the referral relationships she establishes as a result of these efforts?
5. What are other possible referral sources? How would she modify this approach to target them?

ACTIVITY 7.5
A MEDIA ANNOUNCEMENT

Crestview Manor Nursing and Rehab Center will begin offering outpatient services to the general community. Create a media announcement to send to the local radio station to alert the public about this new service. The announcement should include: the name of the organization, address, Web address, name of contact, phone and fax numbers, e-mail address, heading, main announcement in 10 words or less, detailed announcement of 75 words, and a few other less important details that people may want to know.

Social Marketing

The discussion so far has focused on commercial marketing to bring about voluntary exchanges that result in the organization meeting its goals and patients meeting their needs. Social marketing is the application of commercial marketing techniques to services that are designed to influence the *voluntary* behavior of target groups to improve their personal welfare and that of society. Examples include smoking cessation, safe sex, breast cancer screening, family planning, and seat-belt use programs. The key concepts in social marketing include:[2]

- A patient/customer-centered orientation
- Segmentation of target markets
- Accounting for real and perceived barriers that prevent people from adopting a new behavior

- Demonstrating the benefits of the desired change for people in the target markets
- Using a variety of means to reach target markets
- Pretesting and monitoring marketing interventions as they are implemented
- Forming partnerships that enhance credibility and facilitate access to target markets
- Coordinating with other approaches to social change
- Making a long-term commitment to the social marketing strategy

Physical therapy managers must distinguish between traditional marketing efforts directed to meeting the needs of customers and social marketing efforts directed to change the behaviors of a group of people. For example, physical therapists may be involved with a program created by a health-care system to increase the number of at-risk women who are screened for breast and ovarian cancer each year. Social marketing strategies may include asking female patients for the date of their last mammogram as part of the physical therapy admission screening process, reminding them of the importance of screening during therapy sessions, or providing general information pamphlets on the importance of breast cancer screening in the waiting room. Social marketing shifts the emphasis of marketing from what is good for the organization to what is good for the broader society.

A Manager's Responsibility

There are many complex aspects of inbound and outbound marketing. Managers in health-care organizations typically rely on marketing experts who are also employed by the same organization, or who consult with organizations to address particular target markets. Because marketing is about taking risks and decisions often boil down to two plans that are equally attractive, input from specialists is desirable.

Even the best efforts at inbound and outbound marketing may fail. Managers need to be comfortable that they made the best effort to arrive at the best decision particularly as it relates to the needs of people who are often in crisis when they require health-care services. Managers also need to consider the ethical implications of both commercial and social marketing plans, considering whether actions are persuasive or coercive, for example. How the organization addresses these issues so that the target markets are respected and treated fairly is somewhat enhanced by the shift from straight advertising to promotions that emphasize education.

Evaluating the effectiveness of marketing efforts is another challenge because direct relationships between efforts and results may not be obvious, or even measurable. For instance, increased profit margins, satisfaction of staff and patients, increased demands for services, or the number of new patients may be associated with advertising and public relations or not. It may indicate that inbound processes were effective, or not. Managers must be prepared to contribute to both establishing and evaluating marketing efforts. See Activity 7.6.

REFERENCES

1. Thomas RK. *Marketing Health Services*. Arlington, VA: Health Administration Press; 2005.
2. Longest BB. *Health Policymaking in the United States*. 4th ed. Chicago, IL: American College of Healthcare Executives; 2006.

ACTIVITY 7.6
STRATEGIC APPROACH TO MARKETING

Refering to the strategic planning section on pp. 61–62 and the worksheet below, address an inbound or outbound marketing need that a typical physical therapy practice often needs to meet.

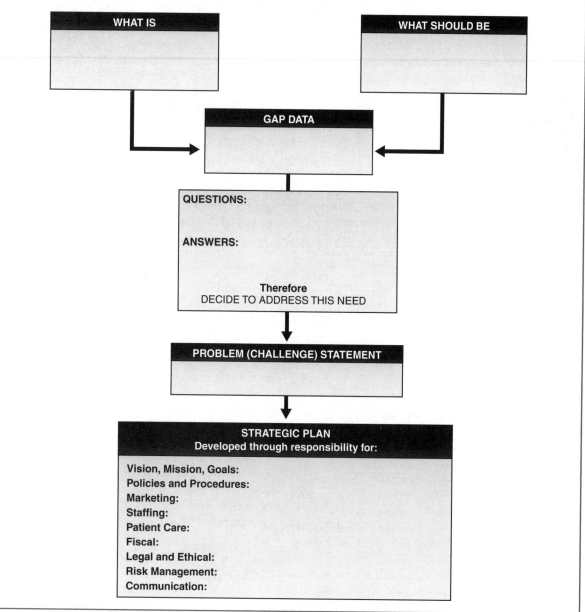

Chapter 8

Staffing Responsibilities

Learning Objectives

+ Identify compensation costs.
+ Compare exempt and nonexempt employees.
+ Prepare a job description for a physical therapist and a physical therapist assistant.
+ Analyze a physical therapist career ladder.
+ Develop a career ladder for physical therapist assistants.
+ Analyze productivity models.
+ Analyze staff mix decisions.
+ Analyze approaches for recruitment and retention of staff.
+ Review hints for interviews.
+ Analyze performance evaluation tools.
+ Set performance goals for a given person using observable behaviors.
+ Discuss approaches to staff development.
+ Discuss management of formal employee grievances.

Overview

In any business, the highest operating cost is staffing. In 2007, an average of 70% of the total costs of employers was for compensation to their employees.[1] Although opportunities may be limited for some people, employment is generally a matter of voluntary free choice, and without staff to accomplish its goals, there are no organizations. Therefore, organizations must add to their high compensation costs the costs associated with the recruitment and retention of their employees.

Managers devote a great deal of their time and efforts to orientation of new employees, work assignments, performance evaluation, and development of the skills of their staffs. In addition, at the heart of the staffing responsibilities of managers in health care is ensuring that employees provide the expected level of quality of care needed to achieve the organization's goals through teamwork and cooperation. Managers must devote attention to the motivation and satisfaction of employees for patients to be satisfied. Patient satisfaction may depend on *how* clinicians and others do their work as much as the actual outcomes of the work they do. For most patients, their interactions with staff members are their impression of an organization. Because of their dependence on employees for meeting such important goals, organizations often consider their staffs their most powerful asset. Each topic in this chapter addresses some aspect of these staffing responsibilities. Related employment laws are presented in the Chapter 12.

Staff Mix

Managers of physical therapy practices may not have a great deal of flexibility in determining the mix of physical therapists, physical therapist assistants, and nonlicensed personnel on staff. In some jurisdictions, the ratio of physical therapists to physical therapist assistants is regulated. Most third-party payers and many jurisdictions recognize that only services provided by physical therapists, and physical therapist assistants under their direction and supervision, can be billed as physical therapy. The role of physical therapy aides, therefore, is as other support personnel. The expectation is that aides are assigned to only very specific tasks that are related more to the operation of the physical therapy practice than patient care. When involved in patient care, they must perform their duties under the direct, continuous, personal supervision of a physical therapist (or physical therapist assistant where legal) who must be physically and immediately available. See Activity 8.1.

Given these restrictions, managers still need to determine what combination of clinical staff can do the most for the least cost. This involves serious attention to job analysis and accurate job descriptions. Managers need to take the time to observe actual work in their setting(s) to determine:

+ What tasks are currently performed by each level of worker?
+ What tasks can each level of worker legally perform?
+ What tasks can be eliminated?
+ What tasks are more easily completed by the physical therapist rather than someone else who will require the time of the physical therapist for direction and supervision?
+ When is work time unproductive?
+ Who is the least expensive worker who can perform each task safely, legally, and effectively?

Any shift in duties and responsibilities because of this analysis needs to be confirmed with the people who actually do the work. A regular re-examination of job descriptions and the number of positions needed may lead to surprising conclusions. For instance, it may not always be the best clinical decision to hire an aide if it means that physical therapists' salaries will be frozen to accommodate that new position. It may be better to hire a physical therapist assistant rather than a physical therapist if the number of new patients per week is low and cancellations are high. Hiring physical therapist assistants when physical therapists prefer a one-on-one, hands-on approach in a specialized practice may result in reduced productivity for the assistants because their patient care assignments will be limited.

Staff mix decisions are never easy. Managers cannot afford to have exempt employees occupied with duties that can be performed by other levels of workers, and they cannot risk the safety of patients and

---

> ### ACTIVITY 8.1
> ### AN AIDE FOR THE SUMMER
>
> Kim Bartholomew's little brother Ken has been receiving outpatient physical, occupational, and speech therapy at Smith and Associates Pediatric Rehabilitation intermittently for all his life—4 years. Kim has approached Anita Smith about a summer job in the practice. She wants to be a physical therapist and feels that a job will not only help her pay for college but give her work experience. Kim feels because she helps to care for her brother and accompanied him to many of his therapy sessions, she has skills that would be of value to Anita.
>
> Anita is short-handed and almost said yes immediately, but she asked Kim to give her a chance to think about it. She only employs licensed therapists and does not have a physical therapist assistant on staff. What does Anita need to consider as she contemplates an aide's position?

quality of outcomes by assigning tasks to workers who are not qualified to perform them. These decisions are further complicated by the fact that not all employees in the same category of work are equally effective. Managers must be fair in expecting the same performance and amount of work for everyone with the same job description. Strong employees become resentful if they feel that managers tend to reward their outstanding performance with more work while mediocre performers receive fewer assignments.

Another staff-mix issue is the ratio of full-time to part-time and contract employees. Particularly if full-time employees are working for salary and those who are not salaried are nonexempt hourly employees. These classifications may be complicated if the hourly rates are significantly higher than salaries for 40 hours of nonexempt work. Full-time employees may become resentful, particularly if there is an actual or perceived favoritism associated with contract status. See Activity 8.2 to explore this issue in more detail. The Fair Labor Standards Act (FLSA) issues may become very complex requiring legal advice in consultation with human resource experts as contracts with registries and other temporary employment companies for placement of workers in an organization are negotiated (see Sidebar 8.1). The potential for associated higher costs in these contracts is another management consideration.

ACTIVITY 8.2
FULL-TIME VERSUS CONTRACT

Candace Peterson has been a full-time staff physical therapist at Wilson County Health Care for 5 years and she is the only one left. She is increasingly unhappy because it seems that her manager prefers to hire contract physical therapists and has not made any efforts to recruit more staff that are full-time employees. Because of the turnover among the contracting physical therapists, Candace feels that she gets behind in her work as she is called upon to help the new contracting therapists with their patients. She also has become resentful because they seem to select only the easier patients when new referrals arrive at the office. She has asked to meet with her manager, Larry Edwards, to discuss her frustrations. She feels that she cannot risk the potential loss of income if she converted to contract physical therapist status should the work available decrease. She needs the health insurance benefit of full-time employment. Role play their meeting.

Job Descriptions

Before recruiting and hiring staff, each position in an organization must have an accompanying job description that serves several purposes:

✦ To establish qualifications and other criteria to recruit the right person for the position.

✦ To classify a position into a pay scale by comparing it with all other job descriptions.

✦ To provide details of duties and responsibilities, physical demands, and other performance expectations.

✦ To serve as the basis for evaluation of work performance.

The creation of new positions and job descriptions is taken very seriously because of the financial implications of the additional costs associated with expanding an organization's workforce. Managers often are faced with a series of approvals to justify the creation of a new position that is aligned with the strategic plans and goals of the organization. Demonstrating how and why a new position is different from those in place is part of this process. Determining if the job description for a contract or part-time employee is different from that for a full-time employee is another important component of this responsibility.

Job descriptions typically include a heading section that includes the job title, grade or level, a unique job code, FLSA status, and implementation date. The body of the job description usually includes a brief overview

---

Sidebar 8.1

Exempt and Nonexempt Employees[2]

Wage-based employees (nonexempt). The Fair Labor Standards Act (FLSA) requires that employees be paid at least the federal minimum wage for all hours worked, and overtime pay at time and one-half the regular rate of pay for all hours worked more than 40 hours in a work week. They typically punch time clocks to determine actual time worked (usually includes all clinical and other support staff who are not physical therapists).

Salary-based employees (exempt). Executives, administrative, professional*, computer, and outside sale employees are exempt from FLSA act if they are paid a salary rather than an hourly wage of at least $455/week. Specific job duties and salary rather than job title determine exempt status. Exempt employees receive a predetermined amount of compensation each pay period (salary) that is not reduced because of variations in their work, and they receive full salary regardless of the number of days or hours worked. As long as they are ready, willing, and able to work exempt employees are paid even if no work is available. Although not stated in the law, employers expect exempted employees to work as long as it takes to get their work and responsibilities done (typically physical therapists are considered exempt employees in full-time positions).

Fee-based employees (may be exempt). Employees paid an agreed sum (fee) for a single, unique job rather than a series of jobs repeated a number of times for the same payment each time are another category of worker. If the fee is at a rate that would amount to $455/week, the employee is exempt from the FLSA. Example: A project that takes 20 hours to complete for a fee of $250 would be equivalent to $500 in a 40-hour week.

---

*The test of a professional is met if the employees make at least $455/week, their primary duty is work requiring advanced knowledge in science or learning that is intellectual and requires consistent exercise of discretion and judgment. The advanced knowledge is acquired through a prolonged course of specialized study.

of the job, essential and nonessential functions, requirements, and other desirable skills or abilities. There is always a statement to the effect that the job description may not be all-inclusive and other duties may be assigned. Practice writing a job description in Activity 8.3

ACTIVITY 8.3
WRITING JOB DESCRIPTIONS

Search for job description templates on the Web. Select one that you think is most appropriate for physical therapists or physical therapist assistants. Complete the template for a generic job description for a physical therapist or physical therapist assistant that could be used in any health-care setting. How would your generic job description change for a particular type of setting? HINT: Go to the Occupational Information Network at http://www.job-descriptions.info/index.html for more information on job descriptions. Also, use resources of the American Physical Therapy Association.

Compensation Costs

When the staff mix and job descriptions have been established, determining compensation for each position and the total cost for all staff demands attention. As a component of inbound marketing discussed in Chapter 7, it also may be risky for an organization to deliberately, or unknowingly, deviate from the going rates for wages and salaries offered by the competition. Underpayment may lead to the inability to fill vacant positions, and overpayment may dip into funds needed for other expenses. For large organizations and independent practitioners, software programs often are used to manage all aspects of compensation and payroll benefits that may include:

- Direct wages and salaries
- Bonuses
- Retirement plans and pensions
- Life, health, accident, and disability insurance
- Vacations, holidays, sick days
- Other leave: jury duty, educational programs, military duty
- Professional society dues
- Journal subscriptions
- Cars and housing
- Club memberships
- Expense accounts

Employers also may arrange for payroll deductions to provide employees the convenience of payment of parking, child care, and other fees; or to make charitable donations. They also withhold social security and retirement contributions and the employees' shares of insurance premiums. Related costs include legal requirements to provide workers' compensation for work-related injuries and unemployment insurance after involuntary termination of employment. Workers' compensation and health insurance benefits are discussed in Chapter 4.

Managers must keep an eye on all of these compensation expenditures in relationship to the accomplishment of the organization's goals. Realizing the value of a given benefit is in the eye of the employee, and because not all employees value the same benefits, many employers have moved to cafeteria plans that allow employees to select those benefits of most value to them. For example, a single worker, in his 40s, may be more interested in retirement options than life insurance, while a married man whose wife has family health-care coverage through her employer, may decline health insurance but take advantage of subsidized childcare at an on-site childcare center.

As long as they are administered fairly and equitably, the opportunity for flexible benefits may make one employer more attractive than another to a potential employee. Employers must be alert to legislative changes that afford tax advantages to businesses that provide certain benefits as they develop these programs. Compensation plans must be accompanied by a strong risk-management program to keep employees healthy and safe to reduce health insurance and workers' compensation costs, to minimize lost workdays, and to increase employee satisfaction.

Most of these details fall to centralized human resources experts in health-care organizations. They interact with managers of units and programs who are responsible for verifying hours worked for non-exempt employees and salaries to be paid to exempt employees. They may provide data to managers on the location and activities for analysis of total personnel costs and cost reporting of per-patient costs. They also work together to determine pay scales and reviews of wages and salaries for adjustments over time based on survey reports of similar employees in other organizations. Adjustments for cost-of-living increases, meritorious performance, seniority, or performance-based incentives also are codetermined, and often negotiated because controlling the costs associated with human resources is a shared organizational goal. Independent practice physical therapists may be at an advantage in recruitment because they have more flexibility in these human resource decisions, but they may not be as competitive in terms of benefits they offer to their employees.

Staff Recruitment and Hiring

Recruiting

Staff mix, compensation policies, and clear and current job descriptions are the first steps in recruitment efforts for all levels of employees. Recruitment requires creativity and the use of a variety of outbound marketing strategies that go beyond newspaper advertisements and professional publications to include the more recent, and popular, online recruiting resources. Formalizing and rewarding current employees with referral bonuses when their efforts lead to a new hire is another recruiting tool.

Other recruitment strategies include promoting the organization's brand with new graduates by attending college job fairs, developing clinical education relationships with schools, and promoting a classroom presence through staff who offer guest lectures. Staff members may think that there is some prestige associated with these assignments, and students may be more likely to work in places that have provided positive clinical and classroom learning experiences.

Managers need to weigh these efforts of staff against a potential negative effect on their productivity. Recognition or reward for these activities that may not be included in a job description (or appear as other assigned duties) may be indicated. Offering new graduates sign-on bonuses or student loan forgiveness programs are other popular recruitment tools.

A common management saying is "find the best, train the rest." In other words, not all recruitment efforts lead to hiring the most qualified person for every job. Recruitment efforts should, however, lead to hiring people who are the best match with the organization who also have the potential to learn the work of the positions they were hired to fill. Determining this ability to contribute requires the identification and nurturing of the important skills, knowledge, and talents of employees that are necessary for patients to have superior health-care experiences. Reviewing credentials and gathering information during employment interviews are the typical means for making these determinations about job applicants. Conversely, becoming the employer of choice requires serious attention from a variety of perspectives. Using the strategic process found on pp. 61–62 may be helpful in clarifying what recruitment problems require solving. See Activity 8.4.

ACTIVITY 8.4
RECRUITMENT TEAM

Mercy Hospital has created a recruitment committee that includes the director of human resources and the managers of each of the hospital's units. Their charge is to develop a new recruitment plan to fill four positions in rehabilitation services, 12 positions in nursing, and six positions in other units. The usual extensive advertising campaigns and contracts with professional recruitment companies have not been successful. Mercy is a good place to work. The other hospital in the city is having similar problems filling vacant positions. Role play this meeting.

Interviewing

Interviews are the opportunity for applicants to learn more about the organization and for the organization to learn more about the applicant. Additional information on interviews is presented in Chapter 13. The more important the position to be filled, the more people who are involved in the interviewing process. The more people involved, the more planning that has to occur so that knowledge gathered about the applicant is thorough, while avoiding duplication of questions by different interviewers. Including potential coworkers of the applicant in the interview process often provides applicants the opportunity to have questions answered by people who are actually experiencing potential work environment. Their impressions of an applicant may give managers information on the person's ability to fit in. Managers should be certain that including potential coworkers in an interview process does not threaten or empower them by clarifying that the final hiring decision is not their direct responsibility.

The manager's goal in interviewing is to confirm that applicants, regardless of the position in question, have the necessary technical skills or competencies, strong interpersonal and communication skills, and problem-solving abilities. Determining if the values of the applicant are compatible with the vision, mission, and goals of the organization is important. Identifying those people with that little something extra that improves patient care and the work environment can be wonderful, too. This is much easier said than done, particularly when managers also must pay strict attention to the legal requirements of interviewing. Because of these complex factors, the interview cannot be left to chance or be conducted ad-lib. Attention to compliance with employment law is another component of recruitment and hiring, which is addressed in Chapter 12.

Managers need to prepare to be effective in the interviewing process. They need to determine beforehand what they are looking for and how they will gather that information. Briefly, only questions that pertain to the person's ability to perform the job should be asked. Applicants should be able to determine how an interviewer will use their answers to the questions to make a hiring decision. To be fair, all applicants for one position should be asked similar questions. See Sidebar 8.2.

Having a standardized evaluation form to rate candidates for positions also helps interviewers stay focused and provides a tool for each interviewer to provide objective feedback on each candidate. Basing the evaluation form on the job description

for the position and the potential to contribute to the vision, mission, and goals of the organization is likely to be all that is necessary to develop an easy-to-complete, one-page form.

When the goals of successful interviewing have been met, managers are prepared, hopefully, to make the applicant an offer and close the deal. Before finalizing employment, required background checks, drug screens, and other legal documentation must be collected, all credentials verified, and any other negotiations closed.

At the other end of employment, exit interviews require that managers engage in the same preparation for the interview, offer plenty of opportunities for the employee to talk, focusing on the strengths and weaknesses of the organization's vision, mission, and goals. Interviewing employees who have chosen to terminate employment may provide insights, which would not otherwise be shared. A supervisor or manager who is not directly involved with the employee should conduct an exit interview.

Orientation

Preparing the new hire for the position is then dependent on a strong orientation to highlight responsibilities and expectations with an emphasis on safety and communication channels. Managers should not assume the level of assistance a new employee may need to transition to a new organization. The needs of someone starting his or her first full-time job are very different from the needs of someone who brings other

---

Sidebar 8.2

Hints for Successful Interviewing[3]

- ✦ Be certain the applicant has all of his or her questions answered. Know the organization.

- ✦ Select the aspects of the resume and reference letters that you want to explore or confirm.

- ✦ Identify characteristics you expect the applicant to have ahead of time. Confirm them because past behaviors predict the future.

- ✦ Make the applicant comfortable and explain the ground rules for the interview.

- ✦ Make sure the applicant understands that the goal is to learn about him or her and the match with the organization.

- ✦ Determine what he or she prefers to be called.

- ✦ Avoid interruptions and follow the applicant's pace of conversation.

- ✦ Maintain control and a logical flow of questions.

- ✦ Only seek answers to questions of interest in decision making.

- ✦ Do not talk too much. LISTEN.

- ✦ Force listening by seeking new questions in the applicant's responses to questions.

- ✦ Do not draw conclusions for 20 minutes to allow impressions to form.

work experience to a position. Managers may make themselves available, particularly during the first few months, to serve as a mentor or appoint someone to mentor a new employee. Employees also should be encouraged to identify their own mentors. In any case, a mentor may facilitate socialization in the new organization and reduce the amount of nonproductive time that accompanies all new work. Providing training to serve as a mentor and rewarding those efforts may relieve concerns about these responsibilities to encourage more participation.

Employee Retention

Some turnover is expected and desired for an organization to remain fresh with new ideas and enthusiasm, and to have new people question the status quo. However, except when employee retirement or expansion of the organization requires it, retention is always preferred because of the time and expense of recruiting. Employees are most likely to remain loyal to organizations that meet their unique needs, while also meeting the general needs of all employees who want to take pride in a safe, fair, and interesting place to work.

Identifying and finding the resources to meet these needs is a primary mana-gement responsibility. Some examples of services to meet the needs of employees include counseling, employee assistance, child care, educational opportunities, social events, discounts on goods and services, etc. that all suggest that the organization values its employees and supports them in the achievement of their personal and professional goals.

Incentives and rewards that supplement basic compensation also may lead to personal job satisfaction and recognition of the importance of work efforts of individuals and groups. Incentives are typically related to contributions to the accomplishment of budgetary goals, but may apply to quality improvement goals as well. See Activity 8.5.

Managers contribute less tangible rewards in their daily interactions with the people they supervise by encouraging, recognizing, and reinforcing actions that contribute to the success of the organization. Some suggestions for rewards that promote a positive, supportive work environment are:

- ✦ Sincerely praising accomplishments and efforts.
- ✦ Presenting tokens of appreciation in celebration of significant actions or performance.

- ✦ Practicing "do as I do" rather than "do as I say" by role modeling expected behaviors.
- ✦ Admonishing in private and praising in public.
- ✦ Relating actions to the vision, mission, and goals of the organization.
- ✦ Encouraging growth and development.
- ✦ LISTENING, LISTENING, LISTENING.

Perhaps the most important aspect of work and therefore the most important retention tool, is providing the opportunity for employees to be heard. In addition to one-on-one conversations, formal surveys and informal employee focus groups may lead to identification of negative factors or employee needs that can be easily addressed if they are identified.

ACTIVITY 8.5
$2,500 REWARD

The hospital's CEO, Jack Belfonte could not be more pleased with the outstanding efforts of Betty Montrose and her rehabilitation staff. They have turned the department around making it a star in the hospital's crown and exceeding their budget goals. To reward these efforts, Jack is presenting Betty with $2,500 to use as she sees fit to recognize the achievements she and her staff of two physical therapists, three physical therapist assistants, a receptionist, and a business office manager have accomplished. What should Betty do with the money?

Career Ladders

Another important recruitment and retention tool may be a career ladder. Career ladders are a series of formal promotions within an organization that are primarily dependent on the size of the organization. In smaller organizations, there may be only one step in the ladder from staff physical therapist to manager that only becomes available when the manager resigns or retires. In large health-care systems, there may be four or five steps in career ladders. Advancement from one step to the next is typically dependent upon years of experience, acquiring additional credentials, and performance evaluation scores. Each step is a higher pay level and typically, the step below is capped at a figure below the base rate of the next higher step. Pay scales may be increased across the board in all steps to reflect cost-of-living and other factors, but the only way for an employee to move beyond these base increases that apply to everyone, is to move up the ladder. See Table 8.1 for a career ladder with some examples of qualifications and responsibilities (not meant to be exhaustive or standard).

Each career ladder step must have an accompanying job description and the career ladder must be shared with new employees so that they understand that climbing the ladder is an expectation of the organization. Managers are responsible for determining the number of positions in each step so that there are positions in place for everyone who is qualified to move up the ladder. Given that there will be turnover of staff, this may not be an issue, but managers need to be cautious to avoid the ladder becoming top heavy while ensuring the opportunity for upward mobility for everyone that seeks it. Career ladders may be very important to some potential employees. Particularly those people who have given some thought to their long-term careers may like a structured opportunity provided by a career ladder, and experienced people may seek a lateral career move to an organization that recognizes their accomplishments through a career ladder. See Activities 8.6, 8.7, and 8.8.

TABLE 8.1 Sample physical therapist career ladder

PHYSICAL THERAPY CAREER STEPS	QUALIFICATIONS	JOB EXPECTATIONS
Rehabilitation Manager	PT SUPERVISOR including 7 years of full-time experience. Advanced graduate degree. MPH, MBA, MHA preferred.	Responsible for all aspects of rehabilitation services. Performance scores of at least 80%. Reports to VP of Clinical Services.
PT Supervisor	PT III or IV including 5 years of full-time experience, completion of in-house management training program.	Direct patient care responsibilities for average of 30 patient visits/week, documentation, and managerial responsibility for clinical or program team. Development, implementation, and evaluation of new program or ongoing management of one in place, including center coordinator of clinical education. Minimal scores of good in all performance criteria. Reports to Rehabilitation Manager.
PT IV	PT III plus board certification in APTA specialty area.	Same as PT III. Reports to PT Supervisor.
PT III	PT II plus 3 total years of full-time experience, clinical instructor for at least three full-time students.	PT II plus assignment to clinical specialty area. Clinical instructor for 24 weeks/year. Mean performance score of 4.0 and at least Good in all CI categories. Reports to PT Supervisor.
PT II	PT I plus 1 year of full-time experience, certified clinical instructor.	Direct patient care responsibilities for average of 75-patient visits/week, timely documentation, direction of physical therapist assistant, present four in-services/year, supervise one full-time student for at least 4 weeks/year. Mean performance score of 4.0 and at least Good in all CI categories. Reports to PT Supervisor.
PT I	Graduation from an accredited physical therapy education program. DPT degree. Current license.	Direct patient-care responsibilities for average of 60-patient visits/week, timely documentation, direction of physical therapist assistant, present four in-services/year. Mean performance score of at least 4.0 Reports to PT Supervisor.

Master of Public Health (MPH), Master of Business Administration (MBA), Master of Health Administration (MHA), American Physical Therapy Association (APTA), Clinical Instructor (CI), Doctor of Physical Therapy (DPT).

ACTIVITY 8.6
CRITIQUE OF A CAREER LADDER

Jonas Marcum is manager of rehabilitation services at Genoa Valley Health Care. He is about to conduct his annual review of the career ladder for physical therapists found in Table 8.1 and the accompanying job descriptions. He is preparing a report to raise the pay scales across the board. What revisions in the career ladder may strengthen his argument for more money for the physical therapists?

ACTIVITY 8.7
PHYSICAL THERAPIST ASSISTANT CAREER LADDER

The physical therapist career ladder at Genoa Valley Health Care has been well received. Liza Crockett is a physical therapy supervisor and Glenda Robertson is a physical therapist assistant at Genoa Valley. They have been assigned to develop a similar career ladder for physical therapist assistants. Role play their meetings and develop the career ladder.

ACTIVITY 8.8
AVOIDING THE LADDER

Liza Crockett, a physical therapy supervisor at Genoa Valley Health Care has met with Leonard Gottlieb, one of the physical therapists on her outpatient team, for his annual performance appraisal. He has 7 years of experience and spent the last 3 years at Genoa Valley. Although his clinical skills and patient rapport are excellent, Leonard has made no efforts to meet the other requirements to advance to the next level on the career ladder (See Table 8.1). He reluctantly supervises one student every year, and really keeps to himself with minimal interaction with his coworkers. He tells Liza that he is happy doing his job and does not intend to move up. Liza asks for a meeting with Jonas Marcum, the rehabilitation manager to discuss Leonard's performance appraisal. Role play this meeting. What action should be taken?

Productivity

Sucessful efforts to recruit and retain staff reduce the efforts of managers to monitor the day-to-day work performed by professionals, which includes work productivity. Some managers feel that productivity goals and outcome measurements are difficult to determine because of the nature of the work of physical therapy. Unpredictable cancellations and no-shows, variations in patient acuity level, and the style and skills of physical therapists and physical therapist assistants all influence their best efforts to reach target goals for number of patients treated or units billed for the services they provide in any setting. Because of these intervening variables, managers have to be careful that setting productivity or outcome goals is neither punitive nor threatening.

That said, managers need to start somewhere and may rely on the history of productivity in their organizations or benchmarking against other organizations. Employees need to have some idea of work expectations so goals expressed in numbers are important in all practice settings. If nothing else, employees may self-assess their own performance by comparing their productivity numbers with the efforts of coworkers. The danger is in focusing on numbers only without putting them in the context of the practice and processes in play. Asking how much do physical therapists work must be followed with asking what they are doing when they are working.

It is not enough only to know the ratio of productive hours to total hours worked. The more productive hours/day the better may sound like a good idea, but it can actually mean fatigued, disgruntled staff and dissatisfied patients. Scheduled breaks should be encouraged even for salaried employees and mandatory for nonexempt employees. At the other extreme, managers cannot afford too much unscheduled nonwork time. Distracters, such as personal phone calls or text messaging, private conversations, and poor patient scheduling among departments, should be minimized so that they do not interfere with the delivery of efficient, effective patient care.

Although not common, professionals with exempt-FLSA status may choose collective bargaining to resolve their employment concerns. Physical therapist assistants and other staff in a rehabilitation department who are nonexempt employees are more likely to be represented by a union that has negotiated productivity, pay scales, and other issues for them. Having employees who belong to a union may lead to adversarial rather than cooperative interactions. On the plus side, a commitment to compliance with negotiated agreements by both sides eliminates the need for managers to negotiate with each individual about assignments, productivity, time off, etc. In those organizations with collective bargaining units, managers should expect that the organization provides them education to function effectively in their interactions with both staff who are members of a bargaining unit and those who are not. See Activity 8.9.

ACTIVITY 8.9
PRODUCTIVITY

At a recent staff meeting, as usual, Janek Breznov, the rehabilitation manager reported productivity statistics for the department as a whole. Hearing mumbling, Janek discovered that his staff is very unhappy about these reports and feel that they just cannot win. Every time they reach a goal, Janek raises it. He says he cannot just eliminate measuring the performance and work of the department because he is held accountable for justifying the costs of their salaries. The expectation of upper management is that the higher their salaries, the harder they need to work. The staff says that there is only so much they can humanly do, and they insist there must be a better way. Are there alternatives for Janek to consider?

Evaluation of Staff Performance

Typically in any organization, a designated probationary period (usually 90 days) gives both the employee and employer an opportunity to test the waters of their new relationship. It typically ends with a formal review at the end of the period and the opportunity to decide to continue in the position as a permanent employee. Should either party decide during probation that the relationship is not as expected, it is typically severed without prejudice on either side.

Employment that continues beyond the probationary period includes formal, regularly scheduled performance appraisals that must be must be fair, objective, and related to set standards. A standard form that aligns with job descriptions serves as documentation of any performance review and becomes part of permanent employment records. Employees should receive regular, formal written performance appraisals, including their affect on the organization, that is presented in a face-to-face meeting. These meetings are typically conducted on a timetable

established by either outside accrediting or licensing bodies or by managers themselves. They may or may not be connected to merit salary increases.

These periodic appraisals include a compilation of all formal, documented evaluations of performance that occurred since the last performance appraisal (typically over the last year). Any actions taken to praise work or to take corrective action when concerns about performance arose in the last year are included. Immediate supervisors who have had the opportunity to directly observe and supervise work performance should complete these reports. However, managers should not let these formal documents stand alone. This ongoing process provides meeting times with an employee that also provides the employee with the opportunity to express concerns, issues, suggestions, and praise for the organization.

Any employee deficiencies or problems should be addressed by setting goals and documenting plans for improving performance. Goals also may be set for professional development or upward mobility in the organization. Assisting employees to adopt a process for setting objective, measurable work goals for themselves rather than setting goals for them, allows managers the opportunity to provide employees with a powerful tool in all aspects of their lives. Managers also have the responsibility to follow up on a regular basis to determine if actions toward established goals are implemented and to assist if necessary. Go to Activities 8.10 and 8.11.

ACTIVITY 8.10
PERFORMANCE EVALUATIONS

In groups, collect and critique existing performance evaluation forms for physical therapy positions. Develop the ideal performance evaluation form to accompany the job descriptions prepared in Activity 8.1.

If job descriptions are well-written, performance evaluations based on them should include interpersonal and problem-solving skills and patient care responsibilities. Managers may need to have the courage to address these important areas and translate impressions into specific behaviors that employees may have the opportunity to improve. For example, asking an employee to be less rude may not result in a change in behavior. What the manager

ACTIVITY 8.11
GOAL SETTING

Frances Newsome wants to help Carol Bradford set some performance goals. She thinks using the following strategic planning worksheet may help. How might Frances and Carol use this tool to improve Carol's difficulty in completing tasks on time? Review pp. 61–62 if necessary.

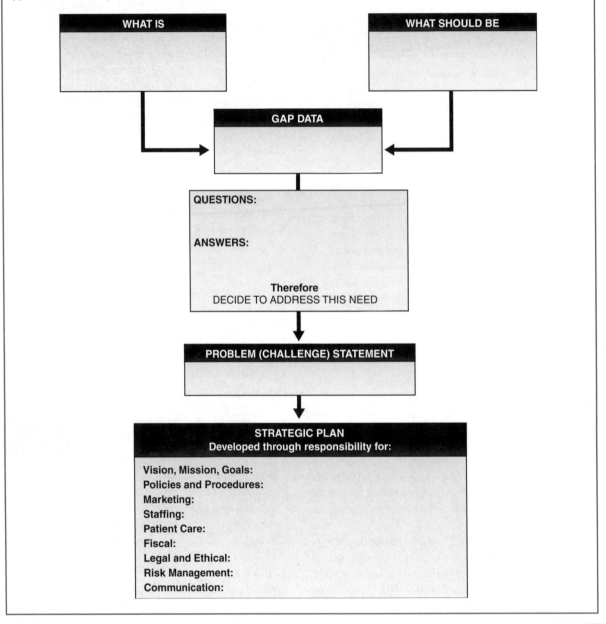

thinks is rudeness, the employee may not. The employee may be even puzzled by the comment. Instead, identifying the behaviors that portray rudeness may lead to goals, such as allowing others to finish their thoughts without interruption, addressing people by their proper names, or responding to people when they ask questions without prompting. See Activity 8.12.

ACTIVITY 8.12
IDENTIFYING WORK BEHAVIORS

Complete the following table by identifying behaviors that reflect the vague goals listed:

INSTEAD OF SAYING:	SAY:
Be less shy	
Improve your attitude	
Work harder	
Take more initiative	
Get along with others	
Work faster	
Be more friendly	
Be more creative	

Staff Development

Staff development programs are where organizations are expected to "walk the talk." If an organization wants to meet its goals and demonstrate the importance of employees to those goals, it needs to support the ongoing job training and professional development necessary to do so. These efforts may take several forms:

✦ In-house sessions on topics related to guest relations, safety, etc.

✦ Support for continuing education courses that support professional *and* organizational goals.

✦ Formal degree programs in preparation for advancement on a career ladder.

In exchange for financial support of an external degree program, an employer may require an employee to commit to continued employment for a specified time. Financial support for travel and tuition to attend continuing education programs or professional conferences that may include paid release time or time off without pay is often provided with no return obligation expected. It is not unreasonable for managers to ask employees to apply for this type of financial support. The application should include justification for the request in terms of the goals of the organization. It is also reasonable for managers to expect employees to present a report on the application of new knowledge attained through the educational experience to an assigned program or task.

In-service programs only take the time of employees but still require an investment on the part of managers to prepare and offer them. The urge to offer in-services on a regular basis just for the sake of offering them may lead to more frustration than learning. Unless it is viewed as important and relevant, employees will tune out as they go through the motions of attending required in-services. On the other hand, employees may appreciate the convenience and opportunity to improve their performance when the programs are well prepared and relevant to their work. In-services also are used to update and inform employees of policy changes and new developments in the organization.

Grievances and Other Problems

Organizations must have mechanisms for employees to have their complaints or questions addressed if they are not satisfied with responses they receive in the regular chain of command. They also must meet legal requirements for processes to address serious issues such as discrimination or harassment. Managers also may do well to have a simpler process for less serious concerns of employees. Resolution of these concerns may involve employees trusting that a manager patiently hears out a disagreement with coworkers, negotiates a vacation schedule fairly, or assists with clinical decisions. Managers typically spend a great deal more time supporting these working relationships and resolving clinical issues than they do serious grievances.

Assuring employees that they are able to present these complaints and problems to a manager who will respond fairly and consistently may relieve a great deal of their job-related emotional stress. Managers help employees realize that they may perform their duties effectively although coworkers may not all be people that they admire or choose to socialize with. Employees are relieved when they can trust their managers to follow through on promised actions.

Coworker relationships that evolve into more personal relationships also may require the attention of managers. Finding a work-home balance is challenging for all employees, but new, evolving relationships that begin in the workplace may become disruptive, and even legally risky if the parties involved are different levels of workers (e.g., supervisor and physical therapist assistant). Managers may need to remind employees of policies related to romantic relationships, while understanding that the workplace is likely to be where many people meet their significant others.

Managerial Responsibilities

Achievement of the organization's goals depends heavily on the selection and retention of people who fit best with its vision and mission. This selection is particularly important for mid-level managers who have a powerful influence on their staffs. Either with the support of human resource experts or consultants, health-care managers bring all of their responsibilities to bear on the most important one, assisting people to perform their highest quality work. Because of the complexity of the legal and interpersonal aspects of these staffing responsibilities, ongoing development is required of managers who must juggle the needs of their staffs with the needs of their organizations.

Managers must seriously reflect on their perceptions of people and their ideas about work to define an approach to their staffing responsibilities that includes patience and fairness. Managers who believe people are eager to do their best and learn approach their staffing responsibilities differently than managers who believe most people need to be persuaded and monitored to work to their fullest potential. Responsibility for staffing is the most complex and challenging aspect of their work for many managers. It also is the most fulfilling and rewarding. Like physical therapists who receive satisfaction in their responsibility for evaluation, goal setting, and outcomes of patient care, managers often express satisfaction in their responsibility for the evaluation, goals, and performance of the people on their staffs.

REFERENCES

1. U.S. Department of Labor, Bureau of Labor Statistics. Employer costs for employee compensation. September 2007. Available at: http://www.bls.gov/news.release/pdf/ecec.pdf. Accessed February 4, 2008.
2. U.S. Department of Labor. Fact sheet #17G: Salary basis requirement and the part 541 exemptions under the FLSA. Available at: http://www.dol.gov/esa/regs/compliance/whd/fairpay/fs17g_salary.pdf. Accessed February 6, 2008.
3. Kanter A. *The Essential Book of Interviewing.* New York, NY: Three Rivers Press; 1995.

Chapter 9

Responsibility for Patient Care

Learning Objectives

+ Discuss the management needs of professional employees.
+ Distinguish between utilization management and case management.
+ Discuss the role of managers in utilization management and case management.
+ Define quality care and its state in current health care.
+ Analyze physical therapy practice for quality defects.
+ Include quality care in given vision, mission, and goal statements.
+ Analyze quality measures and models.
+ Apply the FOCUS-PDCA model to a given problem.
+ Analyze factors contributing to patient satisfaction.

Overview

The amount of direct patient care that a manager engages in varies widely. Solo physical therapy practitioners may spend at least half of their time in patient care while middle-level managers in large organizations may be one or two steps removed from direct patient care. Others may fall somewhere in between. In all instances, managers have indirect responsibility for all of the patient care provided by their subordinates. They must have a plan for monitoring the processes and outcomes of that care. This chapter addresses some common patient care responsibilities of managers that are not included in other chapters: managing professionals, utilization management, case management, quality care, and patient satisfaction.

Managing Professionals

Health-care managers do not have direct responsibility for individual patient-therapist interactions, which are, instead, the professional responsibility of *each* physical therapist and of other rehabilitation professionals. This professional responsibility extends to the other staff that physical therapists direct and supervise. The

Guide to Physical Therapist Practice reinforces the importance of the supervisory relationship.[1] It states that a physical therapist of record remains responsible for *all* aspects of a plan of care although they may direct physical therapist assistants to perform components of that care. Deciding if, and when, to utilize the physical therapist assistant should be based on ensuring safe, effective, and efficient care at each treatment session. They must provide oversight of documentation for all services delivered by support personnel as well.

In all settings, physical therapists currently have a great deal of freedom in day-to-day patient/client management. They are individually accountable for the care of the patients, and the ongoing collaboration and consultation with other health professionals involved in the care of a patient that is necessary to coordinate a patient's goals and the plans to meet them.

Needs of Professionals

It should be no surprise that professionals who assume such a high level of responsibility for the care of others do not really require much management from others to fulfill their clinical responsibilities. They control their own work to a high degree after assignments have been made, and may even have a great deal of control in selecting the patients they will care for in some settings. This autonomy in clinical decision making is confirmed by the recent trend for rehabilitation managers from one discipline to manage professionals from others. The shift to business rather than clinical roles of health-care managers reflects the advancing level of professionalization of rehabilitation specialists who neither turn to supervisors for clinical advice, nor rely on specific physician's orders to make clinical decisions. Instead, professionals (because of their strong technical skills, good problem-solving ability, sound judgment, and sense of responsibility) may need managers only to empower their actions; assist with nonclinical problems; provide performance feedback; and reaffirm the vision, mission, and goals of their organizations.

Managers also play a role in reducing the sources of work stress, such as heavy workloads, interprofessional role conflicts and ambiguity, scarce resources, understaffing, physical strain, emotional labor (maintaining and juggling emotion to present a socially acceptable presence at all times), work/home conflicts, and limited input into organizational decision making. These stressors affect the physical and emotional health of employees. Poor health is costly to organizations in terms of absenteeism, staff turnover, or poor work performance that may lead to clinical errors. Managers may help employees deal with these stressors through several means such as encouraging coworker support as a coping mechanism, arranging flexible work schedules, and rewarding positive efforts to provide quality care.[2]

Rather than micromanaging patient care, therapists want managers to focus on interpreting the big picture of health-care policy, reimbursement, and the organization's goals so that they may care for patients safely, efficiently, and effectively. Managers who clearly delineate the roles and responsibilities of all members of the rehabilitation service and their supervisory relationships are appreciated. That does not mean that they have little to do with patient care. Essentially, all of their other responsibilities—risk management, staffing, legal and ethical, fiscal, etc.—come to rest on the provision of quality patient care. See Activity 9.1.

ACTIVITY 9.1
IS IT AN ISSUE?

During an exit interview with one of her staff who is leaving the profession, Rachel Gibson learns that a major source of her dissatisfaction with her work is the lack of contact with other physical therapists. She tells Rachel she has never felt so lonely. Rachel is taken aback because her impression was that therapists like being independent. She has prided herself in being a leader rather than a manager of her staff. She feels awful that the profession is losing this person. What should she do?

Utilization Management and Case Management

Utilization Management

Another important component of a manager's responsibility for patient care is responding to the efforts of third-party payers to manage their costs and the quality of the care that they pay for. Controlling the utilization of services is now an expected component of health care. Third-party payers may conduct utilization management directly, or outsource it to independent review organizations.

Their reviews are based on written standards for patient care, which are drawn from historical data and typically approved or developed by physician panels in health insurance companies. Those conditions that are the most costly, most utilized, or that result in questionable outcomes receive the greatest scrutiny, but the utilization of any care may be managed.

In any case, the purpose of these reviews is to assess patient care to determine that it is efficient, effective, medically necessary, and appropriate. This means that determining that quality standards have been met precedes payments to providers in essentially all inpatient and outpatient centers.

Each payer addresses the quantity of services, timetable for delivery, and appropriate sources of evaluation and treatment. The decisions of reviewers (typically nurses) about certification or authorization of care is driven by these standards through reviews of medical records and direct communications with providers and billing staff. They are essentially asking if patients received a level of care that was efficient, effective, and consistent with their individual needs and the past needs of patients with similar conditions.

Utilization review becomes territory that lies between the patient care and fiscal responsibilities of managers. They must be familiar with utilization reviews that occur at various points in an episode of patient care. The standards may vary from setting to setting and payer to payer. The types of utilization review are:

✦ Precertification reviews. This process certifies the medical necessity of care <u>before</u> a patient can be admitted for inpatient or outpatient care, and that the anticipated care is provided in the most appropriate setting (e.g., inpatient or outpatient elective surgery). Emergency admissions are reviewed within 48 hours and are based on the same standard guidelines. Managers are involved in the processes necessary for providing required information to reviewers. The purpose of this form of review is to control costs <u>before</u> admission.

✦ Admission reviews. These are reviews conducted after a patient has been admitted for care to determine medical necessity and the appropriateness of inpatient care within 1 working day. Standard guidelines are followed to confirm precertification information, review additional information that has been discovered during admission, and to assess documentation of the planned course of treatment has been implemented to determine the expected costs associated with an episode of care. This review is often conducted on-site in large hospital systems.

✦ Continued stay (concurrent) reviews. These are scheduled reviews, applicable to all admissions and conducted periodically until a patient is discharged. Objective patient data is collected and compared with the standard guidelines or criteria for each patient's diagnosis or diagnoses. The intent of this review is to approve the continuation of care for only as long as necessary to reach the expected outcomes. Identifying options for alternative, less expensive continued care settings are part of this process as a means of controlling costs. The need for intensive case management services for catastrophic conditions and discharge planning are components of this type of review. Typically, these concurrent reviews do not directly involve the patient as decisions are made about lengths of inpatient stays or the duration of outpatient care.

✦ Discharge planning. This is the process of facilitating the transfer of a patient to an alternative, most appropriate, setting when the goals of care have been reached. It begins when the provider or setting receives notification of the certification of a patient's care. Discharge planning includes arranging for any continued care that is needed in advance to avoid delays in transfers, which can be costly to all involved parties. Discharge planning was a component of patient/client management for physical therapists long before utilization management came into being. Including patients in the process has always been important. Managers typically are not involved in this professional decision making unless conflicts arise among the care team engaged in this process.

✦ Retrospective review. This review occurs postdischarge and the same utilization standards used in other reviews continue to be applied. The obvious disadvantage of this type of utilization review is that involved parties do not know until after the fact whether or not the care provided was deemed medically necessary and appropriate. This type of review, which was originally referred to utilization review, has evolved into the broader prospective utilization management.

Managers may represent their staffs during any of these utilization management stages as important decisions are made from pre-admission to discharge of patients. Managers must ensure that staff involved in direct patient care is prepared for the high-level clinical decision making involved in continued stay reviews and discharge plans for particular patients. Rehabilitation staff are expected to be immediately available to provide data when called upon to do so by physicians or utilization review staff. Physical therapists are called upon to determine their patients' ability to walk and function safely and independently, their level of endurance for activity, and their response to exercise. They provide important recommendations for less costly, alternative health-care settings because of their knowledge of function and movement.

Case Management

A parallel process common in contemporary health care is case management. Case management is another cost-control process of hospitals, insurance companies, and employers primarily directed to patients with high-cost medical conditions. It is a collaborative process that includes assessment, planning, facilitation, and advocacy to meet a person's needs through available resources to achieve cost-effective outcomes. Patients may or may not have the option to use case management services. Depending on the setting, the duties of case managers may include:

- ✦ Screening to identify appropriate patients for case management services (e.g., patients with high-risk pregnancy, multiple trauma, or renal disease).
- ✦ Planning and coordinating the delivery of care by the health-care team.
- ✦ Making discharge arrangements and following up with patients.
- ✦ Evaluating the outcomes of care for each patient.
- ✦ Checking benefits available and coordinate with other benefits (e.g., a patient has both Medicare and Workers' Compensation benefits).
- ✦ Recommending insurance policy coverage exceptions where appropriate.
- ✦ Coordinating referrals to specialists and arranging for other special services (e.g., durable medical equipment).
- ✦ Coordinating care with community services.
- ✦ Verifying medical reasons for employee absences.
- ✦ Educating workers with chronic conditions.

Physical therapists and their managers have a long history of professional collaboration with case managers because of their involvement with patients with work-related injuries and other complex conditions requiring rehabilitation. In hospitals, daily collaboration with case managers takes place for discharge planning decisions. Managers may need to intervene to help clarify the roles of case managers and the policies of particular third-party payers because not all insurance companies follow the same standards in their utilization and case management decisions. Managers need to keep abreast of policy decisions and establish strong communication channels with utilization managers and case managers so that they are prepared to address concerns of staff should conflicts arise in these decision processes. In some cases, managers may represent all of the physical therapists as they serve as a "go-between" for them and case managers. See Activity 9.2.

ACTIVITY 9.2
FRUSTRATION AND CONFUSION

Mindy Hanson appears frustrated after 2 months as a staff physical therapist in St. Anne's Rehabilitation Hospital. Joanna Freedman, her supervisor, asks if there is anything she can do to help. Mindy says no because she is generally disturbed about patient policies. She just cannot understand how some of her patients were admitted for an intensive rehabilitation program when they are so sick that they can hardly participate in therapy, and others who have the potential to make significant functional gains are discharged quickly. Mindy is also challenged by the expectation that she provide input for patients' discharge plans when she has barely completed their initial evaluations. What should Joanna do?

Quality Care

The concept of quality has not transitioned well to health care from other types of organizations because the nature of health care is so different from manufacturing and other industries where the study of quality began. The recent report, *Crossing the Quality Chasm*[3] was an effort to span this difficult gap. The report presents a goal-driven definition of health-care quality with six dimensions of patient care:

- ✦ *Safe:* Care should be as safe for patients in health-care facilities as in their homes.

✦ *Effective:* The science and evidence behind health care should be applied and serve as the standard in the delivery of care.

✦ *Efficient:* Care and service should be cost effective, and waste should be removed from the system.

✦ *Timely:* Patients should experience no waits or delays in receiving care and service.

✦ *Patient-centered:* The system of care should revolve around the patient, respect patient preferences, and put the patient in control.

✦ *Equitable:* Unequal treatment should be a fact of the past; disparities in care should be eradicated.

Regardless of the type or size of health-care organizations, these dimensions may serve well to clarify quality so that the concept may be more easily incorporated into their visions, missions, and goals, and serve as a basis for both managerial and clinical decision making. See Activity 9.3.

ACTIVITY 9.3
REVISION OF VISION, MISSION, AND GOALS

Return to the activities in Chapter 5 and revise the vision, mission, and goals developed in the activities as necessary to reflect the six aims of quality care from *Crossing the Quality Chasm.*

The report goes on to classify quality defects as:[3]

✦ *Underuse:* Failure to employ many scientifically sound practices as often as they should be.

✦ *Overuse:* Failure to eliminate diagnostic tests and interventions when they are not indicated.

✦ *Misuse:* Failure to appropriately execute the proper clinical care process.

See Activity 9.4.

Said another way, quality may be defined as the degree to which a health-care organization increases

---

ACTIVITY 9.4
QUALITY DEFECTS

In small groups, identify potential sources of quality defects in physical therapy practices.

---

the likelihood of desired health outcomes, consistent with current evidence about the scientific, interpersonal, and organizational components of health care. Quality depends on the integration of all of its levels: (1) what happens to the patient; (2) the care delivered by health-care provider teams; (3) the organization's management and coordination of all of its units; and (4) the external environment where regulations and policies are made.[4]

Despite efforts to raise awareness and increase the value of quality in health care, attention to quality often is displaced by other urgent priorities, and it is difficult for patients to grasp the concept. However, this has not stopped health-care organizations from gathering data on hundreds of measures related to the complex interrelated components of quality. Some data is required by The Joint Commission and the Centers for Medicare and Medicaid (CMMS).

Fortunately software systems are available that allow analysis of key performance indicators in dashboard formats that are integrated with existing databases. The visual representations of data as dials on a dashboard may facilitate analysis and decision making about financial and clinical aspects of health care. Balanced scorecards can be used as another tool that encourages viewing data from a financial perspective, and balancing that analysis by looking at the organization from the view of its customers, the growth and development of employees, and business processes. Units of an organization or the organization as a whole may use the scorecards.

Perhaps the tools do not matter unless managers have clearly decided what they should measure and for what purpose. Measures of clinical quality remain challenging, but dashboards may serve as links between everyday key operations and strategic goals. They should be shared and discussed with stakeholders. Resources in Sidebar 9.1 provide more information on quality measures. See Sidebar 9.2 and Activity 9.5 for other views of quality.

Sidebar 9.1

Quality Measures

Go to http://www.qualitymeasures.ahrq.gov and http://www.guidelines.gov for resources on quality measures.

Sidebar 9.2

Quality Models

Avedis Donabedian is often considered the father of modern quality assurance. He conceived quality as the interaction of structure (characteristics of systems and providers), process (patient/practitioner activities), and outcome (health status of an individual or community). See his article, The Quality of Care, How Can It Be Assessed? In JAMA, Vol. 260 No.12, September 23, 1988 for a historical perspective.

FOCUS-PDCA is another classic approach to continuous quality improvement that is widely used. The steps in the model include:

FOCUS	PDCA
Find a process to improve.	**P**lan how to implement the intervention.
Organize an improvement team and necessary resources.	**D**o it by initiating the intervention, on a small scale at first.
Clarify current knowledge about the process.	
Understand the process and sources of variation in it.	**C**heck the results of the early implementation, revising as necessary, until it proves itself as an improvement.
Select an improvement or intervention.	**A**ct on what was learned in the check step. If the change was successful, incorporate it on a larger scale.

ACTIVITY 9.5
IMPROVING QUALITY

Jeremy Hines has identified a few quality defects in his private physical therapy practice. Use FOCUS-PDCA to improve these patient care processes:

- It seems that the physical therapists have fallen into the habit of "rewarding" patients who exercise well with a hot pack or cold pack at the end of each session.
- Patients have complained that they often wait almost 30 minutes before beginning their therapy sessions.
- There is a waiting list for physical therapy appointments. On average, patients are scheduled for their first physical therapy visit 14 working days from the time they call for an appointment.

Because quality care is a continually evolving concept that has the attention of licensing and accrediting bodies, its concepts, tools, and terminology seem to change at a rapid rate. Managers must be prepared for modifications in related responsibilities, and develop an approach for keeping abreast of this important aspect of patient care.

Patient Satisfaction

The two aspects of patient satisfaction may be represented on a continuum anchored with content quality and service-delivery quality (Fig. 9.1). All patient care includes both components but depending on their circumstances, patients may lean toward technical excellence and clinical expertise as more important than receiving that care that involves them in a humane and culturally appropriate manner. See the examples in the figure.[5]

Managers must assure the quality in both components of satisfaction. Evaluation and development of staff to maintain skills, learn new approaches as technology advances care, and comply with guidelines is one-half of these responsibilities. The other half is having processes that meet patient expectations for convenience, timeliness, and the development of strong interpersonal relationships with their direct caregivers and other nonclinical support staff.

Many managers value patient satisfaction as highly as they value outcome indicators about mortality and functional status. Because many health-care organizations all reach common benchmarks for clinical outcomes, patient satisfaction is among those factors that may set one organization apart from the others. For example, paying attention to good guest relations in other hospitality businesses can be an important management tool. Avoiding negative

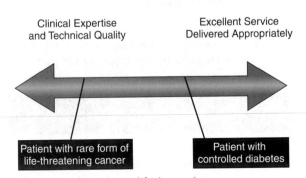

Clinical Expertise and Technical Quality   Excellent Service Delivered Appropriately

Patient with rare form of life-threatening cancer   Patient with controlled diabetes

Figure 9.1 ✦ The patient satisfaction continuum.

impressions is easier than the great deal of time and energy it takes to reverse them at the level of the individual and at the level of the organization. A strong program to address guest relations may give an organization a strong competitive edge.

Managers' identification of the key drivers of satisfaction may include attention to patients' values and preferences, their physical and emotional comfort, and their need for open communication. The only way to know what is truly important to patients is to ask them, and the people who directly take care of them. In large part, satisfaction is dependent on staff that is committed to excellent service throughout all aspects of a health-care experience. Hiring competent people who also seek to serve is a good starting point. Training them to achieve patient service goals is as important as the development of their clinical skills.

Assuming that people have come to their work with these service skills may be risky. It is often easier to determine clinical skills than these important service skills, so formal efforts to address them are necessary. Simple courtesy matters. Employees who smile and introduce themselves, make eye contact, say please and thank-you, knock before entering, explain what they are doing, and maintain a clean, neat environment contribute to a positive health-care experience.

Managers may be working in the right direction if their employees are caring about patients while taking care of them. Empowering employees to eliminate patient disappointments immediately and to anticipate needs may lead to a seamless positive health-care experience for patients. For some employees it may be easier to consider patients as guests. Although difficult in complex, busy organizations making people feel that they are all that matter is an important point in establishing good customer relations. Patients should not feel that making their needs known and having them met is an intrusion in the work of their health-care providers.

Managers also are responsible for creating a welcoming environment that gives the perception of quality, cleanliness, security, and caring. Attention to sights, sounds, smells, and temperatures can promote a sense of healing and comfort. Overloading the environment with too much information may be threatening and confusing rather than helpful. Overdecorating may make it difficult for people to find their way when knowing where to go and how

to get there should be easy. Managers need to scan the environment from the patient's viewpoint rather than their own.[6] See Activity 9.6.

ACTIVITY 9.6
PATIENT SATISFACTION

Amy Allen is pleased in one way and offended in another. She has received a lot of positive feedback from patients on the care that they receive from her staff, but recently she overheard a patient say to another that the place was such a dump. She works hard to keep it neat and clean but has decided that she may need to do more. What other factors should Amy consider? What kind of thing would give the impression that a professional practice is a dump?

The role of patients in contributing to their own health-care experiences and outcomes is also an important consideration for managers. Patients and families who follow instructions for increasing their activities and administrating medications, for example, become coproducers of the health-care experience. Patients and their families may be encouraged to assume increased responsibility for their care by:[6]

+ Training patients with the skills and knowledge they need.
+ Providing opportunities to practice skills.
+ Encouraging patients to monitor employees.
+ Having patients teach other patients.

Handling patients who do not seem to be vested in their care is another management challenge. In the same vein, despite the best efforts of employees, some patients are rude and perhaps even dangerous to employees. Managers need a plan for serving as a buffer between people in conflict. They may need to take direct action to reassign difficult patients to staff with the most patience, or to counsel patients about their inappropriate behavior. Expelling people from the premises may require the support of security or law enforcement officers.

A Manager's Responsibility

Generally patients expect respect and the best efforts of the people who care for them. Although many may be disappointed with the outcomes of their care because their conditions simply do not allow cures or total relief of their problems, few are truly dissatisfied with rehabilitation experiences because they are able to establish strong professional relationships during the process. Managers who are able to make these distinctions in patient expectations may discover that putting out an occasional fire is all that is necessary because of the clinical skills and compassion of the professionals they supervise. It is not surprising then that melding utilization management and quality of care to achieve expected patient outcomes is a critical area of a manager's responsibility for patient care. See Activity 9.7.

REFERENCES

1. American Physical Therapy Association. *Guide to Physical Therapist Practice.* Vol 81, 2nd ed. Alexandria, VA: American Physical Therapy Assoc; 2001.

2. Apker J, Ray EB. Stress and social support in health care organizations. Thompson TL. In: Thompson TL, ed. *Handbook of Health Communication.* Mahwah, NJ: Lawrence Erlbaum Associates; 2003; p 347.

3. Committee on Quality of Health Care in America, ed. *Crossing the Quality Chasm: A New Health System for the 21st Century.* Washington, DC: National Academy Press; 2001.

4. Ransom SB, Joshi M, Nash DB. *The Healthcare Quality Book: Vision, Strategy, and Tools* Washington, DC: Health Administration Press; 2005.

5. Longest BB. *Health Policymaking in the United States.* 4th ed. Chicago, IL: American College of Healthcare Executives; 2006.

6. Fottler MD, Ford RC, Heaton CP. *Achieving Service Excellence: Strategies for Healthcare Management Series.* Chicago, IL: Health Administration Press; 2002.

ACTIVITY 9.7
A STRATEGY FOR QUALITY

Using one of the quality defects in Activity 9.3, refer to pp. 61–62 on strategic planning and use this worksheet to address it. Discuss how to determine the effectiveness of these strategies.

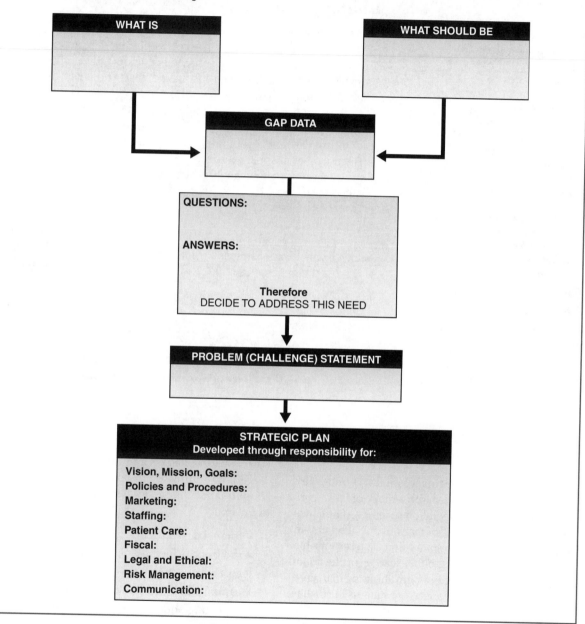

WHAT IS

WHAT SHOULD BE

GAP DATA

QUESTIONS:

ANSWERS:

Therefore
DECIDE TO ADDRESS THIS NEED

PROBLEM (CHALLENGE) STATEMENT

STRATEGIC PLAN
Developed through responsibility for:

Vision, Mission, Goals:
Policies and Procedures:
Marketing:
Staffing:
Patient Care:
Fiscal:
Legal and Ethical:
Risk Management:
Communication:

Chapter 10

Fiscal Responsibilities

Learning Objectives

- Discuss typical fiscal responsibilities of health-care managers.
- For a given physical therapy practice assets, analyze property, location, equipment selection factors, costs, and depreciation.
- Identify fixed, variable, direct, and indirect costs and potential sources of waste or excess that increase practice costs.
- Analyze the effect of employee absences and patient no-shows on fixed and variable costs.
- Compare different payer mixes to analyze their impact on revenue.
- Discuss other possible sources of revenue.
- Analyze factors that enhance reimbursement from third-party payers (i.e., authorizations, coding, billing, contract negotiation, etc.)
- Discuss the use of CPT codes.
- Discuss payroll models.
- Compare and contrast funding sources.
- Identify the components of a grant proposal.
- Discuss the importance of financial statements and budget reports.

Overview

All aspects of health-care finances and accounting are scrutinized for compliance with a range of laws, regulations, contracts, and operation systems. Compliance leads to a standardization of many financial systems in any type of health-care organization. The responsibilities for these systems are either lead by professional financial experts in large organizations or managed with the assistance of financial consultants in smaller organizations.

All organizations have two components to their finances. The first component is financial management, which is a factor in strategic planning that includes funding of assets. The other component includes the controller functions for the day-to-day operations of the business, such as recording all business transactions; setting and achieving costs and revenue objectives; and guarding against theft, waste, or loss of assets and other resources.

To communicate effectively with these experts about finances, upper-level managers should be able to grasp:[1]

- financial statements
- the basic principles of accounting and finance
- cost accounting
- capital and operational budgeting
- reporting and control
- reimbursement and capitation
- databases
- information systems relationship to financial and strategic planning
- basic economics (supply and demand)
- contracts

Health-care financing has become so complex that organizations are compelled to prepare mid-level managers for some of these financial responsibilities as well. This need often leads to an ongoing training program in large organizations because financing is linked to the ever-changing health-care policies and reimbursement requirements. Small private practices face the same challenges in remaining current with these changes, and those related to assets, costs, revenue, financial obligations, and funding.

This chapter is a basic introduction to the complexities of fiscal responsibilities. Outpatient practice is used as the example in all of the activities to demonstrate the interaction of these factors in a straightforward manner. The concepts, however, may apply to any type of practice with consideration for how it fits into a larger organization, its major source of funding, and whether or not it is a cost center (generates expenses but no direct revenue) in the organization. Chapters in Sections 1 and 3 also address some of these reimbursement and policy issues.

Assets

Assets are property like goods, equipment, buildings, installations, land, and money in the bank. Ownership of assets has both financial and psychological implications. People become more vested and committed when a physical therapy practice is connected tightly to their personal funds. Pride in ownership may be a big drive in accomplishing an organization's goals. Real property and equipment assets are the focus of this section. Managers may rely on financial consultants to make decisions about cash, bonds, stocks, and other investments that affect an organization's assets.

Real Property Assets

Particularly for new business owners, owning outright or mortgaging a property (freestanding or condominium) may not be realistic. It is a decision based on the same factors in deciding to rent rather than buy a home. People decide between the investment of ownership and the expense of leasing with attention to the tax implications of those decisions. Determining the square feet of space and how it is arranged is also important. Patient privacy, employee comfort, and safety must all be considered within space requirements of government agencies that license health-care organizations.

Location

Deciding where to place a practice is critical. Location contributes to property value if it is an asset, and whether purchased or leased, location contributes to the value of the practice to its customers. The better the location, the greater the value of the asset to a physical therapy practice. Managers have to weigh the pros and cons of possible locations carefully by answering some questions:

1. How important is public transportation to the target markets of patients and employees? If important, where is the location in relationship to transportation system stops?
2. What are local traffic patterns and commuting times to the location?
3. Is parking convenient, available, and safe?
4. How important is face-to-face interactions with physicians? If this level of interaction is important, what is travel time or distance to these referral sources?
5. Is the location safe? Is the building secure?
6. Do people with physical disabilities have convenient access into the building? Is the location of the practice within a large office building convenient?
7. Is it important to be on the first floor?
8. What are the neighboring businesses?

See Activity 10.1.

ACTIVITY 10.1
LOCATION

For this and the next activity in this chapter, each group of students is to select a physical therapy practice for critique. Begin with identifying the advantages and disadvantages of the location of the selected practice against the list above. Add other identified factors to be included on the list. What does the location say about the vision, mission, and goals of the practice?

Equipment Assets

For convenience, managers may determine that anything over a particular price is capital equipment, $500 or $1,000, for example. Another approach is to classify equipment that is more permanent (lasts more than 1 year, typically) as an asset from that which is more dispensable, expendable, or requires frequent upgrading. For example, a cold-pack machine would be in a different equipment category than the cold packs that are in it. The need for different requests and approval processes for capital and noncapital equipment and supplies partially drives these classifications. Managers want employees to identify and request equipment needs supported by rationale and the potential to generate revenue, but they do not want to be overwhelmed with paperwork to replace expendable supplies and less expensive equipment. More importantly, the classification of equipment has tax implications.

Depreciation

These equipment decisions may require the advice of a tax consultant because of the financial and legal implications of depreciation of *any* asset. Depreciation is an income tax deduction that allows the taxpayer to recover the costs of owned property or other assets placed in service over time that have a determinable useful life. Depreciation preserves revenue and increases profits by reducing tax payments. Because expenses are deducted from revenue when they occur, converting as much as property and equipment as possible into assets defers these losses. Increasing assets for tax purposes is weighed against the costs of either borrowing the funds or depleting funds to obtain them. Another fiscal strategy is reinvesting profits back into the organization to reduce income taxes. To repeat, these are complex decisions that may demand consultation with tax or other financial experts.

Equipment Choices

As real property, equipment, and other furniture may be purchased or leased. Similar to the decision of buying or leasing a car, managers also need to consider the pros and cons of these choices:

1. Will there be frequent new models of the equipment?
2. Is the technology associated with the equipment rapidly changing?
3. Are there classic or traditional pieces of equipment that must be included?
4. Is there a minimal set of equipment required to meet external licensing requirements?

5. What furniture is needed in the staff and/or business offices? Are there special ergonomic needs?
6. What computers, phones, and other means of communication are needed?
7. What furniture and other décor is needed in the reception and waiting areas?
8. What scientific evidence supports the purchase of equipment for particular patient populations?

See Activity 10.2.

ACTIVITY 10.2
EQUIPMENT

Each group of students is to list the equipment assets in their selected physical therapy practice. Determine the pros and cons of purchase or lease of each piece of equipment beginning with the list above. Add other identified factors to be included on the list. What does the equipment say about the vision, mission, and goals of the practice?

Costs

A top priority for managers is determining the cost of doing business, which is usually expressed as cost/patient visit. Without knowing how much it costs to deliver services, managers are unable to determine how much to charge for services to end up with a profit. Negotiating with insurance companies for contracts to provide services may be disastrous if a manager does not know whether the reimbursement rate offered will cover the costs of caring for patients.

Kinds of Costs

The two major categories of costs are:

✦ Direct costs: Expenses for delivering services, which includes salaries, equipment, supplies.

✦ Indirect (overhead) costs: Rent or mortgage payments, utilities, janitorial services, equipment maintenance, office supplies, etc. that underlie the direct delivery of services. Overhead costs are the things that are necessary regardless of the number of patients there are in a practice. For example, even if there is only one patient, the practice needs electricity, temperature control, space, and medical records, etc.

Both direct and indirect costs are either:

✦ Fixed: The same cost regardless of the number of patients who are treated (e.g., rent, ultrasound machine).

✦ Variable: The cost increases as the number of patients increase (e.g., laundry services).

✦ Semifixed: A fixed cost, such as wages and salaries that may vary because of need for overtime, or when work hours are decreased as a patient census fluctuates.

Identifying Direct Costs

Managers may use some historical data to begin to determine a ballpark figure for direct costs. The total labor costs (i.e., salaries, wages, and benefits) divided by the average number of treatment sessions in a unit of time gives an average labor cost/treatment session, which is the biggest cost. Labor costs include other payroll expenses (i.e., workers' compensation, contributions to taxes, etc. at about 2% of total labor costs) in addition to salaries, wages, and benefits. Managers and owners also pay themselves a salary and determine the most appropriate staff mix to control these costs.

Managers strive to occupy as much of the staff time with treatment sessions. Revenue cannot be generated unless patients are being treated. A commonly used standard is that of the 2,080 hours worked in 1 year (40 hours/week for 52 weeks) by full-time physical therapists, they are engaged in direct billable patient care 80% of the time. The rest of the time is paid time off, meetings, breaks, etc. Even with the best attempts to schedule treatment sessions effectively, not all physical therapists work at the same pace so the time to provide the same treatments may not be the same. Experience does seem to count. More experienced therapists seem to work more efficiently and more of the time.

Other factors influencing treatment sessions are patient cancellations and no-shows, which may be due to weather conditions or personal choice. Deciding whether or not one person is assigned the duties of scheduling patients and making reminder calls to patients or whether therapists make their own schedules with patients after they have been assigned is an important management decision. Weighing the cost of the scheduling person against the cost of time away from patient care to do their own scheduling may depend on how well therapists and a scheduler work together and the number of patients to be scheduled.

Double-booking appointments or overlapping the scheduling of patients may be strategies to avoid non-billable downtime. Rushed and harried therapists and unhappy patients must be avoided on one hand, and downtime must be avoided on the other. Unexpected absences of employees often result in this dilemma as well. See Activity 10.3 and Activity 10.11, which appears later in this chapter.

ACTIVITY 10.3
FILLING IN

The issue of "filling in" has become a contentious one for the staff in Rosemont Physical Therapy. Mark Potter has called a staff meeting to brainstorm some ideas to solve the problem of what to do when a therapist or assistant is unexpectedly sick or on planned leave. In the past, the staff simply gathered to review the schedule and divided among themselves the patients of the therapist who was out. However, because they are seeing so many more of their own patients now, it is almost impossible to take on more. Suggestions that are presented are to have another therapist on call who can be available anytime needed or cancel the patients of the therapist who is out. What other options are there? What should Mark do?

Identifying Indirect Costs

Average indirect costs/treatment sessions can be estimated by reviewing monthly expenses, adding them up and then dividing by the total number of treatment sessions held in a month. Although some expenses (e.g., education, bonuses) may only be expended if surplus funds are available, others are embedded in the business. See Activity 10.4.

Other Cost Determinations

This section includes some other considerations in determining costs. Beginning with capital equipment, managers need to be careful to avoid impulse buying

---

ACTIVITY 10.4
CUTTING COSTS

Mark Potter feels that the staff is working as hard as they can and efficiency has significantly improved, but he feels that he still needs to cut costs. He wants to avoid cutting back on continuing education that he is able to support so he has decided to thoroughly examine all potential sources of waste or excess in the practice to reduce expenses across the board. What should he look for?

---

by considering the impact of a large purchase on profits and on the generation of revenue. Having an expensive piece of gym equipment become a rack for drying towels can be disheartening. The final questions to answer are whether the equipment is worth the cost of a long-term loan and what it adds to the value of patient care. Finally, is there evidence to support positive changes in the expected outcomes of patient care because of the new equipment?

A typical formula for predicting the costs of expensive equipment is: Total capital clinical equipment cost/years that the equipment will last X 1 + the interest rate = annual cost / 12 = monthly cost. An example is deciding to borrow $100,000 to buy state-of-the-art equipment, which is expected to last for 10 years. The interest rate on the loan for the $100,000 is 6%. The formula becomes $100,000/10 years × 1.06 = $10,600 annual payments ÷ 12 = $883.33/month for 10 years.

Managers also need to consider the cost of space, which is paid for in cost/square footage whether it is leased or purchased. How much space is needed for effective patient care becomes an important question to control this cost. Some industry minimal standards are 500 sq. ft./physical therapist, 60 sq. ft. for each clerical staff, 100 sq. ft. for waiting room/reception area, 100 sq. ft. for medical records. An example for a practice that includes four therapists, two clerical staff, and a room for medical records would be 2,320 sq. ft. of space. If the cost of rental space were $20/sq. ft./month, this space would be $46,400/month or $556,800/year. The size and arrangement of equipment, patient and employee safety, patient privacy, and health care or business licensure requirements may affect these general guidelines.

Revenue (Income)

Revenue, or income, is the total of all money received for services provided or goods sold during a given period. Managers, perhaps obviously, need to know where the money will be coming from.

Payer Mix

For example, physical therapists and other health-care professionals may be paid in different reimbursement models, such as presented in Table 10.1 (review Chapter 4 for payer sources). The payer mix (the percentage of a target population insured in each model) becomes very important. For instance, if the average cost of treating the mix of patients in Table 10.1 is $50/visit and each of the 4,000 patients in the payer mix averages 12 visits, it would cost $2,400,000 to treat the patients. The physical therapy center would lose $100,000 with the payer mix shown in Table 10.1.

As another example of the impact of payer mix on potential income, see Table 10.2. The facts and figures in this table demonstrate what would happen if a physical therapy practice were to have 4,000 patients in only type of the reimbursement model. The last column suggests the management implications of each single-payment model if the average cost of each visit to the physical therapy center remains at $50.

These reimbursement models have developed in response to concerns about the quality defects—underuse, overuse, misuse—presented in Chapter 9. Insurance companies' preferences, obviously, are for models that reduce the amount of reimbursement they are likely to pay per patient that they insure. Providers of care prefer models that provide the most flexibility in the number of sessions and payment/session they receive to meet the needs of each individual patient. With utilization review methods and models of reimbursement to consider, managers must have a finger on the pulse of income on a daily basis. Attention to contract details in negotiations with insurance companies must be taken very seriously as well.

The other component of payer mix for consideration is the percentage of direct reimbursement in each model of payment. Patient deductibles and co-payments may vary within a model and among models and affect the level of reimbursement, which

TABLE 10.1 Examples of reimbursement models on annual basis with 1,000 patients in each model

FORM OF REIMBURSEMENT	DEFINITION	EXAMPLE	TOTAL REVENUE/YEAR
Fee Schedule Based on Price/Unit of Care	No. of patients/year X No. of visits/patient X No. of units/visit X payment/unit	1,000 patients X 12 visits/patient X 3 units/visit X $25/unit	$900,000
Per Diem or Per Visit	No. of patients/year X No. visits/patient X payment per diem or visit	1,000 patients X 12 visits/patient X $50 flat fee	$600,000
Per Case	No. of patients X payment/patient for 1 year	1,000 patients X $500/patient/year regardless of number of visits	$500,000
Capitation	No. of covered people X premium/patient/month X 12 months/year	1,000 patients X $25/patient/month X 12 months regardless of number of pa- tients who receive services	$300,000
TOTALS		4,000 patients	$2,300,000

is often 80% (for a $100 charge for a physical therapy, the insurer pays $80 and the patient pays a $20 co-payment). Managers would prefer no deductibles, or patients who have already met their deductible amounts before beginning physical therapy to reduce the risk of nonpayment of these out-of-pocket expenses by patients. High co-payments may make it difficult for patients to attend 12 scheduled visits. For instance, if the co-payment/visit were $25, a patient would pay $300 out of pocket for their physical therapy care over a few weeks. Other patients may be uninsured, or they have insurance policies that do not pay for rehabilitation services at all, or only for a limited number of visits/year. Knowing the limits and levels of reimbursement for each patient is critical information for a manager. See Activity 10.5.

Contract Negotiation

Managers who cannot control costs and the number of visits are in a vulnerable position, but negotiating contracts with insurance companies also presents risks. Managers need to know their cost/treatment and desired profit/treatment before entering these

---

ACTIVITY 10.5
CONTRACTS

Most of the patients at Rosemont Physical Therapy work at the regional distribution center at the edge of town. To this point, reimbursement for these patients has been based on a fee schedule. This year the company has offered a health savings account among their health insurance choices, which seems to be popular among the employees. What are the potential financial implications that Mark Potter needs to consider? HINT: see http://www.ustreas.gov/offices/public-affairs/hsa/

---

negotiations. Managers cannot afford to enter into payment contracts that do not cover their costs/treatments, or are at a fixed rate that places profits at risk if the number of patient visits suddenly increases, or if they accept discounted fees and rely on increased volume to make up the gaps created by accepting a lower rate of payment. Managers may need the assistance of attorneys and financial experts to negotiate these contracts and view the big picture

TABLE 10.2 Revenue of each reimbursement model on annual basis when all patients have the same insurance model and managerial considerations

FORM OF REIMBURSEMENT	TOTAL REVENUE/YEAR FOR 4,000 PATIENTS	MANAGEMENT TOOL BASED ON COST/PATIENT VISIT OF $50
Fee Schedule Based on Price/Unit of Care	$3,600,000 ($1,300,000 more revenue)	4,000 patients × 12 visits × $50 cost/visit = $2,400,000 total cost and $1,200,000 profit. To increase profits: increase number of visits and/or number of units delivered/visit. Increase staff to meet demands.
Per Diem or Per Visit	$2,400,000 ($100,000 more revenue)	4,000 patients × 12 visits × $50 cost = $2,400,000 total cost. Break even. To make a profit, increase the number of visits. Determine the needs of target market and how much therapy they are likely to need. Decrease the amount of intervention/visit to be able to see more patients. Profits may not justify adding staff so need to reduce amount of work/patient
Per Case	$2,000,000 ($300,000 less revenue)	4,000 patients × $500 but profits are dependent on number of visits. If each person in this group also has 12 visits/year, the reimbursement/visit is $41.66 but the cost is $50 visit = $8.34 loss/visit resulting in a huge loss/year. Must reduce the total number of visits/patient to 10 to cover costs. Further reduction in number of visits necessary to make a profit.
Capitation	$1,200,000 ($1,100,000 less revenue BUT dependent on number of patients who actually need PT).	4,000 patients × $600/year. At a cost of $50/visit, if each patient receives 12 visits, there are significant losses. However, not each patient may need physical therapy or may not need 12 visits and PT still receives $600/patient. Need to determine the potential need for PT for the target market. If only 2,000 receive 12 visits of physical therapy, then $1,080,000 profit.

of numerous contracts. At least having a checklist of items that need to be addressed in a contract is important to have on hand. Independent practitioners may join networks of practitioners that provide power in numbers during negotiations with insurance companies. Networks also provide services to their members to help implement and monitor these negotiated contracts.

Other Sources of Revenue

Managers may decide that they wish either to supplement revenue from direct patient care or identify other sources of income as a cushion during times of unpredictable patient visits. Selling medical equipment, developing fee-for-service programs that patients pay for privately because they are not included in health insurance policies, or adding services that complement physical therapy (massage therapy is an example) are possible options. Managers must be sensitive to the ethical and legal issues in establishing these additional services so that patients referred to them do not feel coerced into using them. See Activities 10.6 and 10.7.

ACTIVITY 10.6
AVAILABLE SPACE

The space next door to Rosemont Physical Therapy has become available. The leasing office is giving Mark Potter first choice on renting it. Mark thinks the timing is right for expansion of the business, but how? Should he connect the two spaces, add more staff, and expand the physical therapy services? Should he develop a different business? What factors should Mark consider in his decision making? What are the possible alternative business opportunities that might be most appropriate?

Reimbursement Considerations

Depending on the model of reimbursement, managers need to decide whether marketing and increased referrals are really what they want. Increased visits usually mean increased staff to maintain the quality of services provided. Increased staff means increased space. How much growth can a practice handle without increased personnel costs becomes an important

Mark Potter is intrigued but unsure about what action to take. He has been approached by the local arts consortium to exhibit paintings in his practice and offered him 10% of any works that are sold. Neighboring businesses want to place brochures and business cards in the waiting room. A company that sells nutritional supplements wants to set up a display and will pay Rosemont Physical Therapy 10% of sales that are documented as the result of the display. What should Mark do? What are other possibilities for this type of supplemental income?

question. Competition for the most desirable patients (like those who need the least amount of therapy, or those who have the ability to pay) becomes a serious consideration.

Strict adherence to the rules of carriers about authorizations for payment is necessary to avoid payment denials. Business staff and therapists must work together closely so that patients begin therapy services with all necessary pre- and continuing authorizations in place. Therapists need to know the number of sessions that have been authorized and the Current Procedural Terminology (CPT) codes they may use in billing for services for each insurance intermediary or carrier. Procedures for justifying and seeking reauthorizations or extension of services to meet patient goals must be in place. Managers need to be concerned about the time these processes take away from patient care, yet cannot afford patient care that is not reimbursable. Guiding staff to make certain that patient needs are reconciled with insurance requirements is a primary consideration in clinical decision making that cannot be lost in the process.

In addition to bad debts (failure to make out-of-pocket payments), claims for payments may be denied for a variety of reasons like failure to support the medical necessity of the care or technical errors in billing, coding of units, or documentation. Pro bono services also may reduce the profits expected. In some practices, these factors may mean that as much as 30% of the expected revenue is lost—or really, it was never had to begin with. Profit margins, the difference between income and expenses, vary widely in physical therapy as a result. Within a practice, the profit margins may vary from year to year as insurance companies and employers negotiate

contracts that affect coverage of rehabilitation services in the target market of a practice. Congress continues to cut Medicare costs, and intermediaries and carriers adjust their rules to control their payment of claims for rehabilitation services.

Coding and Billing

After contracts that are based on fee schedules are in place, managers need to assure that all services provided are accurately coded and billed for to avoid the potential for fraud and abuse. Accuracy also ensures that they receive all revenue to which they are entitled. To increase reimbursement, clinical and business office staffs typically require outside training for coding and billing, ongoing in-services, other communication methods, and audits to determine accuracy and completeness of billing and documentation of care. The use of computerized billing systems is increasingly required by many insurers and may be integrated with broader information systems, including documentation and scheduling software. These technological interventions are efforts to increase the accuracy of coding and billing and the documentation to support them. They also reduce the time to complete these administrative tasks, allowing more time for direct patient care—and the generation of more billable units.

CPT Codes

Fee schedules used by insurance companies may be based on more than 8,000 CPT codes. Developed primarily as the basis of payment for services provided to Medicare recipients, the system has been adopted by some Workers' Compensation and other private insurers as their fee schedules as well. However, managers should not expect absolute adoption because each insurer may use the codes as they see fit, or may use older versions of the CPT that better suits their purposes.

The CPT codes are established and reviewed each year by a special committee of the American Medical Association that includes other health professionals. This system has provided a uniform language and description for many aspects of medical and other health professional practices, but they are particularly important for reimbursement. For rehabilitation services, about 46 codes in the 97000 set of codes are used most frequently. For example, the code for physical therapy evaluation is 97001, modalities that do not require direct patient contact by the provider are in the 97010–97028 range, and therapeutic procedures that are charged by the minutes are in the 97110–97140 range of codes.

It is important to note two things about CPT codes. First, they are reviewed and modified each year to reflect changes in health-care practice that are determined by surveys of practitioners. Some codes may be deleted and new ones are added. For example, changes in the 2008 version of the CPT Codes include the addition of new codes for non–face-to-face services, such as telephone or e-mail to manage patient care and a code for attending team conferences. The addition of these codes means that other codes have been eliminated or the value of other codes was reduced because CPT coding is a neutral budget system that contributes to controlling health-care costs. The establishment and revision of the codes involves a great deal of negotiation and analysis of practice. See Sidebar 10.1.

Second, just because codes exist does not mean insurers will pay for them. For example, many third-party payers do not reimburse for services that are coded as modalities that do not require direct patient contact by the provider, such as hot packs and cold packs. Many insurers have decided that these passive interventions do not require the skill and knowledge of professionals, and therefore do not pay for them.

Billing for capitated services also may involve coding to track the types and numbers of interventions performed, although this may not be of particular interest to payers. The details of services provided are not a focus of the payers' concerns. Instead, they are more interested in controlling their costs through other means. They leave it up to the provider to determine how to accomplish patient goals within the limits of the payment they will receive and their scopes of practice. See Activity 10.8.

ACTIVITY 10.8
TRACKING BILLING AND CODING

Mark Potter has to come up with a better way. The therapists are taking too much time on determining and coordinating insurance requirements. There are some patient scheduling software packages that include ticklers and alerts and documentation. What should he consider before investing in one? What are less expensive ways to address this problem?

Financial Obligations

Managers must ensure that expenses are paid in a timely manner and payroll is met to avoid the embarrassment of debt collectors or the failure to sustain the services needed to support the practice. Having emergency reserves must be part of the planning conducted with financial consultants. Recognizing the pattern of reimbursement income (how often payments are received for claims submitted) in terms of payment due dates every month is an important consideration. Submitting claims with no errors and no omissions that are supported by detailed documentation helps avoid delays in payment because of denials of third-party payers and the time required to appeal those decisions. See Activity 10.9.

Funding

In addition to reimbursement and other payments for services performed, some larger practices also may receive financial support through local government taxes or bonds. These public revenues may be specif-

---

Sidebar 10.1

Values of CPT Codes

✦ Resource-based relative value scale (RBRVS) is established by the American Medical Association every Fall and implemented each January.

✦ The basic value of each CPT code is set and then modified based on the costs of providing that procedure, test, etc. from one practice to another and from one geographic area to another.

✦ The established uniform relative value is modified by a geographic adjustment factor (GAF) and a nationally uniform conversion factor that changes each year.

✦ For example, payment for code 97110 Therapeutic Exercise may be $26.04 for every 15 minutes of exercise in a rural part of the country and $28.79 in a large metropolitan area where the cost of doing business is higher because of GAF modifications on the RBRVS value for CPT 97110.

ACTIVITY 10.11
DIRECT AND INDIRECT COSTS

Classify the expense items listed on the form in Figure 10.1 as direct or indirect. What other line items should be included?

REFERENCE

1. Ross A, Wenzel FJ, Mitlyng JW. *Leadership for the Future: Core Competencies in Healthcare.* Chicago, IL: Health Administration Press; 2002.

ACTIVITY 10.12
ANOTHER CHALLENGE

Refer to pp. 61–62 on strategic planning and the following worksheet, to address a gap in a physical therapy practice between current payer mix and desired payer mix. Discuss how to determine the effectiveness of these strategies.

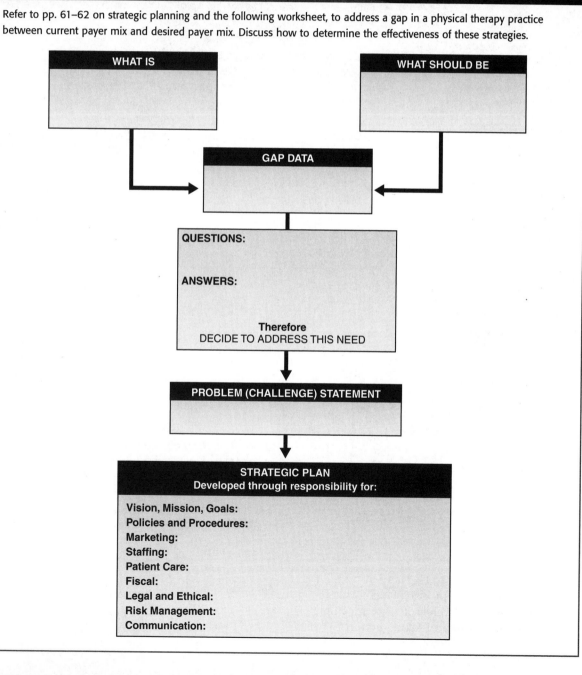

Chapter 11

Responsibility for Risk Management

Learning Objectives

- Discuss insurance as a risk management tool.
- Discuss the categories of potential risks.
- Discuss Occupational Safety and Health Administration (OSHA) requirements.
- Determine strategies for reducing financial risks.
- Analyze strategies for reducing hazard and operations risks.
- Develop a peer-review program to address documentation risks.
- Discuss security of documentation and the environment.
- Develop a strategy to improve a practice's bad reputation.
- Determine the role of job descriptions in reducing hiring and firing risks.
- Analyze strategies for a given human capital risk.
- Discuss the risks associated with the direction of supportive personnel.
- Determine the role of establishing patient rapport in reducing risks.
- Analyze an incident report.
- Apply the Five Whys Approach and root cause analysis to given cases of professional liability.

Special Note

The intent of this chapter is to alert managers to possible risks and related legal duties or concerns as they may relate or their jurisdictions or circumstances. <u>*CONTENT SHOULD **NOT** BE TAKEN AS LEGAL ADVICE.*</u>

Overview

Risk management is the process of identifying potential threats that could severely damage or completely ruin an organization, and taking action to avoid those that are most likely to occur. Although insurance protection (see Activity 11.1) has historically been the tool of risk management, the increased complexity of health-care organizations has broadened its scope and importance to include the following categories of potential risks:[1]

- Hazard
- Market
- Reputation
- Operations
- Human Capital

Glenda Clemens feels that she is at a disadvantage. When she asks her regional manager about the insurance coverage for the Phillipsboro office of the American Rehabilitation Company, he tells her not to worry about it. That corporate office handles all of that. She feels that as the person in charge in Phillipsboro she should not just assume that something as important as insurance is simply "handled." She is meeting with her regional manager next week and has asked for some time to discuss insurance. What questions should she ask about hazard, property, general liability, and professional liability insurance? What levels of coverage might seem appropriate for an outpatient practice that sees about 150 patients/week?

This increase in demand has lead to the creation of risk management professionals in health-care organizations who often report directly to the chief executive officer. See Sidebar 11.1. Using a range of measures and data collection, often supported by computer software, risk managers are at the heart of many decisions related to controlling risks so that losses are minimized. Risk management is about processes to avoid accidents, to decrease liability when incidents occur, and to improve the quality of care. Because of the scope of effort required to accomplish these goals, it becomes evident that risk managers rely on all employees to be attentive and careful at all times.

The roles of mid-level managers in risk management in these larger organizations include providing data to and implementing plans developed by risk managers for the protection of the units they manage. In other types of health organizations, risk management may not be as clearly centralized, or it may be among the responsibilities of the upper management team as a whole. Private practitioners in physical therapy also must consider the importance of risk management to the success of their businesses,

typically assuming responsibilities for these duties themselves. Sidebar 11.2 presents some axioms to begin thinking about risk management.

Managers, particularly in developing program proposals or feasibility studies, may take their risk management responsibility as a "big picture" opportunity to address all components of the business from the somewhat negative perspective of potential losses. This process may identify insurmountable barriers or risks that scuttle an exciting or promising business venture. More likely, it may result in a more impressive, well-thought through plan. Risk analysis leads to a plan that includes possible contingencies and potential ways to address them.

Risk management, with communication and legal and ethical issues, is one of the managerial responsibilities that underlies the others—vision, mission, goals; policies and procedures; marketing; staff; patient/client management; and fiscal. This chapter presents some of the major issues related to these responsibilities and the different types of risks.

Hazard Risks

Because they are beyond the control of managers, the risks of natural disasters demand property damage insurance coverage. Depending on location, managers may identify the need for extra protection against hurricanes, fires, or floods, for example. In areas where hazard risks are particularly high, business interruption insurance that will cover the losses that occur while the business is temporarily

---

Sidebar 11.1

Risk Managers

Go to http://www.ashrm.org/ashrm/aboutus/aboutus.html to learn more about risk managers.

Sidebar 11.2

Risk Management Axioms

✦ Clean Up, Don't Cover Up
✦ Defect Prevention, Rather Than Defect Detection
✦ Inform Before You Perform
✦ Listen, Listen, Listen
✦ No Second Chances
✦ Actions Speak Louder Than Words
✦ Treat Others As You Expect To Be Treated
✦ Under Promise and Over Deliver
✦ Follow Up and Follow Through

unable to operate also may reduce the risk of lack of revenue should the business be forced to close.

Managers in smaller organizations may rely on the skills of insurance agents for these policies and others like professional and general liability insurance that are discussed in other sections of this chapter. Risk managers who are part of the upper management team may negotiate all categories of insurance policies for their organizations. Both types of organizations need to establish ongoing review of their policies to assure compliance with governmental regulations and consistency with any changing needs that may arise.

Another risk in this category is hazardous materials themselves. Although not as critical in outpatient physical therapy practices as in acute care settings, the identification of risks related to infections, bloodborne pathogens, the disposal of sharps and other waste, and the provision of protective devices assures the safety of employees and patients/clients.

Hand washing between patients, disinfecting surfaces and equipment, and supplying fresh or paper linens contribute to a safe healthy environment. Policies and procedures for compliance with universal precautions and required absences for staff who are infectious are equally important for reducing the spread of infections. Patients who are infectious should be rescheduled for outpatient therapy.

Failure to identify and reduce these hazards may result in serious violations of federal mandates under the Occupational Safety and Health Administration (OSHA) and serious disease or injury to staff. Go to Sidebar 11.3 and Activity 11.2.

Market Risks

Changes in the target markets served by an organization may be the biggest financial risk, particularly for independent practitioners in health care.

Defining a market as a specified category of potential buyers, managers of independent physical therapy (rehabilitation) services face the possibility of revenue loses if:

✦ Employers in the community change health-care policies for their employees so that coverage for rehabilitation services is more limited or eliminated.

✦ Insurers reduce the reimbursement for services that are covered.

✦ Physicians who refer to the practice relocate, retire, or choose other providers.

✦ Insurers reduce the number of contracts offered to independent practitioners to control their administrative costs.

✦ Populations shift so the percentage of people who seek rehabilitation services changes. (For example: a factory closes so that patients treated who receive Medicare become a much larger percentage of the total number of patients. Conversely, many older Medicare patients may give up their second homes in retirement areas and no longer make up a large percentage of the patients at certain times of the year.)

✦ Technological advances in medicine reduce the number of people with disabling conditions and diseases who would otherwise require intensive rehabilitation, or the amount of rehabilitation services required is decreased as surgical procedures become less invasive and disease processes are better controlled.

Avoiding most of these risks is beyond the control of managers, and there is no insurance protection for market changes. Managers' ability to develop contingency plans may be critical to the survival of their businesses under any of these circumstances. Diversification of services, new collaborations and partnerships with other health-care providers, and other alternative sources of revenue are some possibilities that may be considered. Consulting with legal counsel may reduce the potential risks associated with the contract negotiations necessary in entering relationships with other organizations.

Cash Flow

Another risk, related to the market that is under the control of a manager is the stability of the

---

> **Sidebar 11.3**
>
> **OSHA and Health-Care Facilities**
>
> Go to http://www.osha.gov/SLTC/healthcarefacilities/index.html for detailed information on the Occupational Safety and Health Administration (OSHA) requirements and recommendations for health-care organizations.

ACTIVITY 11.2
INFECTION CONTROL

Stephanie Morgan is concerned that her therapists do not wash their hands consistently as they move from patient to patient. There is a sink in one corner of the exercise room, in each public restroom, and in the staff bathroom. Staff has reported the locations are inconvenient as the major reason for failing to wash their hands. She is considering mounting waterless sanitizer bottles by each private treatment room and several in the gym. Is this a good solution? What are the alternatives? Refer to pp. 61–62 and the worksheet below to develop a strategic plan to address this need.

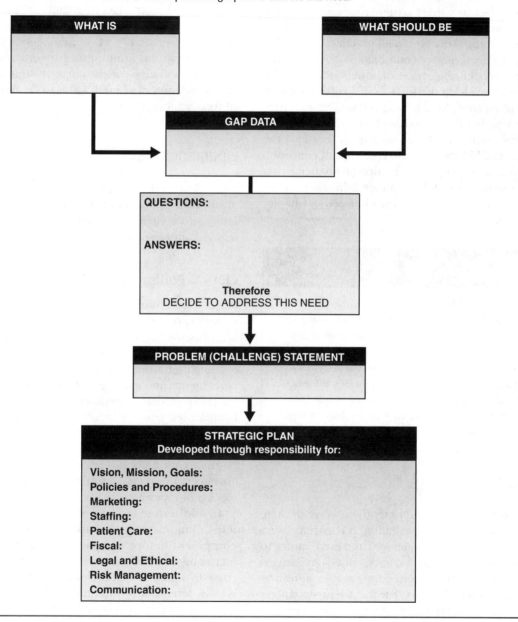

WHAT IS

WHAT SHOULD BE

GAP DATA

QUESTIONS:

ANSWERS:

Therefore
DECIDE TO ADDRESS THIS NEED

PROBLEM (CHALLENGE) STATEMENT

STRATEGIC PLAN
Developed through responsibility for:

Vision, Mission, Goals:
Policies and Procedures:
Marketing:
Staffing:
Patient Care:
Fiscal:
Legal and Ethical:
Risk Management:
Communication:

organization's assets, resources, and expenses. Managers soon discover that hands-on, ongoing, diligent attention to the flow of money in the organization is essential to reduce the risks of spending too much, or not collecting enough, money.

Managers often set "payment due when service is rendered" procedures to reduce the risk of patients who fail to make co-payments or fail to pay their bills on time. Because most patients have to make co-payments, failure of a large number to pay may be ruinous, particularly to a small practice.

These efforts require coordination with an organization's accounting office, or independent practitioners may rely on the services of a certified public accounting firm. Establishing accounting practices and preparing staff to follow clear policies and procedures related to the collection of fees and the payment of bills reduces uncertainty and confusion that also may place the practice at financial risk. Accountants may assist managers in many other aspects of the business that are discussed in Chapter 10. See Activity 11.3.

ACTIVITY 11.3
A FINANCIAL PROBLEM

Walt Cohen, CPA has some bad news for his client Elias Henderson, PT. Although Elias has been doing well in his practice (the number of referrals has exceeded projections), costs continue to exceed budget projections a year after he had projected the practice to break even. Walt wants to meet with Elias to take a look at the books and brainstorm some cost-saving strategies to at least reach the break-even point. What should Elias do in preparation for this meeting?

Reputation Risks

A bad reputation has the potential to severely damage or shut down an organization. It is extremely difficult to earn a good reputation, and even harder to restore one that has been compromised—regardless of the reason. Managers in large organizations may not even know until it is too late that the organization's reputation or the reputation of someone in the organization is tarnished because of poor patient outcomes, suspicious accounting, fraud, false advertising, or unprofessional behavior, etc. Some reasons for a tarnished reputation may be beyond the control of a

manager while others are avoidable. At least the potential negative impact of actions should be identified to reduce risks.

In either case, managers may discover that restoring a reputation requires starting all over—essentially wiping the slate clean. Strategic planning may be vital to tackling this, one of the most difficult managerial challenges. A bad reputation affects interactions with all stakeholders and can be financially devastating. Transforming a "good reputation" into measurable, objective terms takes work. Managers must resist the quick fix and jumping to conclusions without a thorough analysis of the current situation and a clear definition of where it wants to be. Activity 11.4 addresses these issues.

Operations Risks

Operations is the way work is conducted. The risks of operations are most likely to be related to the safety and security of workers and patients/clients that are addressed in this section.

Clinical Equipment and Other Furnishings

Regular maintenance of all equipment used in patient care reduces the risk of adverse effects that are possible, particularly if electrical equipment requires calibration. Managers are responsible for establishing a maintenance schedule and service agreements, and making sure that necessary repairs are completed and documented in a timely manner by qualified people. Operations manuals must be conveniently available for reference by everyone using the equipment, and managers are expected to be the experts who are able to answer or find the answers to questions that arise about effective use of electrotherapy and other equipment.

In addition to routine maintenance, managers must demonstrate the importance of inspecting equipment before *each* use, and using the equipment only as it is intended to be used. Should harm come to a patient because of failure to do so, there is little defense in a potential legal action. It is dangerous to modify exercise equipment or use it in ways other than intended. Wheelchairs, treatment tables, office furniture, and even chairs in the waiting room, require ongoing inspection for signs of instability or wear to prevent breakage. Broken

ACTIVITY 11.4
A BAD REPUTATION

Unfortunately, one of the physical therapists on staff, George Prego, at one of the St. Barnabas Hospital outpatient centers had received a second verbal warning about his unprofessional behavior including rudeness, tardiness, and disregard for patients' concerns and well-being. Before the manager, Sam Zacharias, fired him a week later, George's reputation had already had a negative effect—loss of referrals from several physicians, patient cancellations, and it provoked anger among the staff who felt that Sam should have acted sooner. How should Sam approach undoing the "George effect"? Using the strategic plan presented on pp. 61–62 and the following worksheet, identify and prioritize the needs to move from their current unfavorable status to a good reputation.

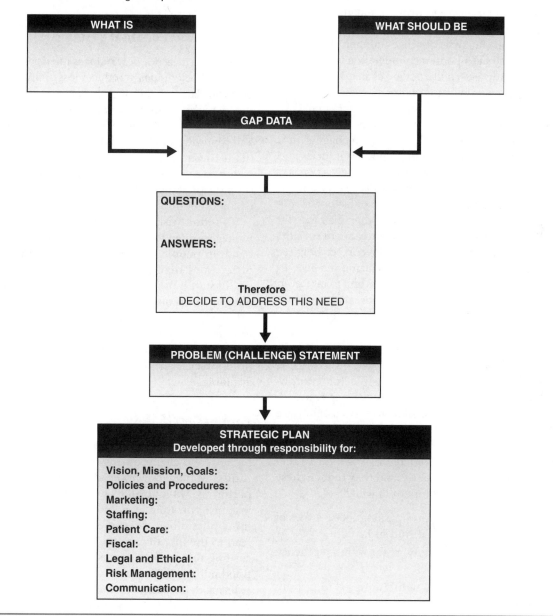

or damaged equipment is better removed than repaired, especially if amateurs are making the repairs. Temporary fixes may lead to permanent losses to the organization.

Not only are frayed electrical cords, loosened connectors, parts held together with tape, and missing parts potentially dangerous, they also project a negative impression that may undermine confidence in the services delivered. Using extension cords are not only electrically dangerous, but extending electrical cords across large spaces presents a danger for tripping and falls.

Ergonomic analysis of office staff and their workspace is another important consideration for reducing the risk of workers' compensation claims or simply loss of work time and pain for injured parties. Depending on the size of the organization, managers may have workers' compensation insurance that defers related costs. With or without workers' comp, managers must be concerned about ongoing repetitive injuries and sudden accidents that may profoundly affect a person's life. Placement of heavy boxes to decrease frequent bending and lifting is one example of factors to consider. Managers also must consider therapists who lift and move patients, or who work at treatment surfaces that are not at the ergonomically correct heights. Avoiding both mental and physical fatigue and encouraging employees to change positions and to take even short walks during the day are activities that managers may encourage to reduce work-related injuries.

Environmental Safety

Managers are not only responsible for complying with the requirements of the American with Disabilities Act for accessibility to services, they are also responsible for safety of the external and internal environment. Managers obtain general liability insurance policies to defer the risk of injuries that may occur on their property, and they reduce these risks through an environment in which:

+ Entryways, streets, and parking lots are free of debris, obstacles, ice, and snow, etc.
+ Commonly used traffic paths within a practice are clear of obstacles.
+ Floor coverings are tightly adhered to prevent tripping or falls.
+ Spills are cleaned up immediately.
+ Adequate space is available for patients and staff

to move about easily without bumping into walls or equipment.
+ Stairways and steps used for gait training are well lit, free of obstacles, with nonslip surfaces.
+ Storage areas include sturdy shelving and other receptacles to clear floor space and prevent falling objects.
+ Fire alarms and extinguishers are conveniently placed and functional.

Security and Personal Safety

Building security not only reduces the risk to personal safety and belongings, it reduces loss of inventory and property damage. Although property insurance shifts the risk, the inconvenience and potential danger compel people to follow procedures for locking doors and reporting suspicious behavior. Of course, it is difficult to know if and which items are missing or stolen, if a complete inventory of equipment and supplies is not maintained. This makes inventory control another important risk management tool.

To reduce risks to both employees and patients, managers need to consider assignments that do not result in people working alone in the building or office, and that paths and parking lots are well lit. All staff must be alert to patients that present a danger to themselves or others. Having a plan to call for assistance is as important for the receptionist as it is for therapist. Emergency numbers should be clearly posted by phones and in other conspicuous places, and first-aid kits should be readily available.

Patient Care Safety

Foremost, managers are responsible for the safety of patients and clients during their care in any organization. Managers who establish procedures to be performed without fail may help reduce the risk. For instance, consistently monitoring vital signs to determine physiological responses to exercise may also lead to the identification of previously undetected cardiopulmonary problems. All staff should be certified in basic life support and the use of automated external defibrillators that are made available in convenient locations. Generally, as the number of patients whom are older increases, and the conditions of many others requiring rehabilitation become more complex, staff in all practice settings also need to be increasingly vigilant and knowledgeable to reduce risks related to things, such as:

+ The effects and adverse side effects of medications.
+ Proper identification of patients.
+ Balancing the use of restraints against the rights and dignity of patients. The use of restraints can lead to injury, but failure to restrain a patient may cause injury to self and others.

Beyond that, managers rely on the skills and decisions of physical therapists and physical therapist assistants involved in patient care to, at the least, do what any other physical therapist would do in similar situations, and, of course, do no harm. Patients expect, rightfully so, that their caregivers are competent and caring in providing care that it is safe and results in a positive outcome. These attributes are discussed in Chapter 12. See Activity 11.5.

Documentation

Documentation of care provided consumes a great deal of time in the operations of clinical practices. The medical record assists in protecting the patient, practitioners, and the health-care organization responsible for that patient's care. It is a legal document that demands managers attend to the production and maintenance of clear, complete records that can meet legal challenges should harm come to a patient.

The medical record serves as the basis for planning patient care and reflects the continuity of decisions and the implementation of those plans. It is the evidence of the course of a patient's care including communication among all caregivers. No one wants to be summoned to give a deposition to explain what happened with a particular patient only to be in the embarrassing position of having incomplete or inaccurate documentation. No one wants to be denied reimbursement because documentation reflecting the medical necessity and goals achieved by patients is missing in the medical record.

Regardless of whether or not the medical record is a hard copy or electronically generated, if some basic principles of documentation are followed, the risk of lawsuits (for any reason) may lessen. These principles[*] include:

1. The patient record is presumed to be true. Licensed health professionals are trusted to be honest in their documentation unless proven otherwise.

2. Documentation of a physical therapist is the single most important evidence of the physical therapist's judgment, actions, skills, and decision making.

---

[*]Based on *The Practical Approach to Documentation* developed but not published by Catherine G. Page and Debra F. Stern, 1994.

ACTIVITY 11.5
A SAFE ENVIRONMENT

Assume the role of an investigator who seeks to identify all of the possible hazard, equipment, environmental, and safety risks in an actual practice. Investigate *all* parts from the reception area to the storeroom (bathrooms, therapeutic gym, entrance, parking, etc.) using the risks presented in the Operations Risks for starters. Identify others.

Create a chart with the following headings to not only identify but make recommendations for preventive measures and assigned responsibility for reducing the risks. Share your findings with the manager of the center you selected.

AREA OF PRACTICE	POTENTIAL RISK EXPOSURE	RISK-CONTROL TECHNIQUES	MANAGERIAL DECISION: WHO, WHAT, HOW?

3. Only the person who delivers care can, and must, document that care. One person cannot write notes for another, or sign notes written by another person.

4. The record must be detailed enough so that another practitioner can assume the care of the patient with no questions to be asked.

5. Information included should clearly identify important characteristics of the patient, support the diagnosis, justify treatment, and establish outcomes reached.

6. All significant information about the patient should be included in the medical record. A parallel set of informal notes are not considered part of this legal document.

7. Entries need to be timely. Writing the note as part of the session is important. Other members of the team may need to refer to the notes written earlier in the day before taking action with a patient.

8. Waiting until later in the day to complete documentation increases the risk that the note may not be accurate because memory fails, particularly after a busy day when the therapist may be fatigued. Also, it is inefficient. Time spent trying to recall what happened earlier in the day lengthens the time needed to complete documentation.

9. Although the use of electronic documentation is increasing, written documentation continues and continues to be problematic. It must be legible to be of value to others as well as the writer. It may be hard to convince others of one's credibility if a person cannot read his or her own writing.

10. All spaces on a standardized form must be completed even if the only thing to enter is N/A or a line through the space. Readers need to know that the person documenting attended to all of the details without having to wonder if the item was addressed and simply not documented. Blanks also provide the opportunity for others to modify documentation in ways that the person who wrote an entry may not intend.

11. Each entry in the medical record must be signed (legible, legal signature) and dated. Many centers also require the time. Managers need to clarify if the time entered is the time

of the treatment session or the time the note is written unless the note is always written at the time of the treatment session.

12. Documentation must be completed by the end of the day, or staff needs to stay until all documentation is completed. Patient records should never leave the facility because the risk of their loss, and the potential breach of confidentiality and privacy are too high.

13. All sources of documentation must withstand audit. Treatment notes, attendance grids, appointment books, billing, etc. must all match. Inaccuracies reduce credibility, and they increase the likelihood of denial of payment.

14. The need for good spelling and grammar may be obvious, but the need for consistent use of abbreviations is often less so. Managers need to adopt a list of acceptable abbreviations for use by all, and a list of professional jargon that everyone should avoid. The fewer the number of abbreviations used, the better the communication.

15. Corrections must be clearly identified with a line through or an addendum to explain the error. Patient records cannot be deleted, erased, or obliterated with whiteout.

16. Keep the content of entries pertinent. Do not include information that is not of value in clinical decision making. Do include *all* information that supports a patient's need for services.

17. Do not complain, criticize, or argue about the patient or other members of the team in the patient record. These entries raise concern about the quality of care provided if members of the team are in disagreement.

18. The patient record also serves as a record of all communication among caregivers including phone calls, faxes, and verbal orders. Missed appointments and the reasons for them need to be noted so that huge gaps in care do not place reimbursement at risk.

19. Documentation must reflect reasonable and necessary care to accomplish patient goals.

20. Treatment notes reflect what care the patient received and the patient's response to it. Progress notes refer back to the initial examination and goals set to demonstrate that the patient is moving towards their accomplishment.

Managers need to identify strategies for implementing these principles, which may include establishing a peer-review program for audit of patient records. The review of others' records is often a good learning experience that reinforces these principles. Even in the smallest organizations, some mechanism for the review of the quality of documentation is important for avoiding reimbursement losses and in preparation for potential legal action. The patient record may be a physical therapist's only defense. See Activity 11.6.

ACTIVITY 11.6
PEER REVIEW OF DOCUMENTATION

Develop a form to be used to review patient records. Decide the key content that must be present and some measure of the quality of each of these key content areas. HINT: Refer to the documentation guidelines of the American Physical Therapy Association either on their Web page or in the *Guide to Physical Therapist Practice*.

Other Important Documents

Patient records are not the only the sensitive material that managers must secure. Patient records storage must comply with state and federal regulations related to access, and the length of time they must be kept available after patients are discharged. If staff takes informal notes to assist their memories of facts gathered during patient care for documentation in the medical record at a later time, these notes also must be secured or destroyed when they are no longer needed. Active records should be accessible only to those personnel who are involved in the patient's care.

Personnel records, contracts, leases, meeting minutes, incorporation documents should be stored in a locked, fireproof box or safe. Passwords for access to computer-based documents need to be protected, and managers need to implement some system to keep both computer and hard-copy files organized so they can be retrieved easily. See Activity 11.7.

Human Capital Risks

Organizations begin the management of human capital risks with current job descriptions that include

---

ACTIVITY 11.7
DOCUMENTATION AND THE LAW

Determine the requirements for documentation in the model practice act found at the Web page of the Federation of State Boards of Physical Therapy. Compare with the actual statutes in selected states.

---

qualifications, duties, reporting relationships, and key indicators of quality performance. Objective performance appraisals that align with job descriptions are the other half of the key documents related to personnel management. Compensation schedules, which are typically based on annual reviews of pay scales and benefits, are often linked to performance appraisals.

Managers must ensure that there are backup people for the critical roles in each job description. Should a person for some reason be unable to perform their duties, another person or persons must be ready to continue the critical functions so that the integrity of the organization is not compromised. To be taken seriously, these backup duties should be formally included in a job description rather than left to the nebulous "other duties as assigned" section. For example, a physical therapist assistant may be the backup for obtaining prior authorizations required for patient care. The business office manager may be the backup for scheduling of patient appointments. The manager of laboratory services may be the backup for the payroll responsibilities of the rehabilitation manager in a large organization. Identifying the key responsibilities that must be sustained is a first, important step.

Managers also determine the inclusion of other duties in job descriptions that go beyond patient care. Input into the business decisions of an organization and quality assurance monitoring are examples. Regular status reports allow ongoing monitoring of performance that help both the manager and employee review and revise job descriptions and discuss performance so that there are no surprises at the time of annual performance evaluations. Status reports also serve as a formal check that additional duties and responsibilities are not deliberately, or unintentionally, built upon until job expectations become unrealistic and performance goals that are impossible to meet.

This section discusses ways to reduce the risk of the impact that ineffective or dangerous employees may have on an organization. Risks associated with personnel begin with the hiring process, continue during employment, and may persist even with termination of employment. Additional staffing information is found in Chapters 8 and 12.

Workforce Shortages

Not enough people to do the work often leads to unhappy, stressed employees and patients who are dissatisfied. Patients on waiting lists for appointments, or those who are simply not scheduled because of lack of personnel, mean lost revenues. More importantly, the risks of worsening patients' conditions because of lack of, or delay in, treatments are a serious concern. Managers may need to identify other actions to take to improve efficiency and effectiveness without additional help. They may decide to limit growth for example. See Activity 11.8.

Contracting with outside agencies to fill positions temporarily is also risky. "Temps" do not often receive the same orientation and they may not have the same commitment to the vision and mission of the organization as full-time employees. They may bring ways of doing things from other experiences that are not consistent with the culture or goals of an organization. Of course, a temp may be reassigned for an extended period and become socialized to a new organization over that time. Should harm come to a patient at the hands of the temp, whether the temp is actually legally an employee of the organization may come into question. The bigger risk is inconsistent care as temps come and go every few weeks. Managers have to weigh the risks of this constant turnover against the risks of a shortage of personnel.

Recruitment

The risk of loss in the recruitment process is the high costs of employment recruiters, want ads (newspapers, direct mail, online), or bonuses to current employees that may not result in placement of a new employee. The risks of workforce shortages are compounded by these additional losses. When the number of additional employees has been determined, the next step may be to shift the analysis to identification of the factors that make the organization the employer of choice. If the supply of employees is small, then encouraging people who are employed in other organizations to change employers may be the only strategy that reduces the risk of loss. Potential employees need to be wary of offers too good to be true, and managers need to be concerned about risks to their reputations that may be result from aggressively recruiting employees from competitors.

Hiring

Managers must determine the accuracy of credentials submitted at the time of hire. One of the greatest risks is staff members who falsely represent their licenses to practice or other credentials. Conducting background checks of all health-care employees has become another requirement in many places to determine any disciplinary actions against a licensee in other jurisdictions, or criminal offenses. Because of this requirement, job applicants are more likely to divulge potential areas of concern than they have been in the past. The risks involved are that billing charges submitted by someone who is not licensed to practice may be retroactively denied, and more importantly, the knowledge and skill required to perform the job may be lacking resulting in harm to patients.

Particularly when there is a shortage of workers, managers cannot risk being hasty to hire any available person. Scrutiny of credentials, may in fact, become even more important. Checking references and work history to verify information is important for solo practitioners as it is for human resource professionals in large organizations.

At Work

Once employed, risks associated with personnel are those related to their failure to perform their professional duties. Costs that incurred as result of malpractice are typically deferred through professional liability policies. Physical therapists who are employees need to determine if they should obtain individual liability insurance policies although the policy of the organization includes their performance. Employers are responsible for the actions of their employees—vicarious liability. This does not mean that the employer will be sued and the employee will not. Attorneys will bring action against both parties. Employers may not support the conduct of an employee and assume no liability.

ACTIVITY 11.8
PATIENT WAITING LIST

Referring to the strategic planning concepts presented on pp. 61–62 and the following worksheet, develop a strategic plan to address the need to permanently eliminate a patient waiting list. How long should a patient reasonably expect to wait for his or her first appointment? Discuss how to determine the effectiveness of these strategies.

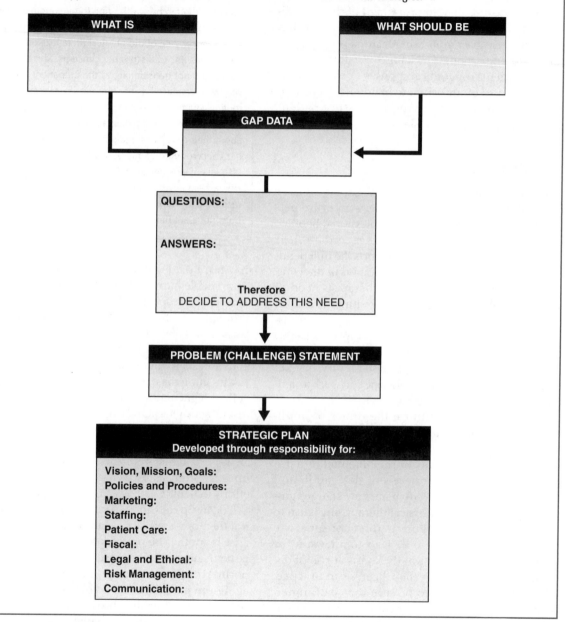

Managers have a responsibility to reduce the potential for harm to patients because employees have failed to perform their duties in a manner expected of professionals.

Although not intentional, injuries to patients in physical therapy may include burns, fractures, or the worsening rather than improvement of their conditions. Typically, these injuries result when staff has failed to identify complicating factors, precautions, and contraindications. The failure of staff to monitor closely patients' ongoing responses to treatment is another cause of unfortunate incidents. Failure to modify or correct interventions to assure patient safety during treatment sessions also leads to injuries.

Direction

The inappropriate direction and supervision of physical therapist assistants or other supportive personnel is another key factor in professional liability. Managers must promote policies and procedures, and an organizational culture that supports the independent decision making of physical therapists in directing and supervising others. Physical therapists need to decide for each patient in each treatment session, when and what components of care may be transferred to the care of a physical therapist assistant. Because the patient's condition and the skills and expertise of physical therapist assistants vary, blanket policies about physical therapist assistant work assignments should be discouraged.

Managers must scrutinize the duties of nonlicensed personnel as well. The type of direction and training they receive must be formalized to reduce the risks of illegal activity or the potential of harm to the patient. Because levels of delegation and supervision are included in many state statutes governing the practice of physical therapy, any harm to a patient because of failure to direct or supervise appropriately may not only lead to a lawsuit for damages but place physical therapists at risk of disciplinary action against their licenses to practice. Managers often need to be sure that staff understands that harm that occurs during care that was delegated to others remains the responsibility of the physical therapists. See Activity 11.9.

Patient Rapport

The most powerful risk management tool is establishing a professional rapport with patients. People

---

ACTIVITY 11.9
DELEGATION

Eric Walters feels fortunate that he was finally able to hire Candace Dumar, a physical therapist assistant with almost 20 years of experience in acute care and nursing homes, although he was hoping to hire another physical therapist in his outpatient practice. After a few weeks, Julie Spencer, one of the physical therapists on staff approaches Eric to discuss her concerns. She feels that Candace is not transitioning to the outpatient setting very well. Candace has been modifying plans of care routinely without consulting with Julie, and she had heard Candace giving patients inaccurate information about their conditions and goals. When Julie discussed her concerns with Candace, she told her she has 20 years of experience and knows what she is doing. Her last employer had insisted that she take on more responsibility for patients that she was assigned and she does not want those duties curtailed.

---

may not take legal action when unintentional or unavoidable harm occurs if they feel they have been treated with respect and dignity in a caring manner, although the physical therapist or physical therapist assistant was obviously not careful enough. The truth is that mistakes happen. Even with the best intentions and skills, unavoidable adverse incidents occur. Taking immediate action when an injury occurs may deflect legal action. Patients expect the truth and resent actions to cover up mistakes. Being honest and calm in developing a plan to manage the recovery from an injury that is the result of treatment is an important first step. Focusing on the patient's best interest often leads to more positive results than efforts to belittle a problem, or attempts to save face.

Follow-up calls and assuring patients that the physical therapist is available at any time should problems arise is another helpful risk management tool. Many patients have increased pain or new symptoms as a normal response to therapy interventions, so encouraging the patient to call if they have any questions or problems after they leave a treatment session is good risk management. Explaining that what they are feeling is expected and normal is often all that they need to reduce suspicions that they have been harmed.

Managers need to be sure that staff is prepared for patients with whom it is difficult to establish a rapport. Conflicts arise despite the best efforts of therapists to establish a professional relationship. Documentation of issues that arise and action taken is important. If conflicts cannot be resolved, transferring patients to another therapist or termination of care may be the only alternative. These situations must be handled carefully to avoid abandonment—unilateral severance of a professional relationship. Should harm come to the patient because of lack of care, there is a risk of lawsuit. Transfer of care or discharge plans must be acceptable to a patient, and therapists need to follow through on these actions to ensure their completion.

Another critical aspect of patient care for physical therapists arises because of their intimate contact with patients. Physical therapy interventions involve a great deal of touching. If not clearly explained, and if permission to touch is not obtained, patients may misinterpret touching as sexual advances. Inform before you perform is a particularly important mantra in physical therapy practice. Patients need to be told where and why they need to be touched, and their permission obtained. Because sexual offenses are taken very seriously, any suggestion of impropriety by the therapist or patient must be nipped in the bud. Discouraging sexual innuendos from patients without destroying rapport must be handled carefully. Transfer of care to another therapist or the presence of others during treatment sessions may be necessary.

Many patients are already involved in litigation because their need for rehabilitation results from work-related injuries, car accidents, or falls in public places. Managers need to pay particular attention to review of their medical records for accuracy and completeness because the records will surely be presented as evidence for recovery of damages in court.

Although managers cannot control affairs of the heart, avoiding personal relationships with patients is critical. They suggest impropriety because of the power role of the caregiver, and give other patients the impression of special or preferred treatment. Managers may need to be alert to these situations and take action to separate personal relationships from professional relationships by transferring the care of the patient to others. Similar relationships among staff may be equally difficult. There is a risk that others on staff perceive these relationships as favoritism or leading to unfair decisions about assignments and performance evaluation. Their concerns may affect patient outcomes and job satisfaction.

Professional Development

Professional development plans that address specific goals of each employee reduce risks because addressing the specific needs of individuals to improve knowledge and skills is more likely to be effective in reducing errors and harm than providing blanket courses directed to all. Employees need to justify their requests for approval of continuing education courses in terms of their professional development and the goals of the organization in order for the costs to be an investment in the organization through its personnel. Managers need to direct attention to courses related to sociocultural issues, reimbursement, and other nonclinical topics. Without this need analysis, the investment in development may have no impact on the quality of care and patient outcomes.

Termination of Employment

Disagreements about promotions, salary increases, harassment, and discrimination may surround the termination of employment. Related lawsuits may be costly and disruptive, as are wrongful termination suits. Most states recognize that employees employment may be terminated at the will of the employer. Personnel policies must be clear and reviewed for compliance at least annually because of these complex legal relationships. Fairness, good faith, and communicating the rights and responsibilities of employees upon hire may avoid disagreeable terminations of employment.

Identifying Risks

Like the care given to keep policies and procedures current and relevant, *all* organizations need to formally review their risks and the effectiveness of efforts in preventing and controlling them, in detail, at least every 6 months. This review should be documented and, of course, actions recommended by the review actually should be implemented. This process may include a retrospective review of documents, such as committee minutes, quality assurance and safety reports, performance measures, peer reviews, benchmarks, qualitative data, process reviews, and submitted incident reports. See Sidebar 11.4.

Sidebar 11.4

A Liability Test

The following questions raise the awareness of managers about potential professional liability risk factors. They may be used to identify areas that require risk management interventions as staff plan their professional development.

Y N   Do therapists limit treatments of patients to those they are qualified to handle?

Y N   Do therapists know their legal duties to their patients?

Y N   Are therapists careful of being overly optimistic when discussing goals or prognosis with patients?

Y N   Do all patients participate in rehabilitation with informed consent?

Y N   Would the organization be embarrassed or prejudicially affected by its patients' records?

Y N   Would the medical records give the organization and individuals maximum protection in a lawsuit?

Y N   Do therapists take special action if a patient does not follow directions or discontinues treatment?

Y N   Are therapists tactful with patients and families?

Y N   Do therapists consult with each other and other health professionals to protect the patient?

Y N   Are instructions to patients and families complete and understandable?

Y N   Are patients notified when therapists will be away and that other arrangements have been made for their care?

Y N   Is expert legal advice sought whenever the possibility of negligence is suggested?

Y N   Do therapist refrain from making any statements about a case unless they have legal advice?

Y N   Is all equipment and environment in the safest condition possible?

Y N   Are all therapists technically prepared to use all equipment?

Y N   Are all employees qualified? Capable? Courteous?

Y N   Do therapists keep current with courses and publications?

Y N   Do therapists refrain from adverse criticism of other health-care workers?

Y N   Are disagreeable misunderstandings about fees avoided?

Y N   Is special care taken in documentation on patients with work-related injuries, who are indigent, and all others who may be involved in litigation?

Y N   How do the professional skills and experience of therapists compare with others in the profession?

Y N   Are patients advised if treatments may be of doubtful efficacy?

Y N   Are therapists always attentive and thoughtful so that patients feel confident and secure?

Y N   Is consideration given to social, religious, economic factors affecting patients?

Incidents, Occurrences, and Sentinel Events

Although these terms may be used interchangeably, Carroll[1] defines an incident as anything that is not consistent with routine care or normal operations. The word occurrence may be used for clinically related incidents. In health care, sentinel events is another term for incidents or occurrences that signals that a death or serious physical or psychological injury or risk thereof has occurred. Any poor outcome may be labeled as a sentinel event to emphasize that health-care organizations are to be held accountable for them.

The problem of course is that the identification of these threats is dependent on people actually reporting them. People may be reluctant to report because of perceived negative consequences to them personally, or because they do not want to be known as whistle blowers or troublemakers. Perhaps they simply do not realize that what happened is an actual incident to be reported. Often significant issues that are nonclinical are simply overlooked.[1] To make reporting easier, organizations typically have a standardized reporting form. The basic content of an incident report is:

1. Date and time of incident
2. Names of persons involved
3. Age, sex, diagnosis, and physician (if patient involved)
4. Description of the event
5. Name and contact information of witnesses
6. Witness's description of the event
7. Treatment offered or rendered
8. Name, title, position of person completing the report
9. Signature and date of person preparing the report

Incidents should include only the facts, very detailed facts, while avoiding personal opinions or judgments. Whenever possible, the actual person involved in the incident should complete the report rather than having it completed by someone who is basing the report on secondary information. The typical procedure is that the report is submitted to the immediate manager first. Managers may find that they must suggest revisions and closely monitor the completion of all components of incident reports so that they are accurate. Immediate action may be necessary, but it should not mean that managers forgo more analysis of the incident. Managers are also responsible for frequently reminding the reporter that the incident should not be discussed with anyone else, whether they were involved in the incident or not, to preserve accurate presentation of facts without bias.

Because incident reports are treated as confidential information to be used internally for quality assurance and other administrative action, they should never be referred to in the medical record. A reference to an incident report may result in an inadvertent disclosure of the incident report during legal proceedings. Confidentiality of these reports is critical to protecting the parties involved and the organization. Most states protect this information as part of an organizations quality assurance process so that people and organizations use the process without fear of repercussions. See Activity 11.10.

ACTIVITY 11.10
AN INCIDENT REPORT

Critique this completed incident report.

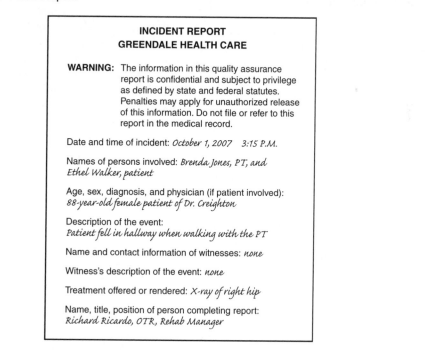

INCIDENT REPORT
GREENDALE HEALTH CARE

WARNING: The information in this quality assurance report is confidential and subject to privilege as defined by state and federal statutes. Penalties may apply for unauthorized release of this information. Do not file or refer to this report in the medical record.

Date and time of incident: *October 1, 2007   3:15 P.M.*

Names of persons involved: *Brenda Jones, PT, and Ethel Walker, patient*

Age, sex, diagnosis, and physician (if patient involved): *88-year-old female patient of Dr. Creighton*

Description of the event: *Patient fell in hallway when walking with the PT*

Name and contact information of witnesses: *none*

Witness's description of the event: *none*

Treatment offered or rendered: *X-ray of right hip*

Name, title, position of person completing report: *Richard Ricardo, OTR, Rehab Manager*

Analyzing Risks

Risk managers are challenged to analyze the data about potential risks and incident reports to arrive at a root cause. The root cause is the factor that if eliminated, the incident or potential risk will not recur. One commonly used, rather simple, method of analysis in other types of businesses is the five whys approach.[2] The risk manager simply asks, "Why did this occur?" In response to the answer, the next question is, "Why did that occur?" The question is repeated until it has been asked a total of five times. Although not a hard, fast rule, five seems to be the average number of required times either to get to the fundamental issue, or an issue that is beyond the control of the committee or organization. The amount of time to answer the questions may take minutes or weeks. See Figure 11.1 for an example of risks of loss at the fictional Buchanan Physical Therapy.

Although the five whys are a good starting point, they are only as valuable as the accuracy of the answers to the questions. For example, if the answer to the first question had been the burglar needed money to buy drugs, the analysis would have taken a totally different track. Because the focus of the five whys is human factors or interactions, it is not as valuable for health-care organizations that typically require a more complex approach to risk analysis that focuses on the many interacting system processes rather than people as the major source of most patient care risks or incidents. Although the format may vary, an expanded root cause analysis is commonly used for more formal, detailed analysis in health care. Figure 11.2 provides one example of the steps involved in flow-chart format.

Not all of the components of the organization may need to be addressed in the analysis of any incident. More likely, some combination of factors, or other factors not included in the figure, may be identified in the process. This multifactor model is also more conducive to examining possible alternative root causes. In health care, the added dimension, particularly for sentinel events, is often to demand evidence to support the identification of the root cause, alternatives, and actions selected. Rather than relying on what may be personal biases in the

---

THE 5 WHYS

Someone entered Buchanan Physical Therapy after hours, stole the computers, television, and other items.

1. Why did this occur? The glass door was easily broken so the burglar had no difficulty entering the office.

2. Why did that occur? All businesses in the complex have the same glass doors.

3. Why did that occur? To make the complex and entrances to all businesses inviting and consistent in appearance.

4. Why did that occur? To add property value and to encourage more business.

5. Why did that occur? To increase the income of Buchanan Physical Therapy and adjoining businesses.

ACTION: Replace glass door and install security alarm by the end of the week.

Figure 11.1 ✦ Example of the five whys.

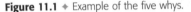

process, a focus on reliable sources of information that support the cause and effect relationships identified increases the power and acceptance of action to be taken.

A Manager's Responsibility

Preventing, reducing and eliminating risks requires managers to be alert to a wide range of possible occurrences and decisions that impact individuals and the organization as a whole. This is a responsibility that underlies all other responsibilities. Managers who view their risk management responsibilities as consultative rather than punitive are more likely to have everyone see risk management as part of their work. See Activities 11.11 and 11.12.

REFERENCES

1. Carroll R. *Risk Management Handbook for Health Care Organizations.* San Francisco: Jossey-Bass; 2001.
2. iSixSigma LLC. *Determine the root cause: 5 whys.* Available at: http://www.isixsigma.com/library/content/c020610a.asp. Accessed January 22, 2008.

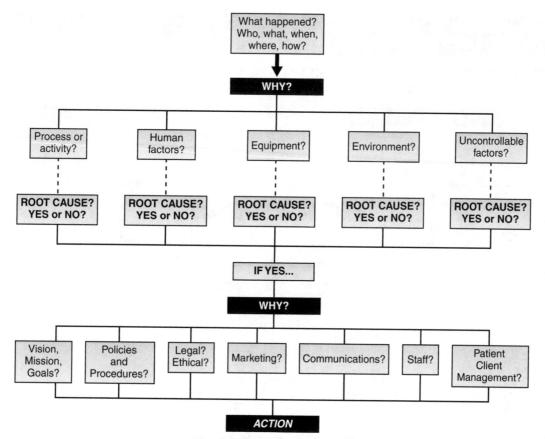

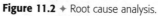

Figure 11.2 ✦ Root cause analysis.

ACTIVITY 11.11
STRATEGIES FOR GAPS IN RISK MANAGEMENT

Identify a gap in managing risks in physical therapy practices. Referring to pp. 61–62 as a guide and using the following worksheet close the identified gap. Discuss how the effectiveness of these strategies will be determined.

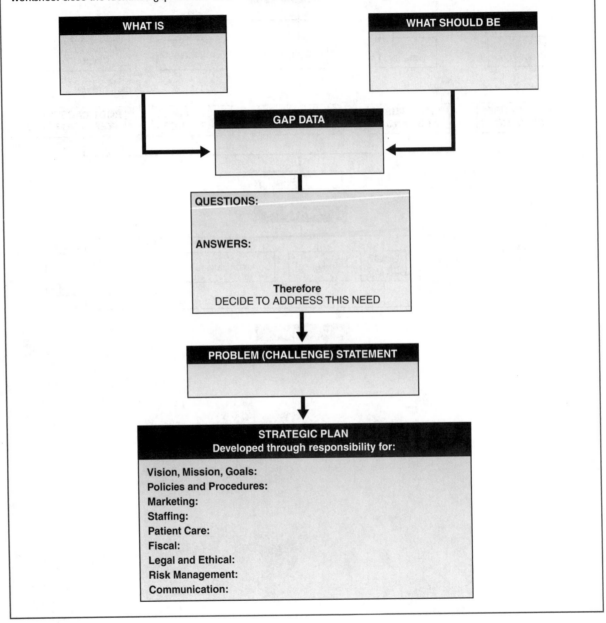

ACTIVITY 11.12
CASE STUDIES

In small groups, discuss the following cases. Determine what elements of each scenario increased the risk of professional liability. The chart in Activity 11.5 may be helpful. Were the therapists involved negligent? Conduct a root cause analysis for each case using Figure 11.2. What risk management interventions should be implemented to reduce recurrence of each incident? What are the legal and ethical issues in each case?

CASE 1

A patient's ambulatory ability at 3 weeks post total hip arthroplasty had improved enough that the physical therapist coordinated with nursing staff to have the patient use a walker with standby supervision anywhere within the nursing home. While walking to the dining room the next day, the patient reported sharp hip pain and began to collapse. The nursing assistant walking with him was able to break his fall and he was seated in a chair. He reported that he was fine.

The next day, his hip pain limited his ability to walk at all. The nursing supervisor ordered an x-ray that revealed dislocation of the hip prosthesis. His recovery period was significantly lengthened because of the need for corrective surgery, and the development of pneumonia during his second hospital stay.

The patient sued the rehabilitation center and the physical therapist for failing to properly instruct and supervise the nursing assistant about the correct gait instructions for the patient.

CASE 2

A woman with a history of osteoporosis was receiving physical therapy for a fracture of the right wrist. Because her function also was limited by back pain, the physical therapist added hot pack and massage to the spine to her treatment plan. The patient reported temporary relief from the back treatments.

The patient called to cancel her 12th appointment and told the receptionist that she had a fracture of one of

her vertebra from the massage and would be unable to continue treatments. The receptionist documented the phone call as "cancellation."

The patient sued the physical therapist because of the new injury, which also lead to her inability to continue therapy for her wrist. She developed contractures of the wrist that severely limited her ability to use her hand. She also claims that the physical therapist violated the practice act because he did not have doctor's orders to treat her back in the first place.

CASE 3

A patient, who has a reputation for making constant demands during her treatment sessions, is treated with hot packs to her right shoulder for pain related to her right hemiplegia. She was given a bell to signal if she needed anything. She was left unattended throughout the treatment session, although several people in the department heard her yelling that the hot pack was too hot and she could not move it. She rang the bell many times. The physical therapist assistant, from across the room, asked her to please be quiet, and reminded the patient that she complained at the last treatment session of not enough heat.

When the physical therapist assistant removed the hot pack at the end of the 20-minute treatment, the patient insisted that she look at her skin because the hot pack was placed over her clothing. The physical therapist assistant discovered a burn that had already begun to blister and applied ice. The patient required a skin graft and sued the physical therapy organization, the physical therapist, and the physical therapist assistant.

CASE 4

A physical therapist asked a new coworker who has just completed a certification in mobilization to consult with him on a patient who continues to have severe pain and limited spinal range of motion after 2 weeks of daily physical therapy sessions. The patient agreed to be seen

continued

by the coworker at the next treatment session. At the beginning of that session, the physical therapist was called away to care for another patient after giving brief introductions and providing the new therapist with a brief summary of the patient's problem. The coworker proceeded with his intervention.

The patient experienced a severe increase in pain during the mobilization procedure. The patient asked that the treatment stop immediately and she left the clinic.

She is suing both physical therapists and the physical therapy corporation because she claims the treatment caused an exacerbation of her problem that required several unsuccessful surgeries. The primary therapist admits that he did not discuss the patient's history with his coworker. The coworker admits that he did not review the medical record or conduct his own history and examination before initiating treatment.

CASE 5

A patient with severe knee pain for an extended period reluctantly agreed to an arthroscopic procedure and he was referred to a physical therapy center for a standardized postsurgical regimen. Because of a waiting list, there was a 2-week delay in initiating physical therapy. The patient did the best he could at home with the exercises the surgeon's nurse gave him to follow.

The physical therapist conducted the initial examination and decided to begin the regimen as if the patient had already had 2 weeks of physical therapy. She assigned the physical therapist assistant to continue the regimen and to report to her every third session.

The physical therapist assistant, new to the center and the protocol, included passive stretching of the knee and continued to stretch, although the patient complained of a great deal of pain and heard a pop in the knee.

The patient asked to see the physical therapist and reported that he had a great deal of pain and that he had never been stretched to that extreme before. Without examining the knee, the physical therapist applied a cold pack and instructed the patient to apply cold several times a day.

The patient never returned for treatment. The patient sued the physical therapist, physical therapist assistant,

the physical therapy center, and the surgeon for referring him there. The patient required additional surgery and extensive rehabilitation to repair the reinjured knee. The documentation includes only checks on a flow sheet.

CASE 6

A child has been progressing well with his exercise program for the last several months and his parents are very pleased. As a reward for good behavior, he is allowed to jump on the small trampoline in the department for a few minutes at the end of the treatment sessions.

During one trampoline play session, although the physical therapist was guarding him, she turned her attention away for a second. The child fell suffering a concussion and fracture of the left humerus. The immobilization of the arm resulted in an elbow contracture and prolonged physical therapy in another center. The care was was complicated by the child's new fears and confusion, although the physician reported no evidence of brain damage resulting from the head injury. The family sued the physical therapist and the center.

CASE 7

A patient reported increased numbness and tingling down the right-upper extremity that had been getting progressively worse during the 2 weeks she had been receiving physical therapy, although her cervical spasms and headaches were reduced. The physical therapist urged her to see a neurosurgeon as soon as possible.

The patient returned to her family physician for a referral to a neurosurgeon. Instead of a referral, the physician told her to just continue the physical therapy.

Physical therapy continued for another week until the physical therapist decided that she should discontinue therapy because the treatment was having no impact on the numbness and tingling. She discharged the patient, again advised her to see a neurosurgeon, and even suggested the name of someone to call.

Two weeks later the patient had an MRI that revealed herniation of two cervical intervertebral disks. Although surgery was successful, the patient was left with residual weakness and numbness in the right upper extremity.

She sued the physical therapist and her family physician for failing to assess her condition correctly and in a timely manner.

CASE 8

A patient signed a financial responsibility form that all patients signed in an outpatient center. He understood that he was agreeing to pay 20% of the total bill and the office manager assured him it would not be more than $20/visit. At the end of his course of rehabilitation, the patient had paid $1,000 for 50 visits and the insurance paid the center $5,000 ($100/visit) as their contract permitted, although the center had billed for $300/visit.

The patient's doctor ordered 16 additional physical therapy visits. The business manager/receptionist advised the patient that the insurance company might not approve the additional visits. He signed an agreement stating he would pay for the 16 visits if the insurance company denied the claim. He was assured a fair payment plan would be established to pay for these additional services as they were for his previous payments.

The insurance company offered to reimburse the physical therapy center for the 16 additional treatment sessions at $57/visit. The PT rejected the offer because it was too low and advised the patient of his action.

The patient has reported the physical therapist to the Board of Physical Therapy Practice in his state charging that the physical therapist committed fraud, which is a violation of the practice act. He claims it was dishonest to charge him the full $300 amount that was billed to the insurance company when the therapist accepted less for the same treatment previously. He feels that he should have been charged the $120 that was collected from him and the insurance company for the first 50 visits. He did not pay, and refuses to pay until this matter is settled. He reports that the physical therapist's business manager is harassing him for the money.

CASE 9

A woman had been receiving the same outpatient treatment for pain relief 3 times a week intermittently during the last 6 months since her spinal surgery after a car accident. One day she received her usual treatment, which included interferential electrical current with the electrodes placed along the lumbar spine and at the right lateral ankle. Her usual therapist had set up the treatment and left to care for an inpatient in the hospital.

Another physical therapist removed the electrodes at the end of the treatment. He noticed more than usual redness at the ankle. He asked the patient if she felt any discomfort and the patient said that she really did not ever feel anything because of the numbness in her leg. The therapist became very excited and said that this electrotherapy treatment should never have been administered.

The patient also reported that her therapist had shown her how to adjust the current and maybe she (the patient) had turned it up too high this time.

A burn was noted at the right ankle during the next treatment session and the patient was referred to the emergency room. The patient eventually required surgical débridement and a skin graft to repair the wound. She sued the physical therapy center and the physical therapists.

CASE 10

A patient had a left total knee replacement, which became infected and was rejected. The prosthesis was replaced and he began a usual regimen of physical therapy. About 8 weeks later, he was discharged from physical therapy because he had met his goals. The office manager told him he would have to pay for further treatment himself because reimbursement for more than 8 weeks of therapy would be denied.

He returned to his physician, who was persuaded by the patient that he could make more gains with additional therapy, which the doctor then ordered. The patient went to a different center to continue treatment.

His new physical therapist noted at transfer of care that the patient continued to have edema, decreased strength and range of motion of the left knee, and an antalgic gait.

The plan of care in the new center included isokinetic exercises, which he had not had before, followed by passive static hamstring stretch and ice application. All interventions in the first two treatment sessions were completed without complaint. Three days after the second session, the patient went to the doctor because of increased pain

continued

that he attributed to the new exercises. An x-ray revealed no problems, but pain was elicited at the lower pole of the patella. The doctor noted how well the patient was walking. The doctor discontinued physical therapy and the patient was advised to swim for exercise.

Two weeks later, the patient returned to his doctor because the pain had worsened and he was unable to walk. There was no loosening of the prosthesis and the doctor told him to come back in a month. Three weeks later, his condition was unchanged and exploratory surgery was scheduled. It was discovered that the patellar tendon was ruptured at the tibial tubercle. The revision and repair of the tendon that was done at that point was unsuccessful because the patient could not tolerate any knee flexion. An arthrodesis was performed 3 months later.

The patient sued the second physical therapy practice claiming that his knee was hyperflexed on the Biodex machine, resulting in the tendon tear.

CASE 11

The patient was an 88-year-old resident in a skilled nursing rehabilitation center at the time of the incident. His poor medical condition (general debilitation secondary to pneumonia) was complicated by dementia for which he was receiving medication. The rehabilitation team reports on the medical record reflect the decision that the patient required restraints except under limited, supervised conditions because of his high risk for falling.

The patient was transported to the therapy room in a wheelchair with a restraint properly applied. The occupational therapist assistant removed the restraint, draping it around the handgrip of the wheelchair, and attempted to work with the patient who was too lethargic to participate.

The patient's occupational therapy was to be followed directly by a physical therapy session. The physical therapist assistant who had been assigned to work with the patient for his session was working with another patient in the same room. The occupational therapist presented the patient to the physical therapist without reapplying the restraint belt and reported that the patient could not be awakened. The occupational therapist then returned to the staff office and the occupational therapist assistant left the room to escort a patient to her room.

The physical therapist immediately tried to awaken the patient, without success, and left the room to report her findings to the nurse. The physical therapist assistant had not yet begun to treat the patient and left the treatment area to transport another patient to his room.

Shortly after, the occupational therapist and occupational therapist assistant in the adjoining staff office heard a loud bang. The patient had stood up and fell to the floor. While in other areas of the nursing home, the physical therapist and physical therapist assistant heard the coded announcement on the loudspeaker indicating a patient had been injured in rehabilitation. They hurried back to the therapy room. The physical therapist's initial examination of the patient suggested that he had broken his hip.

The patient was transported to an emergency room where it was confirmed that the fall resulted in a fracture of the left hip. Surgery to repair the hip was performed. The patient died a few weeks later. The family sued the nursing home, the physical therapist, physical therapist assistant, occupational therapist, and occupational therapist assistant.

Chapter 12

Legal and Ethical Responsibilities

Learning Objectives

- Identify the structure of the U.S. legal system.
- Discuss legal rights, duties, and remedies.
- Discuss a manager's role in contracts, torts, and professional malpractice.
- Discuss selected aspects of employment laws.
- Discuss patient consent, confidentiality, and rights.
- Compare state statutes for patient care responsibilities for selected health-care professionals.
- Discuss the role of managers in addressing the legal duties of organizations.
- Discuss managerial ethics and the role of the American Physical Therapy Association (APTA) Code of Ethics.
- Analyze a given malpractice scenario.

Special Note

*The intent of this chapter is to alert managers to possible legal duties or concerns as they may relate to their jurisdictions or circumstances. CONTENT SHOULD **NOT** BE TAKEN AS LEGAL ADVICE.*

Overview

Managers in health care face a variety of legal and ethical responsibilities. A brief overview of the U.S. legal system is helpful in understanding where health-care legal issues fall. Figure 12.1 shows the four sources of law of the U.S. legal system and their impact on health care. Managers must focus on the legal duties of their organizations and employees as well as the rights of employees and patients. Laws, contracts, and the duties of professionals to behave reasonably and responsibly in meeting the needs of society all impose on the responsibilities of health-care managers.

Rights and Duties

Managers must understand that every legal right includes a duty for themselves and others. The classic example is that the right of free expression does not include the right to scream "Fire!" in a crowded theater when there is no fire. As another example, a person's right to swing their arms ends when one of them touches another person. The person swinging has a duty to take reasonable care to avoid the danger of hitting someone else. As a health-care example, managers may have the legal right to hire and fire employees at will, but they also have the duty to take such actions seriously by following guidelines promulgated to enforce employment laws.

Remedies

Another basic legal principle that managers need to understand is that "every wrong has a remedy."

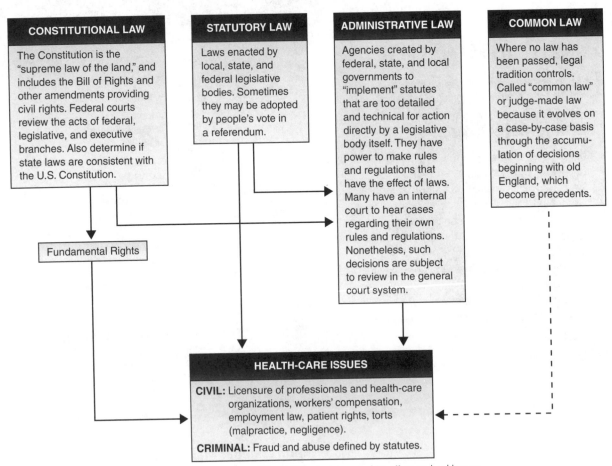

Figure 12.1 ✦ Overview of the U.S. legal system and its effect on health care.

Legal wrongdoing is cured, or relieved, by a penalty of some kind imposed by a court. Courts remedy criminal wrongs by a range of fines and/or imprisonment. Civil wrongdoings involve legal and equitable remedies. A legal remedy (relief) is money for damages incurred, although money may not always be considered an adequate remedy. For instance, in a contract for a unique object, the equitable (fair) remedy may be the delivery of the unique object, not money. A health-care example may be a situation in which a patient "contracts" for surgery performed by a physician with a particular reputation, but the surgery is actually performed by one of the physician's partners or an assistant.

Managers face legal issues across the range of their responsibilities. Selected issues are briefly presented in the following sections to raise awareness of the complexity of these issues.

Legal Concerns of Managers

Contracts

A contract is a legally enforceable agreement created when an offer by one party is accepted by another. It may be oral or written, but the agreement must include some benefit or consideration for each party. Each party in a contract is entitled to the benefit of its bargain under the contract; therefore, managers have a duty to perform exactly as a contract provides. Courts often will find that some provisions are implicit (e.g., each party must act in good faith and deal fairly). A party may be excused from a duty if it becomes impossible, which is referred to as frustration of performance. Otherwise, a court may compel a party to keep an exact promise, to a specific performance, or to pay money damages. Only the court can decide that the substitution of damages is fair.

Based on the actions of the parties, a court may decide if a contract is implied. In the absence of other terms, a party will receive the fair value of its service, which is known as *quantum meruit*. Contracts that are of most interest to health-care managers include:

+ Service and equipment maintenance contracts
+ Contracts for employee benefits
+ Contracts with third-party payers
+ Contracts with registries, placement agencies, or independent contractors
+ Employment contracts
+ Implied contracts with patients
+ Clinical education agreements

Because both oral and written contracts are a legally binding exchange of promises or agreements between parties, enforceable as law; managers should rely on attorneys to negotiate them to assure that their legal interests are protected. For example, restrictive covenants in employment contracts prevent an employee from doing certain things after employment ends. Can the employee work for a competitor? How soon? How nearby? Are any business secrets at risk? Such provisions may invade the employee's right to work and often become an area of contention.

States address the legality of such covenants through statutes that vary widely from one state to another. Attorneys ensure such contracts conform with state law, or in some cases, select which state's laws will be used in contract negotiations. Attorneys also are consulted when employees or others potentially breach contracts; they identify the remedies available to employers.

Managers need to be cautious about promises they make to employees that may be interpreted as contracts. They also need to remind staff about inadvertently making promises about outcomes to patients that may be taken as verbal contracts. For example, physical therapists working with professional athletes may need to be careful in their discussions with these patients, because conversations meant to be casual, could be heard as contracts. For example, when a patient asks if they will be able to win the big race coming up, a physical therapist may think twice about responding, "Sure, no problem, you will be as good as new by Saturday."

Torts

A tort is an injury or wrong—other than breach of contract—committed on another person, their property or reputation, for which the injured party is entitled to seek compensation. For example, damages sustained in an automobile accident may be a tort of negligence because there is a duty to avoid hitting another car. In health care, the duty to respect and protect patients and their privacy is probably the most important duty. Failure to do so is taken very seriously by the law. If reasonable care is not exercised, that failure in duty constitutes the tort of negligence, and creates liability for any resulting injury.

Negligence is the failure to exercise that degree of care, which a reasonable person would exercise under the same circumstances. Other torts may be based on intentional injuries or wrongs, which also may be criminal acts. Distinguishing whether an action was negligent or intentional is important in the law because of the difference in damages that might be awarded. Intentional torts may include additional punitive damages beyond the actual losses that are the direct result of negligence. Intent is sometimes implied from the acts of the parties.

Professional Malpractice

Malpractice is a particular tort based on negligence and of special interest to health-care managers. The tort of professional malpractice consists of the following elements:

+ the duty to conform to a certain <u>standard of care;</u>
+ a failure to conform to the required <u>standard of care;</u>
+ actual injury or damage; and
+ a legally sufficient causal connection between the conduct and the injury.

"Standard of care" is a legal term with a precise meaning. Practice acts that govern professional practices usually include a statement similar to the one below that is the accepted legal definition of standard of care:

A given health-care provider must provide the level of care, skill, and treatment which, in light of all relevant surrounding circumstances, is recognized as acceptable and appropriate by reasonably prudent similar health-care providers.

Although definitions may vary in detail, confusion will result from attempts to paraphrase the term or apply it for purposes other than legal analysis. For instance, most importantly, the legal standard of care does not necessarily equate with professional practices, guidelines, or other clinical "standards."

Because of the variables involved, the standard of care, and whether a physical therapist negligently failed to comply with that standard must be determined case by case. These determinations only can be established by competent expert testimony at trial. Because expert opinions may vary, the result is often a "battle of the experts." For example, it is *not* malpractice if the patient received appropriate care, but the outcome was not as expected because of other factors.

Consider the following scenario: A physical therapist might follow and then modify a postoperative plan of care for a patient with a total hip replacement as necessary to accommodate an individual's current status. That patient may remain unable to walk independently as expected because of circulatory deficits or the patient's fear of falling. In this case, the therapist performed as another therapist would with the same patient and performed carefully so that harm or injury to the patient was avoided during that care. The failure to achieve the patient's goal of independent ambulation is, most likely, not professional negligence.

On the other hand, using the same scenario, if the therapist failed to address the patient's circulatory problems and fears and that failure resulted in the patient's inability to walk, that may be considered malpractice because a prudent therapist, in similar circumstances, would have taken all of these important factors impacting performance into consideration.

Managers and Harm to Patients

Unfortunately, managers may face incidents that result in harm to patients. See Chapter 11 for more discussion on reducing these risks. When an incident occurs, managers must ensure that employees avoid discussions of the incident. The incident is reported first within the organization according to its procedures. In the absence of a risk manager, the organization may report directly to the insurance company that is providing professional or general malpractice insurance, or to an attorney. In many states, organizations also must report any harm to a patient to the appropriate practice board(s) for investigation of potential violation of a practice act(s). Managers must be certain that documentation is thorough, accurate, and held as confidential during these investigative and legal processes.

Receiving subpoenas to provide legal testimony and records can be disruptive to an organization's operations and personally distressing to employees. When an employee with a good performance history is involved in a negative incident, managers may need to be supportive to avoid the devastating effect on the employee. On the other hand, managers have other challenges if there is a history of questionable performance that has now resulted in harm to a patient. Documentation of employee performance becomes critical, and documentation of patient care is equally essential to provide accurate information during malpractice suits.

Lawsuits are expensive and disruptive processes for the people directly involved and the organization as a whole. Managers must attend to the seriousness of these lawsuits while maintaining the smooth operations of the organization. These situations may evolve into adversarial situations as employers and employees each retain their own attorneys to represent them in lawsuits. Managers must continue to uphold their duties to employees and patients in these difficult situations. See Activity 12.1 for more information on practice expectations.

ACTIVITY 12.1
PRACTICE ACTS

Harry Henderson is the manager of rehabilitation services, which include physical therapists, occupational therapists, speech language pathologists, respiratory therapists, massage therapists, and athletic trainers. He feels he must have a handle on the practice acts and administrative rules that govern all of these people. In groups, create a chart comparing the practice acts of these health-care providers (add others of interest) in a state of your choice. Focus on their legal responsibilities for patient care.

Other Managerial Legal Issues

Managers require expert legal advice for many of the complex decisions that they face. In many health-care organizations, in-house legal counsel and risk managers provide advice to managers as issues arise. Independent practitioners also need access to legal counsel for many decisions. This section only serves to highlight some of the legal concerns that most often impact mid-level managers.

Employment Laws

Thousands of federal and state statutes, their accompanying administrative laws, and judicial decisions have been passed or ruled upon to protect employees and their relationships with employers. These include:

✦ *Employment Discrimination Laws.* These laws prevent employers from bias in their decisions about hiring, promotions, assignments, termination, and compensation of employees because of race, sex, religion, national origin, physical disability, age, and in some states, sexual orientation. Forms of harassment also are included in this category.

✦ *Collective Bargaining Laws.* Control the negotiations between an employer and a group of employees to determine the conditions of employment.

✦ *Employment Benefits Laws.* The Employee Retirement Income Security Act (ERISA) is a complicated set of regulations that protects the funds in direct benefit retirement plans.

✦ *Unemployment Insurance* is a federal program that provides cash benefits for eligible unemployed workers.

✦ *Workers' Compensation* is another complex set of state administrative laws that provides monetary benefits and rehabilitation services for employees who are injured or disabled because of their work; or death benefits to dependents of people who die on the job.

✦ *Workplace Safety and Health Laws.* Closely associated with workers' compensation, this set of laws serves to prevent personal injuries and illnesses from occurring on the job. See Sidebar 12.1 for more information on these topics.

Sidebar 12.1

The Department of Labor

In addition to the Web pages of a state's government, go to the following Web pages of the U.S. Department of Labor for more information on employment related laws:

Occupational safety and health at http://osha.gov/

Workers' compensation at http://www.dol.gov/dol/topic/workcomp/

ERISA at http://www.dol.gov/dol/topic/health-plans/erisa.htm

Unemployment compensation at http://www.dol.gov/dol/topic/unemployment-insurance/

Background Checks and Other Credentials

Managers also must attend to the verification of credentials and criminal background checks of potential employees. These responsibilities are directly connected to the protection of the public, and serve to protect patients from caregivers with potential harmful behaviors that place them at risk. For instance, the practice acts governing professions may include measures to be taken when alcohol or drug abuse, mental or physical impairment, felony convictions, failure to meet continuing education requirements, or providing false information to a state occur. Managers are responsible for identifying these unacceptable behaviors, beginning with the application for employment so that they take all appropriate action to protect patients.

Managers in large organizations rely on human resource experts to deal with many of these responsibilities, smaller practices may be legally exempt from some of these legal requirements, but everyone has a duty to protect the public and to treat employees fairly.

Patient Consent

Managers must ensure that therapists seek, receive, and document that patients consent to the care they are about to receive. Managers may need to determine whether a patient simply signing a form during the intake process meets the intent of the legal expectations for consent in their jurisdictions.

Patient Confidentiality

Confidentiality is the right to have personal, identifiable medical information kept private. The importance of confidentiality in health became law in the Health Insurance Portability and Accountability Act (HIPAA) of 1996 that was established to insure the privacy of medical records as information within them is shared among health-care providers and third-party payers. Managers must assure that health-care providers do not disclose the personal and medical information that they hold without a patient's permission.

Creating an environment that discourages casual discussions about patients may be difficult, particularly in small organizations in which patient/therapist relationships are often long-term, and the practices pride themselves on providing a family atmosphere. It is essential that patients trust their caregivers so that a warm and accepting relationship may develop. However, even if unintentional, if confidentiality is breached in any way, patients may have the right to sue if harm is a result of even inadvertent disclosures. See Activity 12.2.

ACTIVITY 12.2
MUM'S THE WORD

Ramon Latoya owns a small independent practice in a rural community. He overhears two patients in the waiting room discussing a third patient who is not there. He is concerned because they are saying that more than one member of his staff has provided them the personal information on the person they are discussing. What should he do?

Patients' Bill of Rights

Health-care organizations develop or adopt statements that reflect their duty to provide patients with information, offer fair treatment, and encourage autonomy over medical decisions that affect them. Many health-care insurers also have adopted a bill of rights for patients enrolled in their insurance plans, which address similar patients' rights and choices in their health care, input on decisions about their care, and access to emergency services. Legislative efforts

to make a patients' bill of rights a federal law continue at this time.

Duties of Organizations

Managers also must attend to laws that apply to the organization as well as persons. Health-care organizations must comply with many federal, state, and county laws that affect a wide range of their responsibilities for safety, payments of taxes, etc. Wrongful actions by health-care organizations may be prosecuted under any or all jurisdictions just like the actions of individuals.

Under the legal theory of *respondeat superior* ("let the master answer"), employers are held legally responsible for the actions of employees during the course of their employment. Patients may take legal action directly against the health professionals who harmed them, and against the health-care organizations that employ the health professionals. This concept reflects vicarious liability in which one party can be liable for the actions of another.

The actions of the employer, conversely, may negatively impact the duties of employees. An employer's failure to provide a safe and secure environment may lead to adverse effects on employees and patients. Professionals who must comply with the rules governing their professions may be in conflict with the financial duties that organizations have in regard to stockholders. Failure to meet an organization's licensing requirements also may affect negatively the safety and health of employees.

Organizations also are responsible for establishing systems to assure patient rights, confidentiality, and the elimination of fraud and abuse. Failure to do so compromises professionals who are required to meet these professional duties. Mid-level managers find themselves at the crosshairs of these decisions in health-care organizations. See Activity 12.3.

Managerial Ethics

Some health-care managers may be former clinical health-care professionals. Their understanding of ethical responsibilities may easily transfer to their new managerial roles. Other managers may adopt codes of ethics developed through professional associations for managers. In either case, expectations

ACTIVITY 12.3
AN UNFORTUNATE SITUATION

Erma Nguyen has heard the rumbling of discontentment among her staff. They are trying to understand how profits of their health-care system have increased 23% in the last year (as reported in the local newspaper) and their salaries remain frozen. What should Erma say or do?

of employees are that managers meet their obligations to patients and other stakeholders as moral advocates and role models for the values necessary for the delivery of quality health care.

Managerial decisions may have more far-reaching implications than individual clinical decisions. For instance, managers have broader responsibilities for enhancing the overall quality of life in a community, the dignity and well-being of patients, and for creating an equitable, accessible, effective, and efficient health-care system. A careful ethical assessment of the impact of their decisions is important to safeguard the rights of patients and employees and the interests of the organization as a whole.

Conflicts of Interest

Managers may need to be particularly sensitive to potential conflicts of interest. Conflict of interest is a matter of degree and often difficult to identify. Because there may be legal implications, managers must be careful to avoid the benefits that result from using their positions of authority to gather information, to use information to adversely affect an organization, or to accept gifts in exchange for influence. Failure to inform their organizations of involvement in, or affiliations with, other organizations that may impact their decisions may raise legal and ethical issues. See Activity 12.4 for more consideration to managerial ethics.

ACTIVITY 12.4
CODE OF ETHICS

Refer to the *Code of Ethics* and *APTA Guide for Professional Conduct* of the American Physical Therapy Association. In a group discussion, determine what parts apply to physical therapists in management positions?

A Manager's Responsibility

In addition to their ethical duties, managers must be alert to the potential legal implications of their actions, the actions of employees, and the actions of their organizations to protect patients. They need to seek legal advice rather than make assumptions that may result in more complex situations than necessary. Although, it may be tiresome and unwise to be on the defensive, it is important for managers to be alert and seek advice as they learn to discriminate red-flag situations that may arise with employees, patients, or managers at higher levels of organizations. Activities 12.5 and 12.6 present the opportunities to address several legal issues.

ACTIVITY 12.5
A DIFFICULT CASE

Carla Morsetti feels that her situation has gotten out of control. Several weeks ago, a patient at Snowy Valley Nursing and Rehabilitation Center was injured while in the physical therapy department. Although she, her staff, and the administration took all appropriate action, the patient died and the family is suing for damages. They contend that the accident in therapy contributed to her death. The staff involved in the incident is not handling the patient's death well, and Carla is becoming increasingly concerned as the person in the middle of this situation.

It seems that the patient's death is all that everyone in the nursing home talks about and she cannot seem to get anything else done. The staff is divided among those who are defending the actions of the therapists and assistant involved in the incident while others are demanding that Carla fire them. The attorney for the nursing home has advised her to avoid talking about the situation, and she has been advised that subpoenas from attorneys for the therapists to appear at deposition hearings have been received by the nursing home administrator. Sorting out the facts of the incident at the time from all of the conversations and rumors circulating since then have distressed her. She is considering submitting her resignation. What legal and ethical issues confront Carla? What should she do?

ACTIVITY 12.6
PATIENT CONSENT

Referring to pp. 61–62 and the following worksheet, take a strategic approach to address the concern that patient consent for physical therapy interventions is not consistently received and documented.

WHAT IS	WHAT SHOULD BE

GAP DATA

QUESTIONS:

ANSWERS:

Therefore
DECIDE TO ADDRESS THIS NEED

PROBLEM (CHALLENGE) STATEMENT

STRATEGIC PLAN
Developed through responsibility for:

Vision, Mission, Goals:
Policies and Procedures:
Marketing:
Staffing:
Patient Care:
Fiscal:
Legal and Ethical:
Risk Management:
Communication:

Chapter 13

Communication Responsibilities

Learning Objectives

+ Review the components of the classic communication model.
+ Determine the most common oral and written communication channels used by managers.
+ Apply strategies for formal and informal meetings.
+ Apply effective strategies for job interview sessions.
+ Discuss telephone communication.
+ Prepare for a business meeting.
+ Prepare for a presentation to a group.
+ Prepare a memorandum, letter, e-mail, and announcement.
+ Prepare a report and a proposal outline.
+ Analyze the content of a Web page for rehabilitation services.
+ Distinguish general literacy from health literacy.
+ Analyze common communication hurdles in health-care organizations.
+ Identify strategies for overcoming gaps in effective communication.

Overview

Because strong communication skills underlie all responsibilities of managers, aspects of communication have been addressed in several parts of this text (Chapter 1 for organization communication, Chapter 2 for intercultural communication, Chapter 7 for marketing communications; see also the communication subtitles in the chapters in Section 3). Communication is a broad and complex topic that is viewed from a wide range of perspectives. Scholars in fields from sociology and psychology to digital technology, art, media, and literature use different lenses to study the transfer of information from a sender to a receiver.

This chapter focuses on a small component of this broad topic by addressing par-ticular oral and written communication skills important to managers as they encode messages and select channels for communication (see Fig. 13.1 for the model and definitions). Many forms of communication also have visual components (the use of slides, graphics, pictures, figures, and the layout of print communication) that require managers to develop those skills.

Effective, understandable communication, formal and informal, is crucial to the life of an organization. Mid-level managers, who find themselves at the crossroads of organizational communication channels, contribute to the success of those health-care

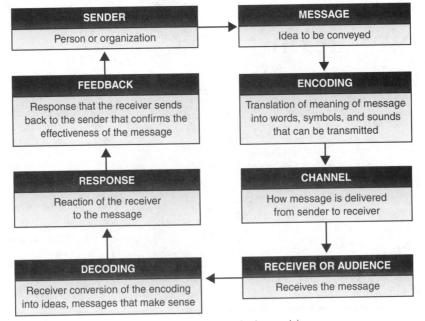

Figure 13.1 ✦ A communication model.

organizations through effective communications. Because communication, at its best, is imperfect, its effectiveness begins with the ability to minimize misunderstandings when encoding messages and the ability to select the most effective channel for the message. Managers also must be able to balance limiting information so they do not overwhelm the receivers of the communication messages while encouraging an open, trusting environment for sharing information. Table 13.1 categorizes communication channels commonly used by managers. They are addressed in the following sections to provide some practical information on common communication responsibilities of managers that are not addressed in other sections of this text.

TABLE 13.1   Classification of communication methods

COMMUNICATION	INDIVIDUAL	GROUP
ORAL	One-on-one formal meetings Informal conversations Interviews Telephone conversations	Presentations to groups Formal meetings Teleconferences
WRITTEN	Letters E-mails Memos	List-serve e-mails Web pages Memos Posted announcements Manuals Reports

Oral Communications

Individual Meetings

Formal oral communication most often takes the form of scheduled one-on-one meetings with an employee in which the message and encoding may be fairly standardized when work performance is good. These meetings may be called when:

- ✦ Regularly scheduled, formal performance reviews must be conducted.

- ✦ Opportunities arise to reinforce and reward employees who are on track with their professional and personal goals that are aligned with the organization's goals.

- ✦ Work performance demands immediate attention because the goals of the organization are not being met.

- ✦ Work performance demands immediate attention because it places the worker or others at risk for injury or other negative consequences.

All of these meetings are documented for the person's employment record. Meetings addressing jobs well done where performance expectations are met, or exceeded, may be one of the highlights of a manager's responsibilities. Meetings held because of concerns about performance may demand more careful planning of the message and its encoding. Standardized guidelines for these discussions and their documentation are important in all organizations, regardless of their size, to reduce the risks of these interactions leading to legal action should employees and managers disagree about the message sent or received.

Managers must prepare in advance for these meetings and establish an environment that reflects their importance. The more that managers limit the discussions in these meetings to performance behaviors related to job descriptions, the more likely the result will be an improvement in work performance and agreement on the issues at hand. Clarifying that it is the behavior and not the characteristics or personality of the person that is the issue helps when the discussion must address a situation in which an employee who is able to perform certain duties, does not.

This performance issue needs to be separated from that in which the person does not know how to perform. These formal meetings typically shift to discussions of clinical expertise or professional socialization issues. They often involve the need for counseling or teaching. In these situations, managers need to be able to identify employee needs that are beyond their skill and expertise and refer employees to others who may be able to help improve performance through professional counseling or other interventions. These difficult meetings are successful if both the manager and the employee feel that they have learned something and can move on without anger. See Activity 13.1.

Job Interview Sessions

Interviews are another form of formal communication that requires advanced planning and development of skills to accomplish hiring goals. Although the messages conveyed are typically consistent from one interview to another, managers may encode them differently from one job applicant to another. A generally accepted rule of thumb is that the person being interviewed should be talking 80%

of the time during an interview session. This requires managers to develop good questioning and listening skills. Asking structured, open-ended questions encourages candidates to talk about their values, preferences, and priorities so that managers can determine if they are a good match with the organization. Some examples of questions to facilitate the other person talking are:

+ Tell me about . . .
+ How important is . . .
+ What do you think the problem is with . . .
+ What will ____ do for you?
+ What prevents you from ____?
+ What would you change about ____?
+ What have you learned about ____?
+ What are your views on ____?
+ Give me your impressions of ____.
+ Please expand on ____.
+ What is involved in ____?
+ What achievements are you proudest of?
+ What is your assessment (opinion) of?

Filling in the blanks above requires interviewers to study applicant resumes and references in advance. They must listen to know which question should follow, and provide the opportunity for candidates to ask questions about the organization at the end of the interview. See Activity 13.2.

Informal Conversations

Informal conversations provide managers with the opportunity to take the pulse of the organization and its employees. They are the means for becoming better acquainted with coworkers and may provide the opportunity to reward performance, meet employee needs, or resolve performance or organizational problems before they need to be addressed formally. These are unscheduled, spontaneous interactions that may become more structured and formalized as the need for more complex problem solving or conflict resolution arises.

Managers may be surprised at how often they become the informal referee in personal conflicts among employees. Disagreements may arise over anything: time-off requests, lunchroom use, parking spaces, tardiness, phone use, patient assignments, etc. Managers need to decide when to intervene

ACTIVITY 13.1
DREADING IT

This is the part of the job as rehabilitation manager than Rafael Ramos hates the most. Judy Waters is an excellent physical therapist with outstanding ratings on her performance evaluations, but she is late again. Although she now calls in when she will be late, her persistent tardiness has upset the rest of the staff who now leave her patients waiting rather than covering Judy's load until she arrives. Rafael is meeting with Judy for the third time to address her tardiness. He is forced to advise her that this is her last chance. The next time she arrives late for work will be her last. He will fire her. Role-play their meeting with consideration for the communication model in Figure 13.1. Refer to pp. 61–62 and use the worksheet to develop a strategic plan for this meeting.

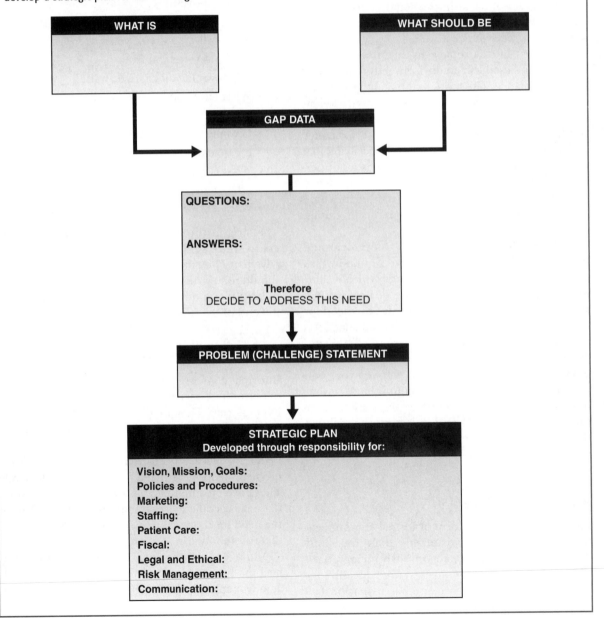

WHAT IS

WHAT SHOULD BE

GAP DATA

QUESTIONS:

ANSWERS:

Therefore
DECIDE TO ADDRESS THIS NEED

PROBLEM (CHALLENGE) STATEMENT

STRATEGIC PLAN
Developed through responsibility for:

Vision, Mission, Goals:
Policies and Procedures:
Marketing:
Staffing:
Patient Care:
Fiscal:
Legal and Ethical:
Risk Management:
Communication:

ACTIVITY 13.2
THE JOB INTERVIEW

Jennie Bakerfield is nervous. She is about to conduct her first job interview ever. The applicant is interviewing for a physical therapist position that was created to meet the needs of Jennie's expanding practice. This is the first and only applicant for the position since it was posted 3 months ago. Jennie feels a lot is riding on this interview. Role-play her interview with Theresa Biscardo. How might Jennie use Figure 13.1 to help her prepare? How might Jennie use strategic planning? See pp. 61–62.

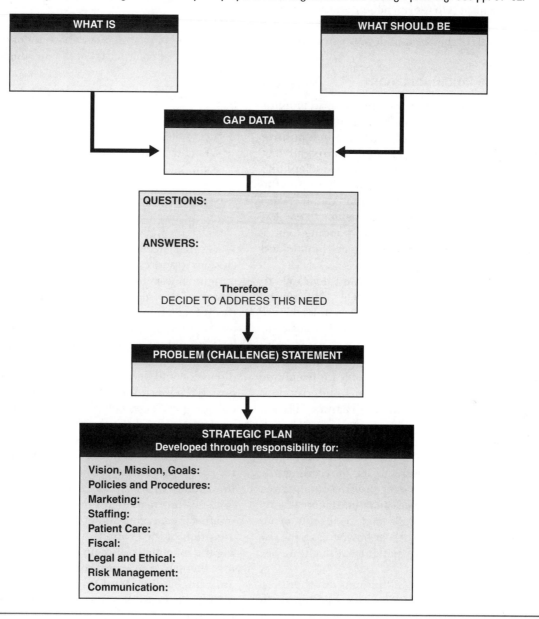

WHAT IS

WHAT SHOULD BE

GAP DATA

QUESTIONS:

ANSWERS:

Therefore
DECIDE TO ADDRESS THIS NEED

PROBLEM (CHALLENGE) STATEMENT

STRATEGIC PLAN
Developed through responsibility for:

Vision, Mission, Goals:
Policies and Procedures:
Marketing:
Staffing:
Patient Care:
Fiscal:
Legal and Ethical:
Risk Management:
Communication:

(typically when behaviors disrupt operations), when to let people iron things out for themselves, and when to accept the fact that people just may not get along but are still able to perform their work. Sometimes employees are simply not a good match with coworkers although they are a good match with the organization. Resolving these interpersonal issues requires managers to remain neutral and stay focused on the impact of these behaviors on performance and the goals of the organization. See Activity 13.3.

Telephone Communications

It is not unusual for large organizations to monitor telephone communications because of their importance in presenting the organization in a positive way. Even the smallest organization may require that employees receive training in effective telephone communications because a phone call is often the first impression of an organization. Managers are responsible for establishing guidelines for all employees when answering the phone, responding to messages received, and documenting calls made and received.

Managers have several important decisions to make about encoding and channels for telephone communications for business. For example, the use of a menu of connections or automatic transfer to a message box often replaces a receptionist, who is responsible for answering and directing phone calls. With a point person responsible for telephone duties, staff and managers avoid many interruptions in patient care and other duties to answer calls and take messages.

Managers must weigh the costs associated with this position against the risks of communication failures. Messages that were not left or receiving confused messages as callers struggle with computerized menus and transfers places an organization at a disadvantage. Returning calls later avoids numerous disruptions during the workday but increases the risk of negatively affecting patient satisfaction. See Activity 13.4.

The use of personal cell phones or other electronic devices during patient care (by both patients and staff) is disruptive and impolite, even if they are used to answer business calls. Managers may be required to establish and enforce policies and procedures limiting their personal use. Patients expect the undivided attention of their caregivers.

Establishing professional relationships with patients may be compromised if they overhear personal phone conversations caregivers are having with family or friends. Having phone conversations about other patients during treatment sessions places patient confidentiality at risk.

Conducting Business Meetings

A basic rule of meetings is to have them only when necessary. The chairperson of the meeting is responsible for:

+ Establishing and announcing the agenda.
+ Following the agenda during the meeting.
+ Focusing discussion on the goals to be achieved.
+ Encouraging everyone's participation.
+ Summarizing decisions and actions taken.
+ Assuring that agreement was reached.
+ Assigning a recorder to take minutes and a timekeeper.

Business meetings bring people together for discussions to address resolution of problems or to work on mutual tasks or projects that require face-to-face meetings on a regular basis. Preparing people with the information they need to review before the meeting reduces the time necessary to present the background information so that more of the available, valuable time of the participants is spent on discussion and decisions. A clear agenda and a purpose is a powerful start for any meeting. Effectively encoding messages before and during a meeting to encourage participation is equally important for effective, comprehensive decision making.

Managers also should provide the opportunity for participants to suggest additions or revisions to the agenda in advance of the meeting. Providing time for informal discussion and socializing before or after the meeting allows managers to call for the attention of the group to address the agenda during the meeting. Follow-up reports on action items may be relayed to staff through memos, e-mails, or announcements. Minutes should be distributed as soon as possible after a meeting to everyone who attended with a deadline for feedback and correction. Typically, the first item on any meeting agenda is approval of the minutes of the last meeting so that accuracy can be documented. See Sidebar 13.1.

ACTIVITY 13.3
THE REFEREE

Rosie and Doris just cannot seem to get along. Coworkers and patients notice their constant bickering, which is disruptive to patient care. Jim Watson, the rehabilitation manager, has tried informally dropping hints that they need to change their behavior because of the effect that it has on others. They simply cannot stand each other and their negative interactions have escalated. Role-play informal conversations between Jim and Rosie and between Jim and Doris. Should Jim meet with them together? Role-play that possible meeting with both of them. How might Jim use the communication model in Figure 13.1 to prepare for this meeting? What component of the communication model is the issue for Rosie and Doris? Use pp. 61–62 and this worksheet to prepare for formal meetings with Rosie and with Doris.

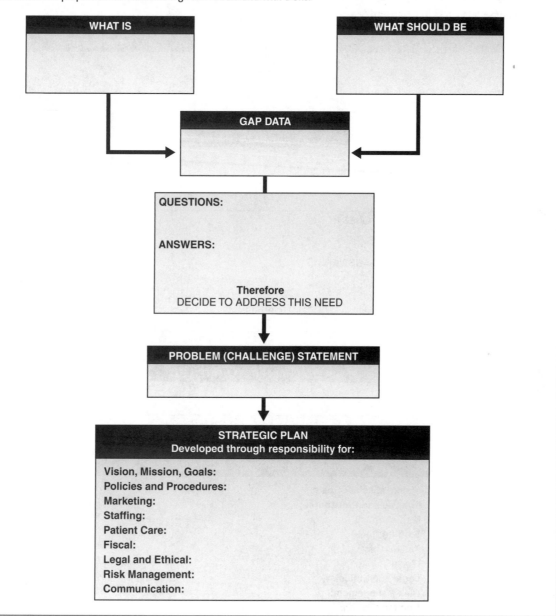

ACTIVITY 13.4
A TELEPHONE PROBLEM

Carterville Physical Therapy receives 25% of its referrals from Dr. Costello. He has just called Barbara Benton the owner of the practice on her cell phone. He tells her that he had no choice because he cannot get through in her office phone system to talk to her or the other staff about patients and referrals. He is very frustrated and does not even bother to leave messages. He admits referring patients to another practice just because it is easier. Her staff requested she put in this new system because they were so frequently taken away from patients to answer the phone. What should Barbara do? Where in the Communication Model found in Figure 13.1 does the problem lie? Role-play a staff meeting with Barbara and her staff to address this issue with consideration for the communication model in Figure 13.1. How should Barbara use this strategic planning worksheet to address this problem? See pp. 61–62.

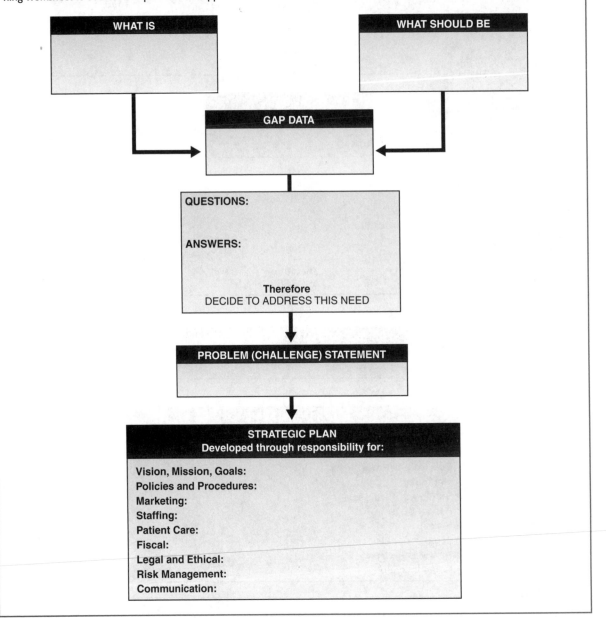

Sidebar 13.1

Meeting Agendas and Minutes

Agendas should:

✦ Be distributed far enough in advance for participants to be able to prepare for the meeting.

✦ Include items for discussion and action, goals to be achieved, time limits, and materials that participants should have with them.

Meeting minutes should:

✦ List attendees

✦ Include date and the time span of the meeting

✦ Focus on action taken and assignments made

✦ Record new items for future discussion

Note: Templates for meeting agendas are widely available in word-processing programs and other sources that are good models for managers new to conducting meetings. A template also can serve as the outline for minutes of the meeting.

Several actions of managers, on the other hand, can limit the effectiveness of meetings. These include:

✦ Holding regularly scheduled meetings for the sake of meeting. This action can be a source of aggravation for staff. It may be wise to block out time on the calendar for meetings to be held so that staff do not schedule patients or other activities during those times. When the meeting time is not needed, these blocks of time can be used for completion of nonpatient care assignments or used for informal socializing or discussions related to clinical decision making.

✦ Taking too much of the meeting time for announcements or reports that people might receive through other channels on their own time (e-mails, memos, bulletin-board posts, etc.)

✦ Requiring attendance of people who become observers because they are not involved in decisions to be discussed.

✦ Giving short notice to attend a meeting that results in a disruption or failure to complete their assigned duties.

See Activity 13.5.

Group Presentations

Managers often are involved in formal presentations that serve to introduce a group to new information or to provide training and education. These presentations require the same attention to the message, encoding, and channels of communication, often enhanced with the use of visual materials. The basic rules of presentations are:

✦ Determine the needs of the audience and the goal(s) of the presentation.

✦ Prepare an outline or guide for the presentation.

✦ Plan what you are going to say, but do not memorize it.

✦ Twenty to 25 minutes is the limit for holding the audience's attention.

✦ Have a beginning (present what you are going to say), a middle (say what you have to say), and an end (tell the audience what you said).

✦ A picture is worth 1,000 words (use slides or handouts). Use them to reinforce, not substitute for, the message.

✦ Use visual material to make a point, rather than to provide as much information as possible.

✦ Visuals should be simple and consistent. Avoid cluttering with a variety of fonts, colors, or other distracters.

✦ Be clear, confident, and friendly to engage the audience.

✦ Get up, say what you have to say, sit down.

Teleconferences

Communication technology has enabled multisite, long-distance virtual meetings and presentations. The same principles of communication apply in the virtual world with additional considerations for effective positioning and use of cameras, microphones, and recording devices. See Activity 13.6.

Written Communication

Memoranda and Letters

Templates in word processing and other software programs are available to format memos for consistency

ACTIVITY 13.5
MEETINGS

Despite his best efforts, Jim Muncie, cannot control staff meetings. First, getting everyone together to start on time every week seems to be impossible. Second, the side conversations, eating during the meeting, and lack of attention is very disconcerting. He does not feel he can get anything done. What should he do? Where in the communication model in Figure 13.1 does the problem lie? Role-play the next meeting in which Jim applies the communication model in Figure 13.1 and hints for conducting meetings in the text.

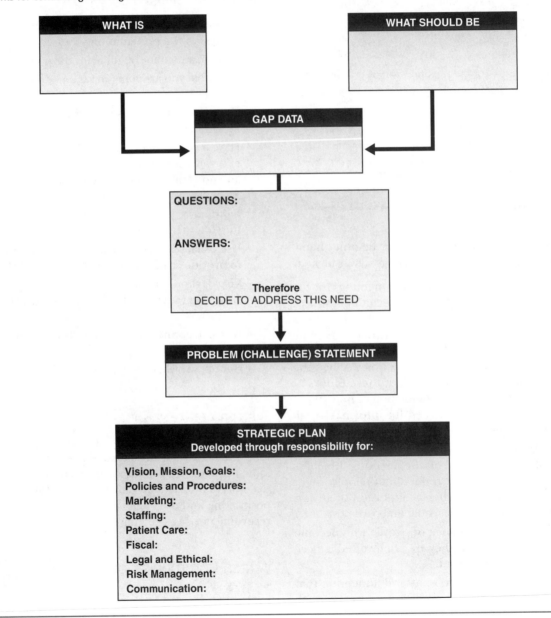

WHAT IS

WHAT SHOULD BE

GAP DATA

QUESTIONS:

ANSWERS:

Therefore
DECIDE TO ADDRESS THIS NEED

PROBLEM (CHALLENGE) STATEMENT

STRATEGIC PLAN
Developed through responsibility for:

Vision, Mission, Goals:
Policies and Procedures:
Marketing:
Staffing:
Patient Care:
Fiscal:
Legal and Ethical:
Risk Management:
Communication:

in appearance. Memoranda (memos) are different from letters, which are more formal and used for external communication of more sensitive and important messages. Memos are used internally to relay messages that are short and direct. Memo formats include lines for Date:, To:, From:, and Subject:, which are followed by the body. The first line should begin with the point of the memo. The rest of the memo should be concise and clear and directed to this statement of the point. If there are attachments, they should be mentioned in the memo. There is usually a heading, MEMORANDUM, which includes the organization's logo or other information. Managers should use memos when they want to inform or recommend something in a concise way that is important but not critical.

Business letters are formal with inside addresses, salutations, and closings. They suggest an important message that demands the attention of the recipient. Because they may typically become part of the organization's records, they should reflect the sophistication and writing ability of the sender. They must be proofread for accuracy of content and adherence to letter writing rules, grammar, and correct spelling. They should be taken seriously and reviewed carefully because they often reflect an important issue that requires documentation of a communication between two parties. Templates in word-processing programs are helpful for new letter writers. Managers may generate letters for a variety of reasons to employees and other stakeholders—a follow-up to an important meeting or an offer of employment are examples. Determining the goal of the letter and rereading to be sure the goal has been met is important in this channel of communication. See Activity 13.7.

E-mails

Electronic communication in business is only meaningful if it is read, and easily separated from the uninvited and unrelated e-mails that appear in an organization. It is helpful for e-mails to have titles (subject lines) that easily enable readers to distinguish business from nonbusiness e-mails. Like memos, e-mails should begin with point of the message and then state the case to support the point.

Managers may be responsible for developing and implementing policies and procedures for e-mails to control what may be an overwhelming interference rather than a powerful communication tool in organizations. Particularly if e-mails are disrupting patient care, managers may find timing the delivery of e-mails so that they are available to be read before lunch and the end of the day decreases a need for staff to engage in ongoing checking for messages during the day.

All managers and staff should be encouraged to be selective about the use of e-mail for communication by asking why the e-mail is necessary, and if it is the best means of communication for the message. They are valuable for distributing announcements and other important information quickly to large groups of people. However, the use of list serves that reach many people at once may not be the most appropriate means for delivering complex or controversial information. Managers should develop a filing system for easy storage and retrieval (electronic or hard copy) of e-mail messages received and sent for documentation of communication to individuals and groups.

Posted Announcements

Managers need to determine when the posting of hard-copy announcements complement or serve to replace e-mail communications. Strategic placement of bulletin boards in public areas for display of information or action to be taken by a group can be an efficient and powerful means of communication of official, general, nonsensitive information. Large organizations typically have policies and procedures for approval of content and appearance of announcements and time limits for their posting. This action keeps boards free from the clutter of outdated or irrelevant announcements. Legal requirements guide the public display of other mandatory information. These required postings may appear in a separate designated space to meet legal requirements. Displaying professional licenses of staff is an example of such a requirement in some jurisdictions.

Managers must attend to the professional appearance of posted announcements because they reflect the organization's culture. Selecting a consistent color and format helps employees recognize announcements that require action. Providing a bulletin board out of the public eye for employees to post informal announcements and information helps managers control the content of official public announcement space. See Activity 13.8.

Reports

Managers are frequently responsible for generating reports on a variety of topics, typically related to fiscal issues. Managers may generate some reports routinely while other reports are prepared in response to a particular request for information. Information is the key word. Reports are about data and their interpretation. The content of report should not be subject to further interpretation.

Preparation of a report begins with determining its purpose and scope, and to whom and how it will be distributed. The next step is identification of the data to be included, and their presentation. If the report includes graphs and charts, managers will need to determine their format. The text of the report should be arranged with bullets and other formatting to improve the chances that the facts presented are not misinterpreted or muddled. Reports prepared on an ongoing basis may follow standardized formats to ease communication. Managers should be ruthless in their preparation of reports so that only information that is needed is included.

Manuals

Chapter 6 includes information on the development of a policies and procedures manual, typically the manual of interest to managers.

Proposals

Proposals include some basic components that are directed to explaining why a program or some other solution is needed, what acceptance of the proposal contributes to the organization, and a plan of action. Managers may take the initiative to develop and submit a proposal, or they may be directed to prepare one following specific guidelines. See Chapter 14 for the development of a special type of proposal—the feasibility study. Depending on the objective of the proposal, a typical proposal outline may include the following components:

- ✦ Title
- ✦ Project Overview
- ✦ Background Information/ Statement of the Problem
- ✦ Project Detail
  - ✦ Goals and Objectives
  - ✦ Clientele
  - ✦ Methods
  - ✦ Staff/Administration
- ✦ Available Resources
- ✦ Needed Resources
  - ✦ Personnel
  - ✦ Facilities
  - ✦ Equipment/Supplies/Communication
  - ✦ Budget
- ✦ Evaluation Plan
- ✦ Importance to the Organization
- ✦ Appendices

Managers need to ascertain the deadlines for submission of proposals and when action is to be taken. An oral presentation also may be required. If so, managers need to realize the goal of the presentation is acceptance or approval of the proposal, which places a selling slant on the presentation. See Activity 13.9.

Web Pages and Other Publications

Depending on the type and size of the organization, managers may have a great deal of responsibility for developing and distributing outgoing marketing materials. At the least, they are responsible for communicating their needs to others with skills in this area. Managers also may use these channels of

ACTIVITY 13.8
E-MAIL AND ANNOUNCEMENTS

Bill Spearman announces the staff work schedule for the next week every Friday by noon. He announces the last week's staff productivity and other patient census information every Monday by noon. Should he use e-mail or posting on a bulletin board for these announcements? Use the communication model in Figure 13.1 in your decision making. Refer to pp. 61–62 and use this worksheet to develop a strategic plan for these communications.

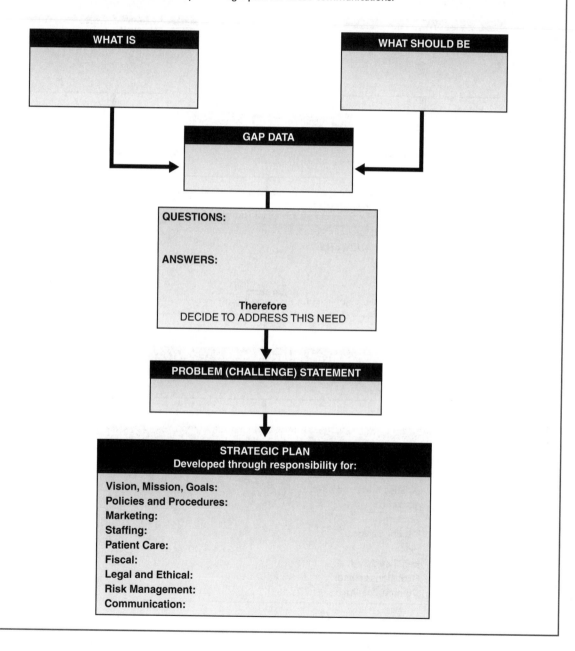

ACTIVITY 13.9
PREPARING A REPORT

Pasha Williams has been asked to prepare a single-page report on physical therapy services each quarter to be included in materials presented to the Board of Directors at their quarterly meetings. What should the report include? What should be the format of the report? Consider the communication model in Figure 13.1 in preparing the outline and format of the report. Refer to pp. 61–62 and this worksheet to develop a strategic plan for this reporting responsibility.

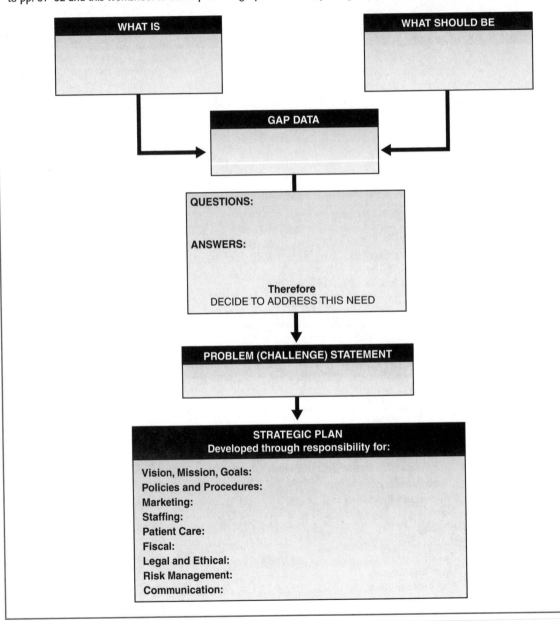

WHAT IS

WHAT SHOULD BE

GAP DATA

QUESTIONS:

ANSWERS:

Therefore
DECIDE TO ADDRESS THIS NEED

PROBLEM (CHALLENGE) STATEMENT

STRATEGIC PLAN
Developed through responsibility for:

Vision, Mission, Goals:
Policies and Procedures:
Marketing:
Staffing:
Patient Care:
Fiscal:
Legal and Ethical:
Risk Management:
Communication:

Sidebar 13.2

Health Literacy

For more information on health literacy go to http://www.iom.edu/?id=19750 and to http://www.hrsa.gov/healthliteracy/ Find a web page with the formula for determining the reading level of materals.

communication for internal purposes, such as staff and patient education. See Activity 13.10.

The same levels of managerial involvement hold true for the development of surveys. Online survey programs, many with standardized questions, make the development and analysis of surveys less difficult than beginning from scratch. Managers may find these tools to be important for gathering data from any stakeholders, even if the online survey is transferred to hard copy for analysis.

Communication and Health Literacy

Managers may be responsible for decisions related to the coding and channels for communicating patient educational information as well. For instance, conducting a cost-benefit analysis of packaged computer programs for exercise instructions is a common responsibility. Reviewing the literacy level of materials purchased or developed to assure their value to the target patient populations may be another important responsibility.

In addition to these basic literacy issues (the ability to read, write, and speak in English), health-care managers must attend to the issue of health literacy. Health literacy is the ability to read and comprehend essential health-related materials (i.e., prescription bottles, appointment slips, discharge instructions) to function successfully as a patient, and to use information to promote and maintain good health.

Health literacy[1] is context specific and can be a major barrier in communication with patients that managers must overcome. People often have difficulty determining what information is important to share and may be incorrectly diagnosed because of providers drawing conclusions without information. Many people do not understand the underlying biology of their symptoms and have unreasonable

expectations about improvement in their conditions as a result, or they may not comply with treatments because they do not have the knowledge to understand their importance.

Because of these issues, managers must determine if communication improves access to and the understanding of the messages that must be conveyed to patients to improve their health and their health care. Because so much information is available to people who are health literate, managers may direct their efforts to those who are not instead. For instance, the reading level of printed materials deserves attention. Using visuals and providing only essential information also may help. Patients are often already intimidated or feeling anxious about their condition which limits their ability to ask and respond to questions. Managers need to make staff aware of signs that may suggest that a patient has difficulty with basic literacy such as: [1]

✦ Taking a long time to sign forms

✦ Relying on others to complete paperwork for them

✦ Asking to take paperwork with them to complete later

✦ Saying their eyes are bad when given something to read

✦ Paying more attention to nonverbal cues than verbal messages

Communication Hurdles

Senders and receivers both compete for attention and time to communicate in busy organizations. Oral and written communications are often blocked, dropped, rearranged, and inappropriately filtered as they travel through organizations in all directions through many levels. The use of professional jargon and the shorthand speech of in-groups complicate communications among interdisciplinary team members as well.

Managers may spend much time in addressing distortions in communications initiated and received by others, if they are committed to open sharing of accurate information. On the other hand, some managers may be an additional barrier to communications as they demand the use of formal channels, make themselves unavailable, withhold or limit time for communications, or disregard messages intended for their action.

ACTIVITY 13.10
WEB PAGE IMPROVEMENT

John Evans is the director of rehabilitation and feels that the Web page for rehabilitation on St. Anthony's Health Center website is very weak. He does not think it represents the rehabilitation services very well and he wants it to become the model for good communication for all of St. Anthony's departments. John's boss has given him permission to work with the director of marketing to come up with a proposal for improving the Web page and told him he has to be reasonable. John is meeting with Susan from marketing next week who is responsible for the center's Web pages. Role-play this meeting. Prepare an outline of the proposal that John should submit to his boss about the improvements for the Web page. Consider the communication model in Figure 13.1 and pp. 61–62 and this worksheet in preparing for the meeting and proposal. HINT: Analyze existing Web pages for rehabilitation services to develop ideas.

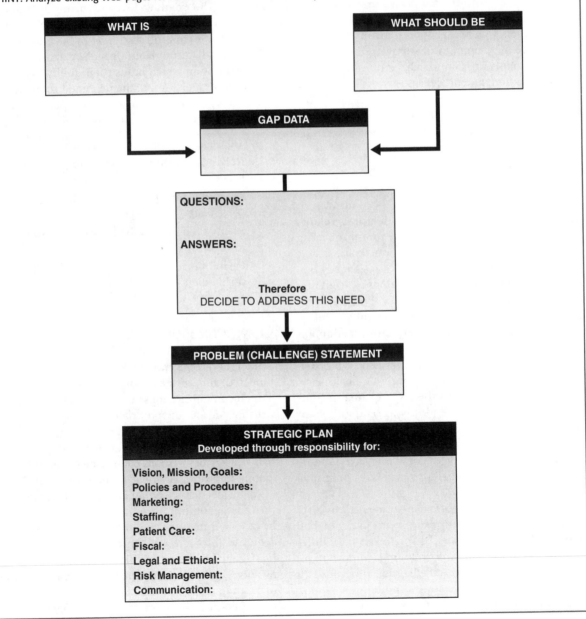

The more individualized the communication, the more likely it will be encoded and decoded effectively, but problems may arise. For instance, when interpersonal relationships are strained or one party provokes negative emotions in the other, it may be difficult to communicate. If people filter messages based on who the sender is, they may not receive it in the first place. Ignoring an important message from a particular sender may result in disastrous consequences for others.

Managers need to assure a work culture that diminishes anger and fear of reprisals and promotes a trust so that people are comfortable disagreeing with managers. Everyone bases their communications on prior experiences that may cover a wide range of socioeconomic circumstances and interactions that make people more likely to be angry, fearful, gullible, shy, jealous, or self-aggrandizing. Managers need to recognize that these behaviors raise barriers to communication.

Other people may simply not understand the message or its frame of reference because they have had no prior experience with the issue at hand. People also bring, intentionally or not, values and prejudices that negatively influence encoding and decoding of messages. Even if all of these factors were equal among communicators, managers must be sensitive to selective listening—hearing what we want to hear rather than the actual message—which seems to be human nature. People tend to filter out the negative and amplify the positive in messages affecting them.

Overcoming Communication Hurdles

Particularly when the message may evoke strong emotions, managers need to review them from the point of view of the receiver(s). Timing and sensitivity may deflect negative reactions so that the message is received. It may be that deferring or leaving a message unsent may be a wise choice when the manager's emotions are high.

The Message

If managers or other message senders are not of the same discipline as the receiver(s), messages should be checked for jargon and abbreviations that may be unfamiliar. Using a common language enhances communication. A good check is to review the message and ask if it contains the fewest number of words and syllables possible.

Employing action words (behaviors) may also result in a clearer message. For example, "great job everyone" may mean different things to different people. Instead, "The team exceeded its goals by 10% this week. Each member of the team will be recognized in the next newsletter. Thank you all for your extraordinary efforts in this important project." is much clearer. Encouraging people to ask for further explanations when necessary promotes communication because the feedback allows senders to improve their future efforts.

Because it is often necessary to send the same message to all members of a team, sending it simultaneously may provide the opportunity for members of a team to seek clarification or confirmation from each other. This interaction may be valuable in saving time because it is likely that more than one person may have the same questions that can be fed back to the sender as one rather than multiple, duplicate messages. Of course, simultaneously sending a poorly prepared message may be problematic, particularly if it arouses anxiety or anger.

The Method

The more important a message is, the more direct it needs to be to a particular person. For example, an e-mail or phone call directly to the person who needs to make an important decision may be more effective than a hard-copy letter that may be handled by one or two other people before arriving in the decision-maker's hands.

Another example is an important or sensitive announcement that is shared with a group of people. The news may be better received and understood by bringing everyone together in person for a meeting rather than sending a simultaneous e-mail to everyone. General information, simple and clear, may be e-mailed or posted in a central location. For example, you may use e-mail for final plans for a holiday party or to announce a simple revision in a policy and procedure related to security. Another message may be so important that managers introduce it in an e-mail, discuss it in a meeting, and follow it up in a memo. Changes in personnel benefits that require action or patient safety efforts are examples of this three-pronged approach.

Listening

Managers not only need to send messages but receive them. Listening is perhaps the most valuable and desirable skill in improving communications. Traditional hints for effective listening include:

- Ask, "What's in the message for me?"
- Do not jump to conclusions
- Fight distractions
- Focus on the message not on the delivery
- Hear tones of voice
- Identify the central idea(s)
- Limit talking to, "I see, uh huh," "go on," etc.
- Make eye contact
- Mentally summarize the message
- Postpone judgment until the message is complete
- Sort facts from opinions
- Take notes to organize not memorize what is heard

Encouraging others to listen can be just as difficult as listening for one's self. Modeling good listening may help. Asking, in a nonthreatening way, the receiver to summarize the message just sent may help them develop listening skills. It also allows managers to regroup and resend messages that were not decoded as expected. See Activity 13.11.

The Grapevine

Informal communication channels and networks evolve from interpersonal relationships and social interaction patterns that occur in all work settings. They occur in parallel with formal communication networks that are established by managers. Although grapevines may lead to difficulties if misused to spread rumors rather than facts, they can be the fastest way to get the word out—much faster than formal channels. For instance, the fact that an organization was just named the best in the country in *U.S. News & World News Report* is exciting news that would spread fast. That staff will be sent home because of a severe weather warning is another example of news that spreads through the grapevine. Even incorrect rumors provide managers with information about communication networks and concerns of employees that are often valuable in decision making. See Activity 13.12.

A Manager's Responsibility

Communication is the fundamental, underlying responsibility of managers that takes a surprising amount of their time. Controlling that time can be challenging. Although, communicating effectively comes more naturally to some managers than others, its importance demands that everyone make efforts to continuing improve both oral and written communication skills. There is no organization without communication. Managers must not only work on their own communication skills, but also guide others in theirs so that the goals of the organization are conveyed and met. See Activity 13.13.

REFERENCE

1. Bernhardt JM. Accessing, understanding, and applying health communication messages: The challenge of health literacy. In: Thompson TL, ed. *Handbook of Health Communication*. Mahwah, NJ: Lawrence Erlbaum Associates; 2003.

ACTIVITY 13.11
I'M LISTENING

Monique LaSalle is the manager of a large rehabilitation staff. She works very hard at communication and is proud that her efforts seem to be effective a great deal of the time. However, Charlie McGill is a thorn in her side. He just does not seem to get it—anything. Whether it is a memo, specific verbal directions, or participating in meetings, it is as if he is in his own world. Monique is beginning to wonder if Charlie has some hearing or cognitive processing problem. She prefers not to think that he just chooses not to listen. When she confronts him or repeats information that he should already have, he always responds with, "I'm listening." What should she do? Where in the communication model in Figure 13.1 does the problem lie? Role-play the next meeting Monique has with Charlie to address this issue with consideration for the communication model. Use this worksheet and refer to pp. 61–62 to prepare for the meeting.

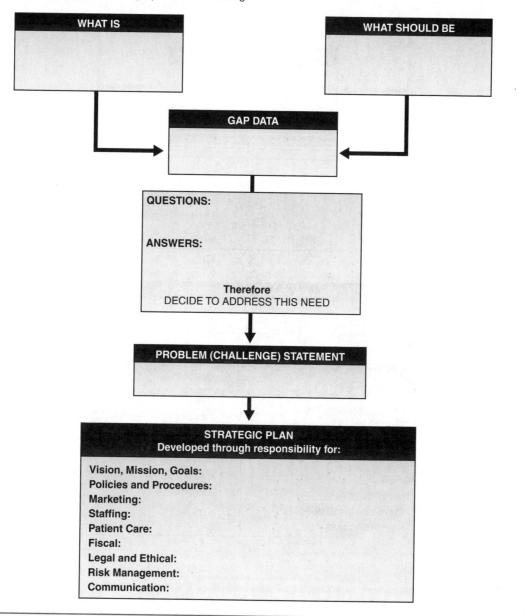

WHAT IS

WHAT SHOULD BE

GAP DATA

QUESTIONS:

ANSWERS:

Therefore
DECIDE TO ADDRESS THIS NEED

PROBLEM (CHALLENGE) STATEMENT

STRATEGIC PLAN
Developed through responsibility for:

Vision, Mission, Goals:
Policies and Procedures:
Marketing:
Staffing:
Patient Care:
Fiscal:
Legal and Ethical:
Risk Management:
Communication:

ACTIVITY 13.12
RUMOR HAS IT

Oliver Hendrix is regional rehabilitation manager for six of All American Rehab Services outpatient centers. One of his center managers has advised him that there is a rumor going around that two of the centers are closing and staff is already looking for new positions. Oliver is determined to follow the trail to the source so the rumor mill may be closed down. What else does he need to do? Consider the communication model in Figure 13.1 and this worksheet. Refer to pp. 61–62.

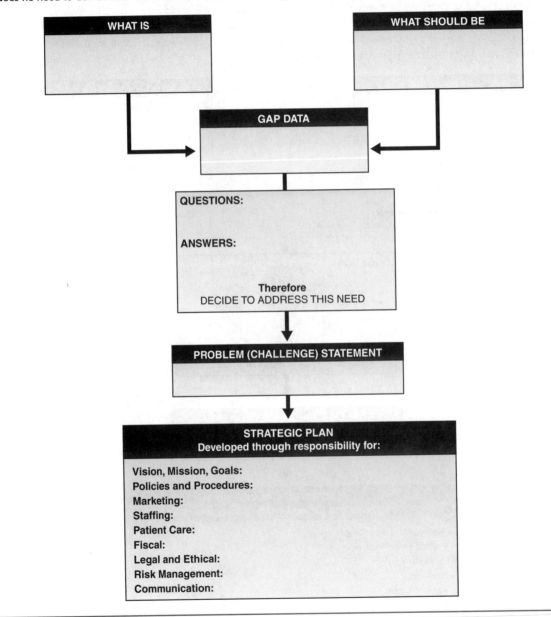

WHAT IS

WHAT SHOULD BE

GAP DATA

QUESTIONS:

ANSWERS:

Therefore
DECIDE TO ADDRESS THIS NEED

PROBLEM (CHALLENGE) STATEMENT

STRATEGIC PLAN
Developed through responsibility for:

Vision, Mission, Goals:
Policies and Procedures:
Marketing:
Staffing:
Patient Care:
Fiscal:
Legal and Ethical:
Risk Management:
Communication:

ACTIVITY 13.13
STRATEGIC COMMUNICATION

Refering to pp. 62–62 and the following worksheet, select another written or oral communication gap in physical therapy practice and identify strategies for closing it. Suggestion: Patient basic and health literacy challenges may be good sources of gaps to be addressed.

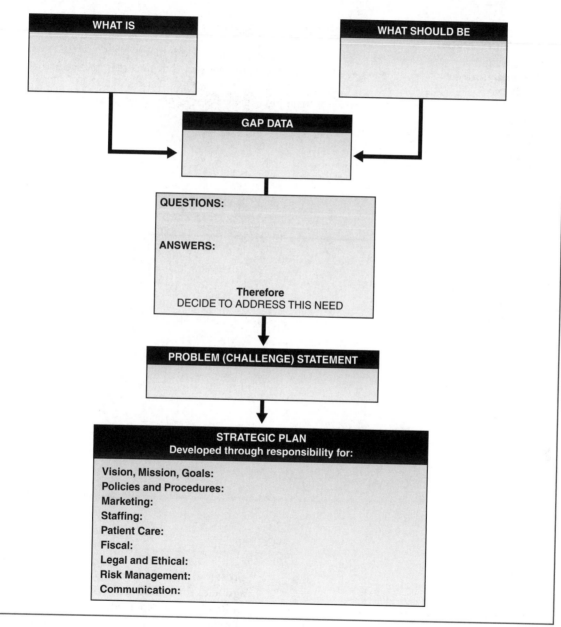

WHAT IS

WHAT SHOULD BE

GAP DATA

QUESTIONS:

ANSWERS:

Therefore
DECIDE TO ADDRESS THIS NEED

PROBLEM (CHALLENGE) STATEMENT

STRATEGIC PLAN
Developed through responsibility for:

Vision, Mission, Goals:
Policies and Procedures:
Marketing:
Staffing:
Patient Care:
Fiscal:
Legal and Ethical:
Risk Management:
Communication:

Conducting a Feasibility Study

Learning Objectives

+ Compare feasibility studies and business plans.
+ Determine the importance of the processes involved in developing a feasibility study.
+ Determine the writing characteristics of an acceptable feasibility study.
+ Prepare a feasibility study.

Overview

This chapter provides a broad outline for entrepreneurs or managers to conduct a feasibility study for the development of a new practice or a program within an organization. As a precursor to a formal business plan, a feasibility study determines the viability of an idea before investing extensive time in producing a detailed, sophisticated business plan for presentation to investors, bankers, or government agencies for funding. See Sidebar 14.1.

Readers are expected *to gather actual data* for the development of a *real feasibility study* for a physical therapy practice as they work through this chapter. They may choose to expand the feasibility study they produce to a formal business plan. Should readers pursue the development of a business plan, they are encouraged to seek additional advice from consultants, the

Sidebar 14.1

Feasibility Studies and Business Plans

✦ The feasibility study is an internal document that only the developer may see. It serves to clarify and verify that a potential business is worth pursuing, or it may lead to alternatives to the original idea for a practice or program. The detailed financial data and associated supporting documents expected in business plans are not included in a feasibility study.

✦ The business plan provides the details for actual implementation of a proposed business (practice or program) and serves to convince potential investors or lenders to support it. Business plans must contain details that reflect that a borrower understands all business aspects of the proposed business and the direction it is headed. The professional and social responsibilities of a health-care practice are *less* emphasized in a business plan.

U.S. Small Business Administration, or other resources. Depending on their prior business expertise, financial and business plan software also may be helpful. All of these tools and resources make planning for a business now much easier. Minor adaptations to make them more relevant for a professional health-care practice often are needed.

Importance of the Process

Both feasibility studies and business plans are essential business processes. They both force entrepreneurs and managers to clarify what they want to achieve and consider potential barriers, risks, and strategies for getting there. Even people who will not have to rely on external funding sources may be foolish to begin a practice without at least a feasibility study. The effort required to supply required financial documents demanded in business plans that may have little chance of success may be avoided if the results of a strong feasibility study have already led to the conclusion that a proposed business is risky.

Many people often conduct feasibility studies on a variety of decisions less formally and perhaps only in a few minutes. For most people the process is as important as the actual product—a written study or plan. The more formal processes and products take time. The actual writing time is typically significantly less than the time required to gather and analyze the data needed to understand the potential place for a practice or program within a community or health-care system, and its potential for success. It often takes several drafts to incorporate new information that is gathered as the process moves along, and to rethink the dream as the reality of a business takes shape.

This is an evolving process, although a step-by-step model is presented here to bring a sense of order to the many factors that need to be considered. As information is gathered in one section, it may be necessary to go back to make revisions in another. The process is similar to the process involved in seeking government or foundation grants for funding of projects or services. The difference is that grant proposals are driven by predetermined dollar amounts and the goals for proposed projects must fall within given guidelines. Managers may also chose to seek such funding opportunities that are a match with the visions and missions of their organizations.

The Actual Writing

Writing the results of a feasibility study is different from other forms of communication. Readers expect a clearly written document that is to the point. The key word is business, not research or prose, so those styles of writing do not easily transfer to business writing. Although the developer may feel passionate and committed to a project, the readers of feasibility studies are only concerned with facts, yet need to know the theme or focus of the intended business or project. Some characteristics of this style of writing include:

✦ Bulleted—Bullet lists make reading easier

✦ Complete—Leaves no unanswered questions so a decision can be made

✦ Concise—Words minimized and short sentences

✦ Crisp—To the point, no emotion

✦ Free of jargon—It distracts rather than impresses, and readers are likely to be from other disciplines

✦ Limited—Who? What? When? Where? How?

✦ Presentable—Neat, correct spelling, proper grammar, and formally presented in a professional-looking binder

✦ Relevant—Include only the facts important to the decision

✦ Reviewed—An objective outsider should review the final draft

✦ Simple—Easy to understand

✦ Sectioned—Divided into smaller topics with headings

✦ Specific—How many and how much are needed are the key questions

The content in this chapter is only one of many basic outlines for a feasibility study. Many other models and outlines are available for review, but developers should not force inclusion of every item in any suggested outline. Since many available models are more often directed to products rather than services, some modifications may be necessary. Specific feasibility studies may not need to address every component, or entrepreneurs and managers may identify others to include during their processes.

For example, an outline of a policies and procedures manual may be included. The contents may be reordered to tailor a report to the particular needs of the expected readers who may have a varying degree of familiarity with physical therapy. Developers should use any outline to stimulate a document that best reflects the information they need for their own decision making, or that meets the needs of others who have the final say on a project. Of course, if the people who will decide to accept or reject a feasibility study provide a standardized format or template to be followed, developers should follow it.

The following sections are a starting point, a sample outline, for conducting a feasibility study. Readers are expected, individually or in groups, to engage in the process by collecting **actual data** about a potential physical therapy practice and producing a feasibility study for review and discussion that will be derived from completion of the activities in this chapter and reference to preceding chapters. Readers should begin an electronic folder on their computers or a hard copy folder to begin collecting the products of their efforts in the following activities. Another folder to begin to collect items to include in the appendix of the feasibility study may also be helpful in organizing this content. Working papers and resources should be collected in another folder.

The major components of a feasibility study to be addressed here are:

I. Summary Statement

II. Market

III. Practice Requirements

IV. Finances

V. Organization

VI. Conclusion

I. The Summary Statement

The summary statement comes first in business writing to give the decision makers reading it the take-home message upfront so they may quickly decide if they are going to invest the time to read the rest of the document. It should only take no more than 60 seconds to read. For example:

(Name of practice or new service) will provide *(type of service)* to *(target markets)* at *(location)* beginning *(initiation date)*, and will be fully operational by *(fully operational date)*. Revenue will be generated through *(list potential revenue sources)* to meet its:

Vision: *(insert vision statement)*.

Mission: *(insert mission statement)*.

Goals: *(insert overall goals of the practice)*.

Presenting the economic and social impact of the proposed practice or project may be another way to address the vision, mission, and goals. The break-even point (discussed later) may be substituted for the fully operational date. Although short and direct, filling in the blanks of the summary statement will take some thought and consideration. The summary statement is often the first part of writing completed, and the last. The first draft of the summary statement often reflects the dreams and ideal of its developer. It may be revised a few times in the development process. For example, target markets and location may change as the developer investigates the competition and alternative locations. Complete Activity 14.1.

II. The Market

Overview of the Profession

Other than themselves, developers of feasibility studies should not assume that other decision makers who will be reading it know much, if anything, about physical therapy practices or the work that

Write the first draft of the summary statement for a selected, actual potential physical therapy practice or new program in a large organization by filling in the blanks in the preceeding template. Expect this process to take some time. At this stage, consider the summary statement as the ideal, dream practice.

HINTS

1. The process for this section may not necessarily follow the order of the blanks in the statement. For instance, determining a name for the potential practice is not likely to be the first thing that needs to be decided. See the branding discussion later in this chapter.
2. Predetermine the time to be devoted to this part of the process. Remember it is the first attempt to set the ideal for the practice, it does not have to be perfect at this stage.
3. Refer to Chapter 5, particularly the information on goal setting for an organization.

physical therapists do. What they do know may not be accurate. This section should include facts, figures, and definitions. Avoiding jargon is important here so official statements from the American Physical Therapy Association and other sources may need to be modified. Think about someone who has never had contact with a physical therapist when preparing this introduction, but keep it short and to the point. Bullet points may work well in this section. This part of the feasibility study is not likely to change. It may be written and put aside for inclusion into the final feasibility study. Managers in organizations developing new programs may spend little or no time on this section. Complete Activity 14.2.

Prepare an overview of the physical therapy profession (i.e., Who?, What?, Where?, When?, and How?). Is it clear and to the point? Are bullets used effectively? Is it easy to understand and free of jargon?

Competition and Demand

Developers may identify the current and potential competitors to a new physical therapy practice using a variety of means. Web searches, Yellow Pages, networking at professional meetings, lists of affiliating organizations with schools of physical therapy, chambers of commerce, and other business associations are all potential sources.

To determine the general demand for physical therapy services takes some effort. U.S. Census data provides information about the demographics for a selected geographic area. Chambers of Commerce usually have economic development services that may be useful. The following questions suggest possible factors for consideration:

✦ Is this a seasonal community?
✦ Who are the major employers?
✦ What percentage of the population is over 65? Over 85? Under age 5?
✦ What percentage of the population is uninsured?
✦ Do existing practices have waiting lists for appointments for physical therapy?
✦ What is the impact of physician-based services in the community?
✦ How far do people currently travel to receive physical therapy? How long does it take them?
✦ What is happening with the hospital(s) in the area?
✦ Are there pending health-care mergers or acquisitions?
✦ Are there plans for expansion of these health-care organizations?
✦ Who are the potential referral sources?
✦ Do unique opportunities for access to referral sources exist?
✦ Is there an advantage because of current visibility in the profession or community?

At this point in the process, the developer of the feasibility study needs to become a sleuth or a spy. It is like an intelligence operation. This information gathering must be accurate and detailed. The developer cannot be shy about asking questions of any potential source of information, while determining how important it is to keep these inquiries confidential. Talking to people who have received services in the competition's practices may reveal additional factors important to potential target markets. Being open and honest about plans for a new business may put up the defenses of others making it harder to get information, or it may encourage people to be helpful. Determining how much of a threat the new practice may be is appropriate at this point in the process. Particularly entrepreneurs, who are new to in a community, need to invest a great deal of effort to this stage of the feasibility study. Determining the mood of a community may be as important as other facts and figures.

Potential Insurance Contracts
Assuming that the major source of revenue (income) will be third-party payers, the feasibility study needs to include information about health insurance following these steps:

+ Identify the types and sources of health insurance for the potential target markets.
+ Identify the model(s) of reimbursement for each of those health insurance policies.
+ Determine the coverage for physical therapy services in those models.

The potential for negotiating new contracts with these insurance companies to provide services is next to be determined. This is a critical step in a feasibility study for practices if they plan to base their revenue on the insurance coverage of patients for physical therapy services. A feasibility study may end here if it is determined that the coverage for physical therapy is not included in most of the policies held by people in the target market, or if insurance companies are not contracting with new practices. If other sources of revenue or other target markets are identified, they may be presented as possible alternatives to the suggested plan, or they may be presented as backup revenue in addition to insurance contracts. Cash payment plans for uninsured or underinsured patients are an example of alternative revenue sources.

Managers in organizations developing programs may be less concerned with this part of a feasibility study because insurance contracts with health-care systems are negotiated more broadly, and managers may need only to confirm that there are no limitations in those agreements that might influence the proposed new service. Complete Activity 14.3.

ACTIVITY 14.3
THE COMPETITION AND DEMAND

After exhausting all resources, prepare this section of the feasibility study. Bulleted lists may be valuable in relating this information under the major headings of competition, demand, and insurance. Include the sources of the information presented to increase the credibility of this section. Developers do not want to be in the awkward position of presenting a completed plan to someone who says, "Oh, didn't you hear about . . .?", which would throw a new light on the feasibility of starting the practice or program.

HINTS:

1. Stick to the facts. Personal opinion or rumors do not form a strong basis for decision making.
2. The information in this section of a feasibility study may need to be double-checked just before its submission to decision makers, or before an entrepreneur decides to open the doors of a practice, if conducting the study has taken a long time. Identifying changes in health insurance that may have occurred during the preparation time span is also important.

Target Market
The information gathered on the competition, demand, and insurance for physical therapy services leads to the identification of a target market(s). It may be foolish to jump to conclusions about the target market without knowing this information. For instance, the target market may be obvious if there is little or no competition, but clearly defining a practice niche in the midst of a lot of competition may be necessary. Although physical therapists with particular experience and credentials may prefer a specialty practice, if there is no demand for that specialty, success may not be realized. Conversely, a developer would not want to overlook a demand that is not being met by the competition. Conducting focused inbound marketing to determine the needs of particular market serves as the basis for this section of the feasibility study. Complete Activity 14.4.

Expected Market Share
Market share is the percentage or proportion of the total sales of a particular product. Health-care entrepreneurs also might want to predict market share of the services they intend to provide as a way to

ACTIVITY 14.4
TARGET MARKET

Identify the target market(s) and provide convincing support for it in this section by relating it to the identified competition and demands, and to the potential unmet needs. Revise the summary statement as necessary.

ACTIVITY 14.5
MARKET SHARE

Determine, if possible, the market share for the proposed practice and either write a description in this section or include a pie chart to reflect this information in this section. Recheck the summary statement to determine if this information should be included.

consider the impact they expect to have on the competition. If they expect everyone in the target market to receive their services in their proposed organization or program, all that is necessary in this section may be a statement saying so. If however, the target market is currently receiving services in existing organizations, a pie chart may be useful.

For example, if the target market is 10,000 patients who have Medicare coverage in a community that has two other private physical therapy practices, a physician-based practice, and a hospital that provides outpatient services, the pie chart might look like the one in Figure 14.1. The value of market share information is dependent on the confidence that a developer has in these figures, which may be difficult to determine in health care beyond a rough estimate. If market share will be of little value to decision makers because of this, this section may be eliminated in a written report. Thinking about market share as part of a feasibility study is helpful, however, to clarify the power of the competition. Developing a pie chart for *each* target market if there is more than one may be more meaningful and assist in further clarifying the potential for business. Complete Activity 14.5.

Branding

At this part of the process, attention to the name of the practice, logos, and other images deserves attention because the data so far should begin to indicate that a new practice or program is possibly feasible. Although for many developers, this is the fun part of a feasibility study, it should not be the most important part, the first task to be tackled, or the process that takes the most amount of time. Entrepreneurs may want to use available graphics or sketch out temporary branding possibilities rather than invest in graphic arts in the preparation of a feasibility study.

Other potential outbound marketing tactics may be presented, in general terms, in bullet format. Plans for acquiring professional marketing services may be included here. For managers developing programs in large organizations, this step may not be included in a feasibility study because marketing staff are in place to address these issues if the proposal is accepted. These managers may only need to suggest some outbound marketing ideas about whom and where they fit into existing plans of the organization. Complete Activity 14.6.

ACTIVITY 14.6
BRANDING

Include the selected name for the practice in the summary statement and include a temporary logo and other examples of branding in an appendix. This is a short section that briefly explains the brand, the image to be conveyed, and potential outward marketing tactics formatted as a bulleted list. Marketing consulting services that will be hired also should appear in this section.

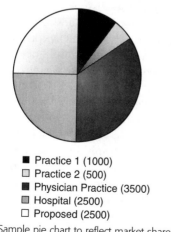

■ Practice 1 (1000)
□ Practice 2 (500)
■ Physician Practice (3500)
▨ Hospital (2500)
□ Proposed (2500)

Figure 14.1 ✦ Sample pie chart to reflect market share for 10,000 patients.

Potential Market Barriers

This section is the opportunity for the developer to demonstrate that they have thought about *all* of the possible factors that may negatively affect their target market(s). Considering worst case scenarios like layoffs in the industry that is the major employer of the target market, or retirees who decide to relocate to be nearer their families as they age may be helpful. It may include possible responses of competitors to the proposed business if it is implemented.

Developers do not want to fail to address an important "what if . . ." identified by other decision makers reviewing their proposals, or to be taken by surprise once a practice has begun. Careful consideration to barriers is important to a feasibility study. Including rough estimates of the probability of these negative impact factors is desirable, particularly if they can be backed up with facts. Complete Activity 14.7.

ACTIVITY 14.7
BARRIERS

Carefully consider all potential market barriers in this section. Lists and bullets may make reading easier. A table that lists the barriers and the potential actions to overcome them is another way of presenting this information. Listing barriers in the order of the likelihood of their happening also is helpful.

III. Practice Requirements

This section of a feasibility study provides decision makers with a picture of the practice or program. They are probably less interested in the aesthetics than they are in the financial impact of these requirements. This section should reflect thoughtful consideration for the relationship between space, equipment, and workforce needed to accomplish the goals of the practice. Exploring these requirements can be fun and developers may seek the assistance of commercial real estate experts and suppliers of equipment and furniture to gather data for this section.

Access

Developers need to consider two types of access. First, physical access to the practice particularly for people with disabilities, such as walking distance from parking spaces to the entrance of the practice, elevators if the practice is not on the first floor, and typical weather conditions. Placing oneself in the shoes of the patients in the target market(s) to maximize their ability to access the services may lead to a potential competitive advantage.

Access also means staff who are able to determine eligibility for physical therapy services in a timely manner and schedule appointments without delay. Including this information on service in a feasibility study demonstrates attention to detail and commitment to customers, which decision makers may look upon favorably. It also helps justify nonclinical personnel. The extra attention to this type of service may be another source of competitive advantage.

Location and Space

It may seem attractive to locate in a part of town where there is no other physical therapy practice as long as the reason for that gap is that no one else has thought about it, rather than some undesirable factor that the developer has overlooked. The dream location may not seem so attractive after more analysis. The pros and cons of locating in established medical complexes that the target market(s) associates with their health care also require consideration. For instance, space in a high visibility location may be more expensive but the need for outbound marketing may be reduced.

The key question to be addressed is how much will the location cost? Providing figures on comparable space in other locations may help decision makers understand your location decision from their primary perspective—money. Adding additional information on the advantages of a location for your target market(s) is important, particularly if the cost/square footage in the selected location is higher than it is in other locations. If public transportation stops, or nearness to interstate exits, or rush-hour traffic patterns are important to the target market(s), decision makers need to know that you have researched and are addressing these issues in the location selected.

Developers also should address why the amount of space is necessary, how it will be configured for patient privacy and safety, and compliance with regulatory demands. Room for expansion and the key terms of the potential lease also should be addressed. Upper management in large organizations may present developers of a feasibility study the limits of space and location from the outset. The challenge for these managers may be accomplishing goals within these limits, or goals may need to be revised to meet these given conditions. All developers may wish to prepare a floor plan to clarify their thinking. It should be included in the appendix of the feasibility study. Floor plans should be drawn to scale when possible. Software is available to generate floor plans.

Equipment

This section may simply refer to a detailed listing of the start-up equipment and supplies with the approximate cost of each item. Preferably, this list is in the appendix rather than the body of a feasibility study to reduce interruption of the flow of the reading. The text in this section should include only an overview of the major categories in the list and total estimated start-up costs for equipment. Justification for unusually expensive or nontraditional equipment should be included. This section includes clinical and office and reception area furniture.

Workforce Needs and Availability

Developers need to discuss the qualifications and expertise expected of clinical and nonclinical staff and the number of people in each category at start-up and when the practice is fully operational. Relating these figures to space requirements is useful. Some assurance that people are available for these identified positions is in order. Developers may rely on potential recruitment methods and national or local labor statistics for this section, and relate them to the costs of recruitment. There is no organization without people so workforce is a critical component of a feasibility study. Relationships with universities and community colleges as an ongoing source of potential employees also may be included here. Complete Activity 14.8.

ACTIVITY 14.8
PRACTICE REQUIREMENTS

Prepare this section and accompanying data for the appendix to support it. Although detailed, this section needs to be concise. The use of charts, tables, and well-organized lists are helpful and should be included in the appendix. Include only information that supports the proposal avoiding personal opinion or biases. Revise the summary statement as necessary.

IV. Finances

Starting this section by presenting the bottom line is often a good idea. For managers preparing feasibility studies in large organizations, the costs involved in a project may be all that they need to provide in this section. Upper-level managers, in the context of the broader organization, then address the financial implications of these costs. Entrepreneurs, however, need to pay particular attention to this section to avoid major financial losses. If the previous sections of the study are strong and impressive, the bottom line (expected profits when fully operational) should lead to a favorable decision because no questions remain, the risks have been identified, and the investment in the practice seems wise regardless of what the bottom line figure is. To arrive at the bottom line, developers need the following data.

Equity and Credit Sources

This section forces entrepreneurs to be brutally honest about their *personal* financial resources and debts. Equity or net worth includes investments and retained earnings. Net worth = assets−liabilities. Assets may include personal cash savings, interest on savings and investments, property, other valuable items owned outright, etc. Liabilities are debts from credit cards, loans, etc. Credit sources may include loans from family and friends, banks, credit unions, etc. This section is not necessary for managers in existing organizations.

It is difficult to borrow money without money so readers who have not yet accumulated much equity or who may not yet have a strong credit history, may want to "pretend" to have $100,000 in equity to continue with the development of a "mock" feasibility study. While pretending however, it is a good exercise to develop a plan for accumulating assets. The beginning of a new career is a good time to take a financial planning course or consult a financial planner whether intending to be an entrepreneur or not. Readers with assets need an accurate accounting of them to determine how much, if any, additional funds are needed to complete this section of a feasibility study for their own use, or to provide information that a potential lender would require. Complete Activity 14.9.

ACTIVITY 14.9
EQUITY AND CREDIT SOURCES

Prepare a list of assets and potential credit sources for this section. Fill in the blank:
net worth = _____ in this section. For educational purposes, $100,000 or some other agreed-upon figure may be used.

Break-Even Analysis

Break-even is the point where revenues equal expenses. It is the point at which there is no profit, and there is no loss. It is the estimated point after which a practice or program becomes profitable. Break-even may not be important for managers in organizations whose financial decisions are based on multiple factors, and that have probably reached their break-even point long ago. Entrepreneurs starting from scratch will find this tool important in a feasibility study.

Break-even analysis is based on estimates that need to be as accurate as possible although the figures may change over time. The break-even point before the practice opens may not be the same break-even point after the business has been running for a few months. Hopefully, the practice has reached the break-even point before expected, but more typically, break-even is pushed back because the best-laid plans are still unpredictable. To determine the break-even point, developers need to determine:

- ✦ **Unit of sale or service:** For physical therapy practice, the unit of service is a treatment session because of most reimbursement model requirements.
- ✦ **Price:** For physical therapy practice, this is the average claim submitted for reimbursement for the average treatment session.
- ✦ **Variable costs (direct):** Those costs that increase as the number of treatment sessions increase.
- ✦ **Fixed costs (indirect):** Those costs that are the same regardless of the number of treatment sessions provided. Costs that exist even if no treatment sessions are provided.

Costs in physical therapy are best determined as cost/treatment session. The question then becomes, how much does it cost to treat the average patient in an average treatment session? This number may not stabilize for a few months—the fewer the patients/month the greater the cost/treatment session. The more homogeneous the patients, the more accurate this estimated cost will be. However, an average cost is often good enough for a feasibility study if the developer knows patients and physical therapy practice even fairly well. Taking the total costs/month and dividing by the number of expected treatment sessions/month provides the average cost/treatment session/month.

For break-even analysis, the question becomes: What is the number of treatment sessions/month at $\_\_\_$/session that will pay for the total variable + fixed costs/month? A simple example for a hypothetical new practice follows:

Example

	10-TREATMENT SESSIONS/MONTH	100-TREATMENT SESSIONS/MONTH
Total Cost	$4,500 + $5(10) = $4,550	$4,500 + $5(100) = $5,000
Gross Revenue	$100(10) = $1,000	$100(100) = $10,000
Profit	$1,000 − $4,550 = (−$3,550)	$10,000 − $5,000 = $5,000
Pfofit margin		50%

The monthly fixed costs for the practice is $4,500. The variable cost/treatment session is $5. The formula becomes:
Fixed Costs/Month + (Variable costs/per treatment session × no. of treatment sessions/month) = Total Costs.
The average revenue/treatment session is $100.
Revenue/Month = Revenue/treatment session × total number of sessions/month.
Profit = Revenue − Total Costs.
Profit margin = revenue − expenses ÷ total revenue and is expressed as a percentage.

The break-even point for a practice lies where the expenses = revenue. Break-even is typically represented in a line chart as shown in Figure 14.2 in which revenue is $50 X number of visits. For this practice, the break-even number of visits is when the total revenue is about $4,000 or 80 visits per month, which is expected to happen in June if projected referrals, contracts with insurance companies, and other factors occur as expected. The major rule of business becomes obvious. Keep cost/treatment session low and the number of treatment sessions high. Profit is the business goal.

Determining Total Start-Up and Operational Costs

In feasibility studies, rounded numbers and best estimates are all that may be necessary. The question to be answered is how much money is required to open the practice on the first day and how much more will be needed to keep the practice open until it becomes profitable (meets the break-even point). Good "guesstimates" are acceptable but omissions of costs are not. This process must be carefully undertaken so that all costs are identified. Failure to recognize and consider costs may be the source of more early business failures than any other factor.

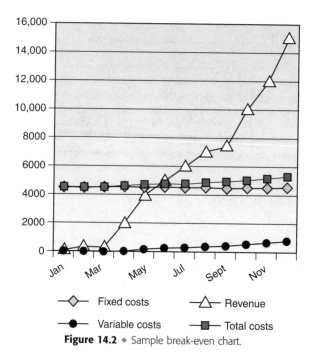

Figure legend:
—◇— Fixed costs   —△— Revenue
—●— Variable costs   —■— Total costs

Figure 14.2 ✦ Sample break-even chart.

In health care, the first reimbursement checks from third-party payers may take time as contracts are negotiated and reimbursement systems are put in place, so although treatment sessions are provided, actual money in hand may be delayed. Other sources of income may be slow in starting. Without proper planning, these can seem like scary times. This is a period in which entrepreneurs are essentially paying to go to work, so they must be comfortable with this concept. For managers developing new programs, costs may be low if existing facilities and equipment are to be used. The development of a new freestanding center will take the same attention as entrepreneurs devote to starting a new practice. Complete Activity 14.10.

Revenue
Revenue is primarily dependent on reimbursement models of the health insurance companies that are paying for the services that patients receive. Regardless of these models, the average cost/average treatment session that is determined above is held constant for financial planning purposes. The projected revenue/month for each type of model may be very different. See Table 14.1 for a brief comparison of revenue models.

These comparisons demonstrate the importance of contract negotiation and the need to consider the developer's tolerance for financial risk. The worst case scenarios in each model need to be considered.

The ethical challenges presented by each model also require attention. Realizing that this process is about averages rather than actual costs also is important. Not all patients are the same so cost/treatment session may vary widely among patients, and vary for one patient who improves during the course of their treatment sessions (they may need less therapy as time goes by, or may be able to tolerate more therapy as they improve).

Developers may also consider other sources of revenue. Patients may pay directly depending on their deductibles and co-payment rates at each treatment session. Cash payment for other services or by patients who have no insurance is another source of revenue. Complete Activity 14.11.

Cash Flow
Understanding cash flow is an important management tool. Although exciting to focus on income, its relationship to expenses is critical. Although a practice may be making money, whether it has enough cash to pay all of its expenses and loan payments is the more important question. Cash flow is analogous to a checking account. Determining if there are deposits to cover the checks written is a type of cash-flow analysis. For managers in health care who are dependent on third-party payers, cash flow is

TABLE 14.1 Impact of reimbursement models on profits

MODEL	IMPACT ON PROFITS
1. Fee Schedule	The more units of service provided in a treatment session, the greater the revenue.
2. Based on value of CPT codes/unit.	Requires provider of care to be efficient and fill scheduled treatment sessions so there is no downtime. The number of treatment sessions and the number of units/treatment session are both important to profits. Preauthorization by third-party payers for the number of sessions and/or number of chargeable units to meet patient goals is common.
e.g.: Average three units/treatment session @ $25/unit = $75/session	
3. Per Case	Payment is a flat fee/person regardless of the number of treatment sessions that person receives. The fewer the number of sessions a patient needs to meet goals, the greater the profits. If the total costs of the number of sessions needed exceed the payment/case, the provider loses money.
Number of cases/month × average payment/case each month.	
e.g.: 8 × $600 (each case = about 12 treatment sessions)	
4. Per Visit	The payment/treatment session must be greater than the cost of the treatment session. The more visits, the more profits. Controlling the costs/session becomes especially important (staff time, for example, or the cost of the person providing the services) to increase profits.
Number of visits/month × payment/visit.	
e.g.: 100 × 50/treatment session	
5. Capitation	The provider receives a flat sum of money/year to take care of all of the patients in a particular group. Profit is dependent on the number of patients in the group who actually receive physical therapy. The more people who need physical therapy, and the more physical therapy each of them needs, the less the profit.
Number of covered lives × premium/month.	
e.g.: 2,000 lives × $5/life/month	

ACTIVITY 14.11
TOTAL REVENUE AND PROFIT

Project the total revenue for the first year of the practice by completing a chart in which months go across and the models of reimbursement are listed in the first column.

critical because the check to pay for services provided may arrive weeks after the services have been delivered. Depending on the reimbursement model, some claims may not be submitted until the patient's entire plan of care is complete.

Cash flow is typically determined on a monthly basis by simply comparing the money received with the money expended. Including a month-by-month projected cash-flow chart in a feasibility study may be useful. The two major categories are "cash flow from operations, investments, etc." and "use of funds." The bottom line is the net increase (decrease) in cash.

Expected Balance Sheet When in Full Operation
A balance sheet is another tool that may be valuable in a feasibility study. It is a documented report of a company's assets and obligations, and the residual ownership claims against equity at any given point in time. A balance sheet is a cumulative record of business to date. Balance sheets are used for comparisons to determine the changes in the value of the organization and if debts and capital are increasing or decreasing. A balance sheet for an organization includes its:

ASSETS

✦ Current Assets (cash and items that can be converted to cash)

✦ Accounts Receivable (amounts owed to the practice)

✦ Inventories (goods available for sale) *if applicable*

✦ Prepaid Expenses (insurance, rental fees)

✦ Investments (stocks, bonds, retirement funds) *if applicable*

✦ Practice Assets (land, buildings, equipment, etc. used in operations)

✦ Intangible Assets (franchises, goodwill expenses, legal costs)

✦ Other Assets (funds for special purposes, advances to owner)

LIABILITIES

+ Current Liabilities (those that will be paid in the next year with current assets, e.g., loan payments, income taxes, payroll taxes, wages and salaries, utilities, etc.)
+ Long-Term Liabilities (debts not due for more than a year)
+ Deferred Revenues (money paid in advance of services rendered)
+ Owner's Equity (amount invested by the owner, retained earnings)

Complete Activity 14.12.

ACTIVITY 14.12
BALANCE SHEET

Prepare an expected balance sheet as it might look on the first anniversary of opening day of the practice. Put the balance sheet in the appendix of the feasibility study. Remember that a balance sheet should balance. Assets − liabilities = 0. Simply refer to the appendix in this section of the feasibility study. Developers may wish to seek consultation or software to complete a balance sheet. Understanding of assets and liabilities may take additional sources.

Underlying Assumptions and Summary

The final paragraph of the financial section of the feasibility study should summarize the assumptions that underlie the information presented. It is a place to bring all of this financial information together in a clear, concise statement. Complete Activity 14.13.

ACTIVITY 14.13
SUMMARIZING

Prepare the final section of the finances portion of the feasibility study by clearly summarizing this information. Bullet lists may be helpful.

V. Organization

Legal Structure

Entrepreneurs need to establish a new practice as a separate legal entity that in the eyes of the law has the capacity to engage in contracts, assumes the obligation to pay its debts, and is responsible for its actions so can be sued. The practice may be an individual, partnership, proprietorship, corporation, association or other organization. Developers should seek legal advice in the preparation of this section because of the complexity of the tax implications of this decision. Managers in large organizations may exclude this section.

Decision-Making Flow

This section of the feasibility study may be represented by an organizational chart or narrative that includes a chain of command, if there is one. If the practice is small, this may be only a brief description of the relationships of its members and stakeholders.

Key Individuals and Qualifications

This section should include the projected position titles and descriptions of these positions. Job descriptions should be placed in the appendix. The names of the people expected to fill them are listed in this section if they are known, and their resumes should be included in the appendix. Complete Activity 14.14.

ACTIVITY 14.14
THE ORGANIZATION

Prepare the organization section of the feasibility study and include information in the appendix as needed.

VI. Conclusion

Complete Activity 14.15.

ACTIVITY 14.15
THE SUMMARY STATEMENT

Take one last look at the summary statement and revise as needed to reflect the best possible picture of the proposed practice or program before writing the conclusion.

At this point developers need to reread the feasibility study and take time to reflect. This section is the conclusion of their work. It should include a statement, such as:

Based on the information gathered in this feasibility study this practice is (feasible not feasible).

Developers need to answer the following questions in this part of the feasibility study:

+ Should a formal business plan be presented for funding?

✦ Should the idea be totally scrapped?

✦ Are there alternatives that may be more attractive?

✦ Are the alternatives presented in detail?

Complete Activity 14.16.

ACTIVITY 14.16
CONCLUSION

Prepare the conclusion of the feasibility study.

A Manager's Responsibility

The development of a feasibility study is the first and most important responsibility for any entrepreneur seeking to develop a health-care business. For managers in large organizations, the importance of this process and the ability to present a feasibility study may be no less important in meeting the goals of their organizations. Managers should not be hesitant to call upon consultants or other people within their organizations to develop a strong proposal that is well supported with accurate facts and figures.

Management in Specific Physical Therapy Settings

This section provides the opportunity to take a more detailed look into the range of practice settings of physical therapists, the many managerial opportunities that they present, and some of the common issues that managers in health care can address to influence quality patient care. Each chapter in this section is devoted to management of physical therapy (or rehabilitation) services based in one of the major practice settings:

✦ Long-term care
✦ Outpatient centers
✦ Special education units of public schools
✦ Home health agencies
✦ Hospitals and health-care systems

In some settings, such as outpatient centers, physical therapy managers are the chapter's topic because it is less likely that managers in that setting will have responsibility for other professionals. In other settings, such as long-term care situations, it is more likely a rehabilitation manager (who may be a physical therapist) has responsibility for staff from other health-care disciplines. Although managers in any center may head a discipline or an interdisciplinary team, only one or the other is addressed in each chapter for easier reading.

Each chapter in this section is divided into two parts. Part 1 of each chapter addresses contemporary characteristics and common issues in the setting that affect the work of physical therapists. Part 2 identifies the potential managerial roles in the setting and addresses the eight areas of managerial responsibility presented in Section 2 of the text—vision, mission, goals; policies and procedures; marketing; staffing; patient care; fiscal; legal, ethical, and risk management; and communication. At the end of each chapter are activities that provide the opportunity to develop managerial decision-making skills in the context of each setting. Although many of these decisions arise in all practice settings, they are placed in a particular setting and not repeated in other chapters. For example, one activity addresses decision making related to a patient's fall that occurs during a transfer. This challenge was placed in the long-term care chapter although it may be a challenge in other settings.

The final chapter presents challenges to the physical therapy profession as they address the issues surrounding physical therapists as managers in health-care organizations.

Chapter 15

Management Issues in Long-Term Care

Learning Objectives

- Discuss components and characteristics of contemporary long-term care.
- Analyze key licensing, accreditation, and reimbursement requirements.
- Analyze the work of physical therapists in long-term care.
- Determine the role of the care team, particularly certified nursing assistants, in the accomplishment of patient rehabilitation goals.
- Determine the importance of family education in long-term care.
- Determine the managerial roles and challenges to managerial responsibilities.
- Analyze managerial decision making in given situations.

Part 1
The Contemporary Setting

Overview of Long-Term Care

The provision of social and medical services are intertwined tightly in long-term care to meet the needs of people with complex, multisystem problems across the life span. Only 53% of the people who require long-term care are elderly. Many of the younger people have long-term care needs because of cognitive deficits and mental illnesses. The focus of long-term patient care shifts toward the ability of a person to function rather than on their diagnoses and treatment of their diseases.[1]

Long-term care may be best represented (as shown in Fig. 15.1) as a continuum of care, which is anchored with skilled care at one end and nonskilled care at the other end. Long-term care can occur in a variety of settings represented by the circles in the figure. Note that home care (provided in the patient's home) is a unique form of _intermittent_ long-term care that may be skilled, or nonskilled, or a patient may receive both levels of services at the same time at home. Home care is discussed separately in another chapter. Since the need for skilled interdisciplinary care is a requirement for admission into skilled long-term care, most patients are admitted directly from an acute care hospital.

Nonskilled residential care may be provided in many types of long-term care and assisted living facilities under a variety of names that may overlap and confuse. These facilities are inconsistently and variably regulated from one jurisdiction to another, but their services attend to the personal needs of their residents using nonskilled employees to help them with self-care. Some residential facilities may cater to particular populations, such as adults with mental retardation. Often there are restrictions for admission related to a required level of mobility. The patients may need to be, minimally, independent in wheelchair mobility to live in some centers, for example.

A special type of residential care is the adult (congregate) living facility in which people maintain a private or semiprivate residence within a large building while sharing common areas for meals and activities. Transportation and housekeeping services

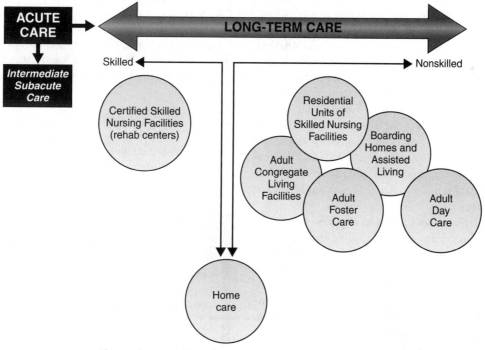

Figure 15.1 ✦ Health-care continuum.

are typically available. Nursing supervision 24 hours a day is available to monitor and assist with residents' medication and other health-care needs. Typically, residents need to be ambulatory. They may receive intermittent physical therapy as outpatients or through home care services for short periods, and nonskilled home care for assistance with activities of daily living or homemaking on a long-term, intermittent basis.

A nursing home may have units that are Medicare-certified in which the patients (often referred to as residents in these settings) receive skilled interdisciplinary care, and a separate unit that is not Medicare-certified where residential long-term care is provided. Although they are in the same building, they are managed as separate entities because they are regulated differently.

Residents in a residential unit may develop a new problem that requires a formal transfer to a certified bed in the Medicare unit in the same building—a person who falls and fractures a hip, for example. They remain there to receive skilled interdisciplinary care through the acute and subacute stages of recovery. Conversely, residents admitted from a hospital to a nursing home for skilled rehabilitation services may be discharged to the residential care unit if their improvement is not enough to discharge them to their homes—for example, a person admitted after a stroke whose rehabilitation goals are not met, or a person whose family support system is not adequate to return to home.

People in the residential care units of a nursing home may qualify for Part B Medicare or Medicaid-intermittent skilled rehabilitation services as outpatients as if they were living in their private homes, although they are residents in an inpatient facility. An example might be a patient with a rotator cuff tear who requires physical therapy. Another example is a patient who is transferred from the skilled to the residential unit who continues rehabilitation or nursing services intermittently as a patient receiving Medicare Part B services.

The level of assistance a person requires in the components of long-term care may range from general supervision for safety or administration of medications to maximum assistance for all activities of daily living. These needs may change over time. The concept of continuing long-term care bridges all of these needs. It typically takes the form of a campus-like retirement community with private homes, opportunities for many leisure activities, an assisted

living facility, a skilled nursing facility, outpatient care, and a residential care home. Residents of the community buy a private home and contract for lifelong care within the community that includes transfers among the community's facilities as their medical and social needs change.

It is also important to note that an intermediate (subacute) level of care (between acute care and long-term care) is defined as a short period (normally no longer than 6 weeks) of intensive rehabilitation, treatment, or intensive care that may be provided in subunits of hospitals, skilled nursing facilities, or in patients' homes, typically after discharge from the hospital. Subacute care is discussed in Chapter 19. The aim of intermediate care is to make sure that people who are able to become as independent as possible do so to reduce or delay the need for long-term care and to improve the chances of returning to their homes and independent living. It also may be used to deter admission to a more expensive hospital whenever possible.

At the other end of the spectrum, long-term care includes nonresidential adult day-care centers, which provide a range of skilled and nonskilled services to people who are brought to the centers on a daily or intermittent basis by their families because they cannot be left alone safely. They provide social and physical support, freeing family members to work or take care of other family responsibilities. Table 15.1 summarizes the characteristics of the major types of long-term care and the role of physical therapy in them. Go to Sidebar 15.1 to learn more about current issues facing long-term care organizations.

Skilled Nursing Facilities

Skilled nursing facilities (SNFs), which also may have "rehabilitation center" in their names, are clearly defined by certification requirements of Medicare

---

Sidebar 15.1

Current Issues in Long-Term Care

Other data about contemporary long-term care and current policy issues can be found at the Web pages of the American Health Care Association at http://www.ahca.org/about/profile.htm.

Table 15.1   Levels of long-term care and the role of physical therapy in them

TYPE OF LONG-TERM CARE	LEVELS OF SERVICE	ROLE OF PHYSICAL THERAPY
Skilled nursing facilities (rehabilitation centers)	Skilled nursing and rehabilitative services are an integral component of care. The length of stay may be shorter than the 100 days available for those needing intermediate levels of rehabilitation before transferring to a lesser level of care. Longer lengths of stays are common for people with complex chronic conditions.	Member of the interdisciplinary rehabilitation team to return people to the safest, optimal level of function.
Residential care homes	Provide nonskilled personal care and supervision for people unable to meet their personal needs independently. The care may range from minimal to maximal assist for activities of daily living, medical management of chronic diseases, etc. There may be nonskilled units in SNFs.	When a residential care unit is in a SNF, physical therapists may treat residents as if they were Medicare B outpatients for brief periods, a few times a week (e.g., a resident receives physical therapy 3x week for 3 weeks after hospitalization for viral infection). Establishing restorative programs and functional maintenance programs to promote optimum quality of life and independence of residents is another responsibility. Physical therapists may treat residents of boarding and foster homes as home care patients in these settings.
Adult (congregate) living facilities	Provides meal services, organized activities, and supervision of medical status to residents who live independently in their own units. May also include lockdown units for patients with dementia to assure patient safety.	Physical therapists may provide home care services to residents, residents may travel to outpatient centers for physical therapy, or there may be an on-site therapy clinic.
Continuing care communities	Provides services on a campus that may include apartments or homes where people live independently, a SNF, an adult congregate living facility, and a residential care home or unit. Residents buy into a program to meet their needs for the rest of their lives. They move from one type of care to another as their needs demand in a continuous manner.	Physical therapists may be employed by the community or contract their services through other agencies to provide inpatient services in the SNF, outpatient or home care to people who are living in their own homes on the campus or in the assisted living facility, and intermittent care to residents in the residential care units. They may have educational responsibilities for nursing staff development and resident educational programs. They may assist in the development of health and fitness programs for members of the community. It may be that different physical therapists or physical therapy companies provide services in different components of the community complex.
Adult day care	Provides assistance with personal care and social activities in a community-based center on a regular basis. Clients return to their own homes at the end of the day. May address the needs of particular groups like patients with Alzheimer disease.	Physical therapists may serve as consultants to develop group exercise programs. They may treat individuals requiring skilled outpatient services in the centers although treatment resources may be limited.

and Medicaid. They are the most tightly regulated health-care setting and the focus of this chapter. The importance of this component of health care is reflected in the following skilled nursing home statistics from 2004: [2]

+ There are more than 16,000 certified long-term care facilities with more than 1,750,000 skilled nursing beds in the United States for Medicare and Medicaid beneficiaries.

+ More than 5,000 nursing homes are proprietary.

+ More than 4,000 are *neither* Medicare nor Medicaid certified.

+ About 5,600 are *both* Medicare and Medicaid certified.

+ Occupancy rate of nursing homes is more than 80% in the United States, and more than 90% in 11 states.

+ 1.4 million people are permanent residents of nursing homes and an almost equal number have shorter stays for rehabilitation after hospitalization for acute care.

+ More than one-third of residents are dependent in mobility and eating and also are incontinent.

+ 6% of U.S. health-care expenditures are for nursing home care.

+ The average monthly charge per resident in skilled nursing facilities is $5,690.

Because the acuity level of patients discharged from hospitals has increased, the number of people who require skilled nursing care at discharge has increased at the same time that reimbursement reductions and financial constraints have been imposed. Many nursing homes have closed or currently operate under bankruptcy protection. Frequent changes in ownership, management, and organizational structure have also resulted.[3] The trend toward large, national chains that allow the shifting of resources among buildings may be one outgrowth of these health-care policy and reimbursement decisions.

Nursing Home Regulations and Quality Management

Omnibus Budget Reconciliation Act (OBRA)

The 1987 Federal Nursing Home Reform Act, which included OBRA, was the primary catalyst for change in long-term care. It included the requirement that *each* resident "attain and maintain her highest practicable physical, mental, and psycho-social well-being" for the facility to receive Medicare and Medicaid funding. National standards of care and rights for residents were established that include:[4]

+ Emphasis on a resident's quality of life and the quality of care.

+ New expectations that each resident's ability to walk, bathe, and perform other activities of daily living will be maintained or improved absent medical reasons.

+ A resident assessment process leading to development of an individualized care plan.

+ Rights to remain in the nursing home absent nonpayment, dangerous resident behaviors, or significant changes in a resident's medical condition.

+ A right to safely maintain or bank personal funds with the nursing home.

+ Rights to return to the nursing home after a hospital stay or an overnight visit with family and friends.

+ The right to choose a personal physician and to access medical records.

+ The right to organize and participate in a resident or family council.

+ The right to be free of unnecessary and inappropriate physical and chemical restraints.

+ Uniform certification standards for Medicare and Medicaid homes.

+ Prohibitions on turning to family members to pay for Medicare and Medicaid services.

+ New remedies for certified nursing homes that fail to meet minimum federal standards.

The importance of rehabilitation services in meeting these standards becomes apparent. The shift to skilled care to restore and maintain function from nonskilled care to simply take care of people with functional deficits became a major philosophical and managerial challenge for many nursing homes. OBRA led to a focus on compliance with regulatory mandates on all aspects of the management of skilled nursing care. Staff/patient ratios, mixes of licensed and unlicensed personnel for the full 24 hours of care, and the development of the Minimum Data Set (MDS, which will be discussed later) are the result of this legislation. Burdensome reporting requirements to demonstrate the efforts made to improve the quality of care and quality of life for residents continue to detract from the actual provision of that care.

Regulatory Surveys

Compliance with OBRA legislation is determined through an annual state survey and certification process established by the Centers for Medicare and Medicaid Services (CMMS). The survey involves unannounced on-site audits of all nursing homes. It includes interviews of staff members, residents, and family members after a review of established quality indicators has been completed. The purpose of the survey is to assess whether the quality of care provided is in compliance with given standards and the needs of individual residents. Noncompliance with Medicare and/or Medicaid regulations, and/or state certification laws may result in penalties, such as denial of payment for new admissions, fines, revocation of certification, and transfer of residents. Any identified deficiencies must be addressed promptly.

In addition to survey and other administrative data requirements, the CMMS also monitors nursing homes through the MDS that is used to comprehensively report the status of each individual receiving care. The data are aggregated, analyzed, and then converted to specific indicators that cover all aspects of the quality of interdisciplinary care, and compliance with residents' rights. All of this information is available to the public to assist in their decision making when selecting a nursing home for placement of family members. As such, it provides another incentive for nursing homes to continually improve the quality of their care. Go to Sidebar 15.2 to learn more about specific nursing homes.

Sidebar 15.2

Data on Nursing Homes

Data from state surveys and the MDSs on each resident can be found on each Medicare/Medicaid nursing home at http:// www.medicare.gov/ NHCompare/Include/DataSection/Questions/ SearchCriteria.asp?version=default&browser=IE% 7C7%7CWinXP&language=English&defaultstatus =0&pagelist=Home&CookiesEnabledStatus= True. Read the detailed information on two or three selected nursing homes of similar size.

Accreditation of Long-Term Care

Long-term care organizations have the opportunity to seek voluntary accreditation from two organizations. The Joint Commission of Accreditation of Health Care Organizations, referred to simply as The Joint Commission, expanded its accreditation activities to include health-care organizations other than hospitals. This credential is probably more important to, and more feasible for, larger nursing homes or those that are part of a larger health-care system. The Joint Commission's gold seal does reflect a commitment to certain quality standards that may exceed those required in the SNF certification process.

The Commission on Accreditation of Rehabilitation Facilities (CARF) recently acquired the Continuing Care Accreditation Commission (CCAC) and became the only accrediting body for continuing care retirement communities (CCRCs) and other types of aging services networks. This accreditation may be more important than that of skilled nursing facilities because the government's regulation of retirement communities and other networks of aging services are inconsistent.[5] Gather more information about these organizations at Sidebar 15.3.

Unique Features of Physical Therapy Practice in Skilled Nursing Facilities

Although the regulatory mandates they must follow are similar for most nursing home administrators, they may be for profit, nonprofit, or governmental organizations whose organizational structures vary widely from small, freestanding, proprietary homes to large, national nursing home corporations that include hundreds of nursing homes in many states. In those large multisite organizations, the value of the support provided by regional managers and

---

Sidebar 15.3

Accreditation of Long-Term Care

Go to the Web pages of The Joint Commission (http://www.jointcommission.org/Accreditation Programs/LongTermCare/) and CARF-CCAC (http://www.carf.org/) to learn more about their standards and goals.

corporate experts must be weighed against demands for conformity that affect decision-making authority, work incentives, the monitoring of operations, and the selection of employees. These issues filter down to the mid-level managers in each building.

These managers need to consider those factors that make the work of physical therapists and other professionals fulfilling and rewarding in long-term care, a setting that presents unique challenges related to the clinical management of elderly residents with chronic diseases, residents' needs for sophisticated postacute care, and complex regulatory demands. See Sidebar 15.4.

These large organizations provide upper-level management opportunities that may not be available in other health-care organizations. Perhaps more than any other setting, career ladders for advancement of rehabilitation professionals present themselves frequently in long-term care. Opportunities to assume responsibility for interprofessional teams that extend beyond the typical rehabilitation team also are possibilities.

The Care Team in Skilled Nursing Facilities

Probably the most striking characteristic of SNFs is the shift in the major responsibility of the care of residents from a physician to the professional caregivers. All residents have a physician of record who certifies the decisions of the team, and there is a medical director hired by the SNF (often a part-time position) with administrative and leadership responsibility for the provision of quality clinical services.

A physician or physicians' group with responsibility for many residents in a particular nursing home,

---

Sidebar 15.4

Characteristics of Work in Skilled Nursing Facilities

✦ Involvement with comprehensive care in interprofessional teams, which presents many opportunities for professional interaction and mentoring within and among disciplines.

✦ Focus on residents' functional abilities and their independence to maintain quality of life.

✦ Rewards associated with accomplishing significant outcomes with complex residents who are appreciative of the work of the rehabilitation team.

✦ Focus on education and assistance for paid and family caregivers to establish specific programs for residents. Extended interactions often lead to a sense of being part of the family, particularly during discharge planning.

✦ Challenges of transferring resident care to family members who may be either unwilling or unable to assist with a person's complex conditions.

✦ Ability to implement and follow through a comprehensive plan of care from beginning to end with a great deal of autonomous decision making.

✦ Opportunities to raise awareness of the importance of patient safety and optimum aging.

✦ Many opportunities to expand clinical expertise with complex patients, develop new programs, and improve marketing skills.

✦ Demanding paperwork and documentation of patient contact time.

✦ Spurts of high activity and downtime over the course of a day because of difficulties in scheduling treatment sessions, because of the high demands placed on nursing staff to ready residents for therapy sessions and conflicts with other patient activities.

✦ High-productivity demands while meeting multiple guidelines for compliance and reimbursement that may seem to conflict.

✦ Dependence on CNAs and activity coordinators for carryover of rehabilitation programs into daily routines.

✦ Challenges of caring for residents with dementia whose behavior may be disruptive.

✦ Time required to meet strict regulatory demands to assure that the environment and care are in compliance.

✦ High-staff turnover across all disciplines.

may assign either a nurse practitioner or physician assistant as the person who coordinates the care of their residents on a regular basis and reports back to the physician(s). Physicians who have been conspicuously absent in the day-to-day management of residents in nursing homes may now conduct weekly rounds in a building. Involvement of medical directors in direct patient care beyond mere attendance at quarterly meetings of the board of directors continues to increase.

Along with nursing managers, managers of rehabilitation services use care plan meetings to represent their staffs in making interprofessional decisions about each resident's care. In larger centers, managers may monitor and evaluate the decisions of their staffs in this care planning. Despite the many regulations that are often restrictive and burdensome for the organization, physical therapists have high levels of autonomy in their clinical decision making with regard to the levels of care provided and the details of the daily management of residents—many of whom are acutely ill with complex problems.

Therapists also have increased responsibility, either independently or in consultation with nursing, for clinical decisions about immediate actions to be taken when unexpected responses to care occur, or when there is an unexplained decline in a resident's medical status. Managers have a major responsibility for assuring that therapists are prepared for these higher expectations and demands for their expertise. Important decisions about residents' overall potential for rehabilitation and their safety are at stake. Therapists in these settings are less likely to be able to rely on rapid decision making of physicians when clinical concerns or medical emergencies arise. Instead, physicians rely more heavily on the expertise and daily contact that therapists and nurses have with residents as they make their medical decisions.

Managers also have an important role in evaluating information on applicants for potential admission to a facility. Making judgments about who gains admission to the SNF is probably a more important managerial responsibility here than in any other type of health-care setting. The people who are admitted influence all aspects of resource management. An accurate prediction about the resident's potential utilization of those resources is crucial in accomplishing positive clinical outcomes with the least financial impact on the organization.

Regardless of the organizational structure, nursing home operations rely heavily upon dependable staff members who are flexible and responsive to regulatory changes, particularly because of the punitive nature of their regulatory system. The increase in regulatory demands combined with limited reimbursement opportunities result in a lack of resources to pay competitive wages for the direct caregivers. Performing a difficult, demanding, nonglamorous job for low compensation does not reflect the value of these caregivers in health care. This workforce issue is one of the major management challenges of long-term care.[3]

Rehabilitation Professionals and Certified Nursing Assistants

Another important responsibility of rehabilitation service managers in skilled nursing facilities is establishing strong working relationships with certified nursing assistants (CNAs) who, under the direction of licensed nursing personnel, interact with residents at a higher frequency and intensity than any other care provider. Underestimating the important role that CNAs play in the management of the facility, and in the lives of the residents they care for, may result in major setbacks in meeting the goals of the rehabilitation services and the planned outcomes for residents.

CNAs can make or break a nursing home because the care they provide determines the carryover needed to achieve the optimum level of care for each resident, which leads to financial success for the organization. The reported feelings of CNAs that they are undertrained, overworked, and underappreciated seem incongruent with their importance. This incongruence is likely to be reflected in their dissatisfaction and decreased efforts, not to mention the high turnover among this staff. The secondary effect is, of course, lack of continuity of care and dissatisfied residents and families that may have serious repercussions for the SNF.[6]

Particularly as the acuity level of residents in SNFs increases, rehabilitation managers may play an increased role in preparing CNAs for their expanded responsibilities. These responsibilities often involve increased emotional and physical work demands with residents who have more complex medical, emotional, and cognitive problems. Recommending and participating in programs that encourage increased involvement of CNAs in identifying barriers to their work and encouraging their recommendations should be considered. Having CNAs participate in discussions to solve problems rather than listening to lectures to be told what to do about problems alone may be an effective strategy. The involvement of rehabilitation staff in collaboration agreements with local technical schools and the development of in-house training programs are other options for strengthening the care team.

Rehabilitation professionals are dependent upon CNAs to reach their patient outcome goals in two important ways. Without the efforts of CNAs to assist them in bathing, dressing, and feeding, residents are not ready to participate in rehabilitation sessions. If residents are not attending therapy, the ability of therapists to reach their frequency and duration goals for reimbursement is compromised. Without the cooperation of CNAs, patient follow-through of exercise or activities to reinforce their rehabilitation progress is not accomplished and clinical outcomes are not achieved.

Realizing the physical effort required of CNAs to lift and bathe many residents who may be hostile and confused and resistant to the care they need, physical therapists can establish a mutually beneficial relationship. Helping CNAs understand and redirect behaviors based on cognitive and functional ability may dramatically affect outcomes. Assisting CNAs to care for *specific* residents through demonstration and education enables them to contribute more effectively to the quality of care and rehabilitation of their assigned patients.

CNAs often face constant demands and even abuse from some residents with severe cognitive limitations. They may be so involved with behavior issues that it is no surprise that time and attention to established protocols or new interventions often is not available. Physical therapists can play a major role in making their jobs easier. Simply by asking their opinions and including them in decisions made about the people they care for can dramatically affect their difficult work.[6] This collaboration leads to CNAs who are able to work smarter, not harder and physical therapists with access to important information about residents that only CNAs know because of their intimate 24/7 contact with them.

Rehabilitation Professionals and Family Education

Perhaps more than any other setting, family involvement is a critical component of rehabilitation in SNFs. Often the key determinant for whether the patient returns home or transfers to a residential care setting is the family. The following factors influence the affect family education may have on the achievement of rehabilitation outcomes:[7]

+ Family's knowledge, attitudes, and skills including physical capabilities
+ The physical therapist's ability, willingness, and skills to involve family members
+ The family's relationship with the patient before the injury or disability
+ The availability and opportunity of family members to be involved
+ The cognitive status of the patient (the more impaired, the more family involvement required)
+ Multiple formal and informal avenues for family training (support groups, home visits, "open-door" policy visiting hours, and scheduling changes)

Although these factors are evident in any practice setting, rehabilitation managers in SNFs perhaps face the greatest challenges in family education because their patients rely on it the most. Residents in SNFs often have cognitive deficits and complex medical problems requiring them to have more assistance from family members, whether they return to their homes or they are admitted to residential care. These family members, particularly spouses and adult children, may also be elderly with cognitive and physical challenges of their own that can limit their ability to assist. Convincing caregivers of the residents' limitations, as well as their own, is often the most important first step. Managers are responsible for assuring that the abilities and limitations of family members are accurately assessed to reduce the exposure to lawsuits because of inappropriate discharge planning.

If family members have the cognitive and physical ability to assist, they are often available and likely to be involved in family education and the direct care of residents in SNFs. Managers need to be aggressively proactive in creatively establishing a variety of means for including family members in the rehabilitation process at every opportunity, and advocating for the inclusion of rehabilitation staff in educational programs in other services. The start-ing point may be staff development to improve the skills of therapists so they effectively include families in their interventions and goal setting for residents. In return, therapists may feel gratified by the effect they have had on a family's ability to care for a loved one.

Part 2
Management Issues

Overview of Management in Long Term Care

The number of SNFs with less than 50 certified beds is about the same as the number with 200 beds or more.[2] (Note: Bed is the term used to identify the space available for a patient who will be admitted for Medicare services under Part A.) More than any other factor, the size of the nursing home and the number of beds certified by Medicare and Medicaid determines the model for rehabilitation services in a SNF. Because of the increased need for skilled care for elderly, complex patients, it is now more common for a nursing home to have all of its patient beds certified as Medicare beds rather than a mix of skilled and nonskilled units. Some examples of managerial roles for physical therapists in SNFs include:

✦ Traditional director of physical therapy services in a larger SNF (rarely seen because the number of discipline-specific managers has decreased).

✦ Interprofessional director with responsibility for all disciplines in a rehabilitation service of a SNF. The director may be a physical therapist assistant or occupational therapy assistant in efforts to reduce costs, or because therapists are simply unavailable.

✦ Area manager for rehabilitation services with responsibilities for several staffs and patient care in multiple facilities (5–10) of a national chain of SNFs. Regional managers may have similar duties as area managers but for more buildings (15–20). As part of the management team, responsibilities also may include contributions to decisions related to the organization as a whole and interpretation of outcomes and other data. They may report to a vice president who is the manager for several states. Clinical specialists for each rehabilitation profession at the corporate level may advise and consult area and regional managers about clinical issues.

✦ Solo physical therapist, employed in a smaller SNF with all patient care and managerial responsibilities.

✦ The director of rehabilitation in a large teaching hospital who is responsible for all aspects of physical therapy services provided in the hospital's SNF and all other inpatient and outpatient units. The larger the organization, the more likely unit supervisors manage the day-to-day operations of these units. They may have some flexibility in shifting staff among units, as staffing needs demand.

✦ Owners of private practices who contract with nursing homes to provide services and coordinate assignments of physical therapists who may have a mix of outpatient and SNF care duties.

✦ Managers of contract therapy service companies whose responsibilities may include negotiating contracts for assignment of physical therapists in any of the above settings.

✦ Physical therapists who are consultants to groups of SNFs. They monitor physical therapy or rehabilitation services, train staff in interprofessional models, and advise administrators.

Managerial responsibilities, because of the organizational differences in SNFs, may vary widely. They may include responsibility not only for clinical outcomes but also for budgets, quality control, marketing, and customer satisfaction in one or more buildings. The availability of managers and their contact with the staffs they supervise may range from constant and predictable to long-distance and intermittent. Their level of involvement with direct patient care also contributes to the extent of their managerial role. Managers in long-term care may be in the trenches of patient care, which may reduce the time they have to spend on managerial responsibilities.

At the other extreme, managers may be so far removed from observing or participating in direct patient care, that their managerial role becomes top-down rather than bottom-up as they focus on profitability, the oversight of budgets, and the development of managers in their assigned buildings rather than direct patient care. Striking the balance of these two extremes is often a challenge for SNF managers in their responsibilities for high-quality rehabilitation services that comply with all regulatory demands.

Management Responsibilities

Mission, Vision, and Goals

Rehabilitation managers need to participate in the creation, or regular review, of the mission and vision of SNFs so that the role of contemporary rehabilitation practices is soundly incorporated. As health-care policy changes, opportunities for identifying and clarifying the role of rehabilitation in the goals of SNFs lie with managers. They must collaborate with nursing home administrators and directors of nursing as SNFs take on these regulatory and philosophical challenges.

Managers may need to identify a variety of means for transforming the mission and vision into action and for demonstrating the link between the goals of the organization and the day-to-day responsibilities of rehabilitation professionals. Particularly at times of organizational change, managers need to be particularly diligent in transitioning changes in mission and goals into the behaviors of staff. Reconciling potential conflicts between professional responsibilities and the demands that set the culture of the organization may be of particular importance to managers in SNFs, particularly for those in for-profit corporations.

In a typical scenario, a large national corporation purchases a small, independent nursing home that is providing private, residential care. All of the beds are converted to certified Medicare beds, which immediately places higher demands on all of the staff for documentation and a high level of quality of care as required by the newly implemented Medicare regulations. A rehabilitation manager in this situation needs strategies for transitioning from the former philosophy of care (nurses taking care of people) to a rehabilitation philosophy of setting care plan goals for the highest level of function for each resident. Managers need to take the initiative to identify regulatory changes and modify policies and procedures, often before the ink is dry on those just implemented. As visions and missions are revised, resolving potential conflicts between corporate directives and professional practice guidelines also may require close monitoring by managers.

Policies and Procedures

Policies and procedures that clarify roles and responsibilities become especially important when care is interdisciplinary. Implementing regulations rather than establishing policies and procedures is more of the role of managers in SNFs. Again, being held accountable for regulations and rules for which they had no input during development can lead to managerial frustrations.

If the SNF contracts with an outside agency to provide rehabilitation services rather than hiring its own staff, those contract managers may have additional burdens in sorting out competing or contradictory priorities of the contracting agency and the SNF. The agency's policies and procedures that bind their employees regardless of where they are assigned, must be reconciled with the policies and procedures of the SNF, and with the less formal culture of the organization. Identifying where loyalties lie, and should lie, may be difficult.

Marketing

Rehabilitation managers may have many opportunities to contribute to program development in SNFs that are part of large corporations, or they may have to take the initiative in program development in smaller SNFs. Identifying niche markets to target particular groups of patients for systematic, well-defined programs to meet their specific needs is one commonly used marketing strategy. People with memory deficits are one example of a target market. SNFs may also focus on marketing their homelike environments with attention to meeting individual needs. In either case, rehabilitation managers are usually considered part of the marketing team. They need to be prepared to market rehabilitation services and their centers aggressively because of the competition with other SNFs and other types of long-term care services.

Even if initially driven primarily by health-care policy changes, nursing home administrators increasingly rely on rehabilitation managers. They assist the SNF in attracting appropriate patients for skilled care through promoting strong relationships with referral sources, optimizing patient outcomes, and identifying niche markets. Managers need to advocate for appropriate utilization of rehabilitation services and, as importantly, identify new services that may be offered.

Nursing personnel have traditionally dominated long-term care, so managers of other services need to take every opportunity to consider nursing staff as a target market as well. A great deal of progress has been made in SNFs as nurses, who are very comfortable in the medical model of care because of its focus on treatment of disease, transition to a rehabilitation way of thinking and decision making. Shifting to care that centers on improving patients' function regardless of their diagnoses becomes critical. Rehabilitation managers are better positioned as key players in skilled nursing care as a result.

Staffing

Staff turnover is probably the biggest issue for SNF managers. The cost of recruiting, selecting, interviewing, checking credentials, and orienting a new employee may far exceed the monthly salary of an employee. Therefore, managers are compelled to retain employees as much as they need to hire additional employees. Retention becomes increasingly important during growth periods. When competition for qualified employees is high, workforce demands and turnover increase simultaneously.

Avoiding turnover is especially crucial in long-term care because of its effect on elderly residents who come to rely heavily on their caregivers. They do not tolerate changes in personnel very well. New employees face the additional challenges of attempting to adhere to the routine of the usual, consistent care that many people depend on to function at their optimal levels.

Meeting workforce needs with temporary workers may be more problematic than helpful in long-term care because these employees lack the history of care and knowledge of the complex conditions and idiosyncrasies of residents. This places the SNF at a higher risk for errors in judgment in caring for residents. A vicious cycle of losing personnel because of the errors that occur, followed by more errors made by their replacements, can be difficult to break.

Rehabilitation professionals accepting positions as traveling therapists is common during times of workforce shortages. They are offered short-term assignments (e.g., 6 to 13 weeks) that offer high salaries and the opportunities for a wide range of experiences. Because managers know that the end of their assignment is always near, any professional and behavioral performance issues may not be addressed effectively. The added expense of fees paid to agencies to be able to provide these services may be high but unavoidable. The alternative—recruitment costs for full-time, permanent staff—is another important financial consideration for nursing homes as they seek to provide the quality of care and the quality of life that the residents deserve.

Supportive Personnel

State statutes guide administrative rules about the role of licensed physical therapist assistants and other supportive personnel in SNFs. In some states, physical therapist assistants may work in a SNF without a requirement that a physical therapist be on-site. Although this level of direction and supervision may be legal, managers need to determine the roles of assistants by considering the levels of complexity and acuity of patients' conditions, and the expertise of particular assistants. The more unstable and unpredictable a patient's condition is, the less appropriate it may be for physical therapists to direct others to perform interventions independently. Having responsibility for decisions about each resident at any point in time, therapists must know and trust the skills and knowledge of the assistants that they direct and supervise, particularly if they are not always on-site when the physical therapist assistant is.

At the same time, to remain efficient and control costs, determining the appropriate utilization of physical therapist assistants, and hiring them, is critical to managing physical therapy services. Clarification of the duties and responsibilities for provision of care and reporting of that care to the physical therapist of record is necessary to reduce the risk of adverse physiological responses of patients with complex conditions. The strengths and weaknesses of physical therapist assistants should not be assumed any more than the strengths and weaknesses of physical therapists should be assumed.

Because of the risks inherent in the SNF population, the direction of lesser level personnel than the physical therapist assistant should be limited to non-treatment responsibilities like maintenance of the environment, transport of patients, running errands, filing, and assisting with other managerial requirements. Should they be included in patient care, considering them as an extra set of hands to assist during treatment sessions is probably the most appropriate view of these tasks.

Managers should consider how valuable the physical therapist assistant might be in family education and teaching CNAs and other caregivers. Providing one-on-one instruction and classroom instruction may be a vital role for assistants. These assignments result in the ability of therapists to attend to the complex clinical decisions that need to be made in one-on-one direct patient care.

Perhaps more than any other setting, SNFs provide physical therapist assistants a wide range of upward career opportunities as they engage in other administrative duties, and the opportunity to develop strong clinical skills with complex patients in what may be considered a specialty practice for them. For instance, because of workforce shortages, it may be that assistants are the managers of rehabilitation services because of their administrative skills and expertise. Perhaps they may be the most senior person on staff because of the turnover of therapists or the percentage of staff who are temp or traveling therapists.

These managers who are assistants may have the administrative expertise but lack the clinical expertise for some difficult decision making about the care of patients. They must assure that physical therapists and other therapists are *not* deferring these important clinical decisions to them just because of the positions they hold. Assistants in these positions need to stop and check that they are not practicing physical therapy without a license by consistently separating their managerial duties from their patient care duties, which must be under the direction and supervision of a licensed physical

therapist. Shifting from "being the boss of" clinically to "being bossed by" the same person requires physical therapists to clarify roles and responsibilities carefully.

This unusual dynamic may be another reflection of the change in health-care managers who are expected to deal with financial and staffing rather than clinical practice issues. Managers in positions that include supervision of staff from many professions are required to be health-care–discipline neutral in their managerial decision making. It may be helpful for physical therapist assistants to remain neutral as well in physical therapy clinical decisions. The potential for gaps in the need for professionals to have role models and mentors in their clinical decision making is at risk in these models.

Patient Care

Reimbursement is tightly intertwined in patient/client management in SNFs, resulting in patient care decisions that have a direct impact on tight financial circumstances. In addition to this complicating financial factor, managers have to be certain that therapists are well prepared for evaluating the physiological effects of their direct interventions on the complex conditions of their patients. Close monitoring during treatment sessions is essential to reduce the risk of harm to patients. Therapists in SNFs also must be cognizant of the impact of their choice of interventions on the psychosocial needs of patients who may find it difficult to learn new motor tasks, or who may be struggling with the losses they experience because of a serious illness. See Sidebar 15.5.

Prospective Payment in SNFs

Assuring that evidence-based interventions are used to achieve patient goals efficiently, within a discipline

---

Sidebar 15.5

MEDQIC

Explore this Web page for more insight into quality issues in SNFs and other health-care settings at http://medqic.org/dcs/ContentServer? pagename=Medqic/MQPage/Homepage or among disciplines that provide care to a resident, is paramount because of the prospective payment system imposed on SNFs. Complying with established plans of care and projecting the number of minutes/day that patients must receive skilled therapy services are required for payment of services. Plans of care are based on standardized assessments of patients using the MDS. The skill involved in compliance with regulations in this process is as important as the delivery of appropriate, effective interventions themselves. Additional information on this complex payment system can be found on the Web pages referred to in the sidebars. They should be referred to frequently because of ongoing modifications that require new action. Current highlights of this complex payment system are presented here.[8]

✦ The Medicare Part A prospective payment for care provided by SNFs is based on a per diem rate/patient admitted. This base rate bundles the payment for all services. The rates are established and reviewed regularly by the federal government to cover *all* costs of the nursing home, not just patient care. There are different rates for urban and rural nursing homes. See Sidebar 15.6.

✦ The base per diem rates are adjusted for each patient based the results of the Resident Assessment Instrument (RAI) that includes the MDS triggers, Resident Assessment Protocols (RAPs), and utilization (treatment time) guidelines. The RAI is intended to be completed by an interprofessional team (i.e., dieticians, therapists, nurses, pharmacists, etc.). The RAI scores determine the case mix for each patient and

the wages for providers at the level of skilled care (time) required to provide the care a particular patient needs.

✦ The case mix and time adjustment is based on a classification system, the Resource Utilization Groups III (RUGs). Each patient's RUG is determined by the data generated by each member of the care team as entered into the standardized MDS that must be signed by a nurse—typically with the title of MDS coordinator. The MDS data may trigger one or more of the 18 resident assessment protocols (RAPs) that lead to more assessment of potential problem areas. Typically, different sections of the MDS are assigned to different members of the team. Go to the Web page in Sidebar 15.7 to gain a better understanding of this important documentation.

✦ This MDS reimbursement requirement also affects the quality of care by requiring a thorough evaluation of each patient (resident) with this standardized, comprehensive, and reproducible assessment. It improves communication within the facility and among facilities because everyone is speaking the same language. This reimbursement/quality approach is designed to prevent the avoidable decline of patients and build upon their current strengths to improve their quality of life through high-quality care.

✦ Assuring that there are no inconsistencies or contradictions in the MDS among the data generated by different team members is critical for accurate determination of each patient's case-mix RUG group. Rehabilitation managers are included in this decision making for each patient admitted to a nursing home. Identifying all factors that may qualify patients to the highest RUG level is important to the financial stability of the nursing home. They cannot

---

Sidebar 15.6

Prospective Payment in Skilled Nursing Facilities

To learn more about the complexity of prospective payment, see http://www.cms.hhs.gov/SNFPPS/ and the chart at http://www.cms.hhs.gov/SNFPPS/Downloads/3ruralchart.pdf, which presents the services that Medicare pays for and how they must be billed in rural hospitals. This information reflects how hospitals deal with designated swing beds, which may serve as nursing homes within the hospital.

Sidebar 15.7

MDS

Go to http://www.cms.hhs.gov/NursingHome QualityInits/downloads/MDS20MDSAllForms.pdf to view the MDS with particular attention to Section G and the list of RAPS.

afford to provide more care than they will be reimbursed for, so the determination of the level of care that will be required must be accurate. The skill and knowledge to contribute to this process is important for managers to develop.

✦ The 53 RUG III classifications that are most important to the nursing home because of their higher levels of per diem rates of reimbursement just happen to be those that involve the patient's need for rehabilitation services. See Table 15.2 for examples of RUGs.

✦ To which of the 53 levels of the RUG classifications a patient is assigned determines, for example, the services a patient will receive and the number of minutes that must be met for each therapy service. This assignment has serious implications for rehabilitation managers who are responsible for staff compliance to these reimbursement requirements. The Centers for Medicare and Medicaid developed the Data Assessment and Verification (DAVE) project to determine the accuracy of data submitted. See Sidebar 15.8 for tips on coding and documentation compliance issues related to therapy minutes.

✦ The data from individual patient MDSs is transmitted to centralized databanks in each state that are then forwarded to a national database at the CMMS and analyzed and used in the measurement of outcome-based quality improvement criteria. See Sidebar 15.9.

Sidebar 15.8

DAVE

Go to https://www.qtso.com/download/mds/DAVE_TipSheet_Section%20P1b%20Therapies_March%202005.pdf for information on therapy minutes.

Sidebar 15.9

Quality Outcomes

Go to http://www.cms.hhs.gov/NursingHome QualityInits/01_Overview.asp for more information on quality initiatives.

Nursing Rehabilitation

At the other end of the spectrum of long-term care is the managerial responsibility for nursing rehabilitation (restorative care services) that are provided to individual patients in residential care. The rehabilitation manager has responsibility for assuring that all patients in residential care are walking and exercising to maintain their maximal level of performance for as long as possible. Educating CNAs to perform these activities as part of their routine care of patients, and reinforcing the need for group physical activity as part of the center's activity programs are other ways that rehabilitation managers have a major impact on positive patient outcomes. As the medical management of chronic diseases increases in importance, the sophistication and consistency of restorative care must improve accordingly.

Fiscal

Historically, reimbursement policies have shaped the delivery of therapy services in all practice settings. SNFs may face some unique challenges in assuring that documentation of care matches the billing for that care. The care is very interdisciplinary yet the documentation and billing are discipline unique. In addition, *actual* time spent in treatment *must* be accurately reflected in the documentation because billing is based on time to meet current Medicare requirements. Regulatory surveys include review of billing documentation that leads to review of clinical documentation to support the claims for reimbursement.

To assure consistency and accuracy, decreasing the number of different providers who work with any particular patient increases the likelihood that there will be agreement among treatment notes, weekly progress notes, and billing sheets; and better coordination of care among disciplines. Management accountability for accurate reporting may require ongoing audits of documentation and billing. This important responsibility reduces the risks of payment denials and provides the opportunity to identify treatment activities that may not be assigned easily to a particular billing category. Avoiding documentation of activities that overlap with that of other professions is another possible area of concern that calls for clarification so that records and billing forms are both accurate. Therapists expect, rightfully so, that managers will assist in these important responsibilities because accountability for documenting and billing stops with the individual providing the care.[9]

TABLE 15.2   RUGs Examples

RUG LEVEL REHABILITATION/ NURSING	PATIENT REQUIREMENT	REHABILITATION MINUTES AND DISCIPLINES	TYPICAL PATIENT	ACTIVITIES OF DAILY LIVING (ADL) INDEX AND RUG CODES FROM MDS*
Ultrahigh/Extensive	IV, tracheotomy, ventilator, or suctioning in last 14 days. Feeding tube, Nil per os (NPO) orders, parenteral fluids in last 7 days.	720 minutes or more of rehabilitation/ week. One rehabilitation discipline 5 days/ week and another 3 days/week.	People with neurological diagnoses who were independent with excellent rehabilitation potential to return home or to lower level of care.	16–18 RUX 7–15 RUL *If ultrahigh without extensive nursing then:* *16–18 RUC9–15 RUB* *4–8 RUA*
Very High/Extensive	Same	500 or more minutes. At least one rehabilitation discipline for at least 5 days.	People with cerebral vascular accident, joint replacement, new condition that required limited assistance with very good rehabilitation potential to return home or lesser level of care.	16–18 RVX 7–15 RVL *If very high without extensive nursing then:* *16–18 RVC* *9–15 RVB* *4–8 RVA*
High/Extensive	Same	325 or more minutes of rehabilitation/ week. At least one rehabilitation discipline 5 days/ week.	Cerebral vascular accident, hip fracture, elective surgery who will likely be discharged to long-term care.	16–18 RVX 7–15 RVL *If very high without extensive nursing then:* *13–18 RHC* *6–12 RHB* *4–7 RHA*

* Go to http://www.cms.hhs.gov/SNFPPS/downloads/RUGDesSch.pdf for definitions of RUG codes.

Their fiscal responsibilities require that rehabilitation managers remain current in their understanding of Medicare/Medicaid rules and the frequent changes that occur. They must share this information not only with their staffs for implementation, but also with upper management to advise them of potential areas of risk— fraud, abuse, underutilization or overutilization of services.

Rehabilitation managers may not have responsibility for financial planning, but have input into budgeting decisions, particularly about capital equipment (typically for the expansion of services) and space allocation. They are often more accountable for implementing a budget than they are for developing it, and most frequently face decisions calling for a reduction in resources that have been allocated. Controlling costs, particularly workforce costs,

becomes a focus of managerial efforts. Finding the resources to cover important patient care–related functions that are directly billable also causes pressure, particularly in for-profit corporations, to maintain certain profit levels.

Legal, Ethical, and Risk

Long-term care is a high-risk environment because patients often have both cognitive deficits and complex medical conditions that require extended periods of care during which many variables impact their well-being or recovery. Attention to the rights and dignity of patients is paramount regardless of their ability to participate in their own care and decisions. This demand is the basis of the high level of responsibility that the staff in SNFs often holds for the care of the most vulnerable people in society. From the use of restraints to control patient mobility to living wills, the staffs in SNFs face major legal and ethical issues on a daily basis. Managers have a responsibility to question and understand the values of the people they supervise and thereby avert the potential for a failure to respect the dignity of or to violate the rights of the individuals they care for.

Delegation of skilled care to family members and other nonskilled paid helpers increases safety risks. The ramping down of therapy intervention toward discharge to a safe environment presents a variety of opportunities and legal challenges for managers. Managers are responsible for representing the rehabilitation perspective in comprehensive, interprofessional discharge planning that is needed for a smooth, *safe* transition to the next living environment. Identifying the potential risk factors and assuring that safety requirements can be met is a major responsibility.

Remaining rational and objective about safety when patients and family bear pressure because of their strong desire to return to their prior living situations often takes courage. Creative planning and the desire to help people with many barriers go home again make rehabilitation in SNFs rewarding and exciting. Managers who are able to convey the importance of this role and the satisfaction of these accomplishments may have one of the most powerful recruitment tools.

Communication

Because of the fast pace of the work in SNFs with residents who have needs that seem to never end, opportunities for informal conversation among staff may seem to occur rarely. Formal communication about patient care, however, is often mandated and documented in detail. Depending on the size of the SNF, staff may be grouped into teams that work in particular units with the same residents throughout the length of their care. This team model is effective in improving formal and informal communication. Because of the individualized, long-term needs of most residents, it is more effective for everyone taking care of a patient to meet about that particular patient than to gather caregivers together to discuss global, generic issues about patient care. These team or utilization meetings are formalized so that each discipline is represented as interprofessional decisions are made and documented about each patient's care.

Managers often feel that all they do is attend meetings. With the MDS coordinator, social worker, business office manager, admissions coordinator, and perhaps others, rehabilitation managers attend daily, supposedly brief, stand-up meetings. The topics for discussion typically include a review and updates of the census in the building (admissions and discharges), 24-hour nursing reports to report any patient incidents or problems, and reminders of days remaining in patient benefit periods. These meetings demonstrate the importance and urgency associated with controlling those factors that affect the finances of SNFs. Other meetings are necessary to assure accurate interprofessional completion and revision of the MDS for each patient.

Rehabilitation managers may have a great deal of interaction with the director of nursing (DON) in SNFs. They face many of the same issues. For instance, both are responsible for efficient utilization of staff and management of financial resources to provide care. They both are responsible for the day-to-day staffing and overall operations of their services. Developing and implementing plans of care are also shared responsibilities. DONs are often the right hand of nursing home administrators who may defer a great deal of decision making to them. Rehabilitation managers who establish a strong professional relationship with DONs may find that they are part of a powerful managerial team, particularly when the clinical problems are many and common to both disciplines.

Rehabilitation managers also may meet formally every day with the nursing home administrator. This frequency may vary depending on the role of the DON and the presence of assistant administrators in certain centers. Managers should not assume they would have the same direct working relationships with each nursing home administrator as they move from one building to another. These meetings typically include review of Medicare statistics, authorization for care of indigent patients or others with special needs, budgeting, marketing plans, and census building. Rather than direct responsibility for individuals in a nursing home, the administrator typically has the broader responsibility for the outcomes and profits of the nursing home as a whole.

As the size of SNFs continues to grow, managers have more opportunity to interact with larger staffs to monitor their performance both formally and informally. With the increased number of therapists in a building, new therapists can also receive a higher degree of mentoring and assistance with clinical decision making. Although inter-professional teams are paramount in long-term care, managers have more opportunity to facilitate the development of discipline-specific teams. These teams are able to apply and contribute to the evidence for patients with complex conditions and for chronic disease management expected in their professions. Promoting these professional interactions (e.g., journal clubs) either within a building or within an area where there are several facilities may be an important management tool.

Conclusion

Long-term care, more than any other component of health care, provides many management opportunities for physical therapists because of the breadth of services provided and the anticipated growth in the need for high quality services to manage chronic diseases among the elderly. The management of skilled nursing care today is similar to the management of acute care hospitals in the past in terms of the variety of clinical learning experiences and opportunities for upward career mobility. Managers may need to focus on the transfer of these exciting characteristics to the long-term care setting to improve the recruitment of therapists who often have negative preconceived notions to overcome.

Either through internal corporate-management programs or self-directed professional development, physical therapists and assistants may prepare themselves for careers in long-term care at a variety of levels of care and management. They may anticipate new approaches in aging services that will continue to broaden the scope of physical therapy services. Such approaches are limited only by the imagination and initiative of managers. Activities 15.1 through 15.17 present scenarios for working through some long-term care management challenges.

REFERENCES

1. Pratt JR. *Long-Term Care: Managing Across the Continuum.* 2nd ed. Sudbury, MA: Jones and Bartlett Publishers; 2004.
2. National Center for Health Statistics. Health, United States, 2006 with chart book on trends in the health of Americans. Hyattsville, MD: Centers for Disease Control; 2006. Available at: http://www.cdc.gov/nchs/fastats/nursingh.htm. Accessed September 12, 2007.
3. McCarthy J, Friedman LH. The significance of autonomy in the nursing home administrator profession: A qualitative study. *Health Care Management Review.* 2006;31:55–63.
4. National Long-Term Ombudsman Resource Center. OBRA '87 Summary. Available at: http://www.ltcombudsman. org/ombpublic/49_346_1023.cfm. Accessed September 12, 2007.
5. Commission on Accreditation of Rehabilitation Facilities. Who we are. Available at: http://www.carf.org/consumer. aspx?content=content/About/News/boilerplate.htm. Accessed November 1, 2007.
6. Hill RD. *Geriatric Residential Care* Mahwah, NJ: Lawrence Erlbaum Associates, Inc.; 2002.
7. Ryan NP, Wade JC, Nice A, et al: Physical therapists' perceptions of family involvement in the rehabilitation process. *Physiotherapy Research International.* 1996;1(3), 157–179.
8. Department of Health and Human Services. Prospective payment system and consolidated billing for skilled nursing facilities-update-notice. Available at: http://www.cms.hhs. gov/snfpps/downloads/cms-1530-n-display.pdf. Accessed November 16, 2007.
9. Erhart A, Delehanty LM, Morley NE, et al: Consistency between documented occupational therapy services and billing in a skilled nursing facility: A pilot study. *Physical & Occupational Therapy in Geriatrics.* 2005:24(2), 53–62.

ACTIVITY 15.1
PATIENTS OR CLIENTS

Are the people who receive rehabilitation services in skilled nursing homes more like patients or clients as defined by the American Physical Therapy Association? Defend your answer in a group discussion. What difference does it make?

ACTIVITY 15.2
THE MANAGEMENT TEAM IN SNFs

Pleasant Valley Care Center is a 200-bed skilled nursing facility with one wing of 30 beds for nonskilled residential care. Sam Simmons, administrator; Rebecca Romano, director of nursing; and Louise Lopez, director of rehabilitation, meet every Monday for 1 hour to brainstorm and solve one selected problem.

The issue that continues to be unresolved is the decline in the quality of care on weekends. Despite efforts to provide consistent weekend staff from their per diem pool and to improve in the transfer of information from the weekday to the weekend staff, they have not been very successful. Resident, family, and staff complaints continue about what seems to be every aspect of care delivered on Saturdays and Sundays.

Sam is very concerned that these complaints will lead to noncompliance in several areas during the next state survey. He asks Rebecca and Louise to join him all day next Saturday and Sunday to identify the sources of this discontent. They agree that 24/7 means 24/7 consistently. Each of them agrees to develop a list of things to look for or ask during all three shifts on Saturday and Sunday. They will fine-tune and share their agenda on Friday before they gather data on the weekend. What should be on their final list of things to look for? What should be their approach for gathering information?

ACTIVITY 15.3
CMMS AND PHYSICAL THERAPY

Go to the CMMS Web pages and find the requirements for physical therapy services in certified SNFs at http://www.cms.hhs.gov/default.asp? How do they affect the management of rehabilitation services?

ACTIVITY 15.4
THE JOINT COMMISSION AND LONG-TERM CARE

Sam, Rebecca, and Louise at Pleasant Valley Care Center are at their weekly meeting (See Activity 15.2) discussing the pros and cons of seeking Joint Commission accreditation for Pleasant Valley. What are some of the questions they should ask? What other considerations they should take into account? Hint: Go to The Joint Commission Web page for more information.

ACTIVITY 15.5
THE WORK OF PHYSICAL THERAPY IN SNFs

Louise Lopez, the director of rehabilitation at Pleasant Valley Care Center, faces the challenge of high turnover among the rehabilitation staff with an average stay of only 6 months. Applicants often tell her that they would like to work in nursing homes because they like old people. However, she finds that they just do not understand the complexity of their patients' conditions and of the regulatory demands on their care. What should she do?

ACTIVITY 15.6
CNAs AND PHYSICAL THERAPY

Louise Lopez does not know what to do. Although her staff is scheduled to work 8-hour days, it seems that all the patients receiving therapy are treated between 10 a.m. and 2 p.m. The therapy areas are crowded and noisy during these hours and empty otherwise. Both patients and therapists feel rushed and the therapy rooms look like therapy mills rather than therapeutic settings. Her staff reports that patients are not ready to come to therapy any earlier and they are scheduled for other social activities in the afternoons. What should she do?

ACTIVITY 15.7
FAMILY EDUCATION

Louise Lopez, rehabilitation director at Pleasant Valley Care Center, has another issue to resolve. Although she sees many family members in the therapy rooms during treatment sessions, they seem to be observing rather than participating. She believes this contributes to the low rate of discharges to home. She is trying to decide whether to focus her energy on intensifying one-on-one family education or on developing family education classes. Which should she do? Why?

ACTIVITY 15.8
OWNERSHIP CHANGE

Robert O'Reilly has been the manager of rehabilitation services at Mountain Top Nursing Center, a SNF in rural Montana with 20 skilled and 30 residential beds, for 3 years. As the only physical therapist in the SNF, he has been responsible for all physical therapy services with the help of a full-time physical therapist assistant. He is also responsible for hiring and evaluating the occupational therapist and speech language pathologist who work on a per diem basis. He places great pride on his achievements in the development and incorporation of rehabilitation services in the SNF and on his strong work relationships with the nursing staff. Things could not be better.

The administrator/owner of Mountain Top calls a general staff meeting to announce that he has sold Mountain Top to All Nation Care, a nursing home corporation. Effective the first of the month, All Nation Care's transitional team will be at Mountain Top to conduct the transition process to the new ownership. He assures the staff that all changes will be for the better including across-the-board salary increases in anticipation of doubling the size of the facility. After the shock wears off, what questions should Robert prepare for his meeting with the All Nation Care's corporate coordinator of rehabilitation?

ACTIVITY 15.9
A PATIENT FALLS

Robert O'Reilly receives a call at home on Sunday morning from the licensed practical nurse (LPN) charge nurse on the north wing. She reports that while the physical therapist assistant and CNA were performing a transfer of Mrs. Langdon, requiring the maximum assist of two people from bed to chair, the patient fell. The LPN thinks that Mrs. Langdon's hip is fractured and wants to know what she should do. Fill in the blanks: Robert should_____immediately. He should also_____to prevent a similar incident in the future.

ACTIVITY 15.10
DUPLICATION OF SERVICES

When conducting his monthly audit of rehabilitation records, Robert O'Reilly notices that physical therapy and occupational therapy goals, interventions, and billing for several patients appear to be overlapped. How should he resolve this duplication of services? Why does it need to be resolved?

ACTIVITY 15.11
A NEW OPPORTUNITY

Seashore Pavilion is a 200-bed SNF that is completely Medicare/Medicaid certified. Tina Tirelli has just begun her position as director of physical therapy with a staff of 10 physical therapists and 10 physical therapist assistants. One of her challenges is the 16-bed state-funded pediatric unit for children with complex medical needs. None of the current staff is either willing or able to provide services to children and there is a hold on new hires. State funding of the unit is at risk if they do not comply with regulations regarding the provision of rehabilitation services to these children. What should she do?

ACTIVITY 15.12
A FULL RANGE OF SERVICES

Moonlight Bay is a large retirement community with a full range of social and medical services for its residents. Rehabilitation services are of concern to Janet Blackstone, the administrator. Although the staff in the SNF are employees of Moonlight Bay and residents of the community can receive outpatient rehabilitation services there, they often choose to go to other outpatient centers in the nearby town. Residents of the adult congregate living facility receive home care rehabilitation services through City Home Health, although home nursing care is provided by Moonlight Bay nursing staff. Concerned about the promise of continuity of care to the residents, she asks Robin Blessing, the director of rehabilitation at the SNF to explain how they reached this state of affairs and to propose a plan for keeping all rehabilitation services within the community. What should Robin's report include?

ACTIVITY 15.13
PATIENT PROGRESSION

Inez Roberts, PT is on the verge of tears as she meets with Robin Blessing, rehabilitation director. Inez reports that Karl Smith, the Physical Therapist Assistant, is impossible. Despite her warnings to Karl, he has often progressed a patient's exercise or weight-bearing without consulting with Inez first. None of the other therapists seems to have a problem with Karl.

Today was the last straw. Inez just received a call from an orthopedic surgeon who is outraged that his patient has been instructed to walk with more weight bearing than he ordered. As a result, the patient will require surgery to revise her total hip replacement. Karl has provided all of the patient's care in the last 2 weeks and only reported to Inez that the patient was doing well. Inez says she has had enough and plans to submit her resignation. What should Robin do?

ACTIVITY 15.14
PATIENT DIGNITY

Joanna Barnes is a physical therapist assistant with 6 years of experience in a large medical center where she rotated among inpatient and outpatient care. She accepted a position at Moonlight Bay Nursing and Rehabilitation Center. Robin Blessing, rehabilitation manager, has been very pleased with her clinical skills but is concerned, however, because Joanna, not in a malicious or hurtful way, often makes fun of patients with cognitive problems or who appear or behave oddly. The remarks and mimicking are funny, and her presence has lightened the mood of the rehabilitation department. Everyone really likes her. Robin, though, is concerned that she often crosses the line with some of her comments, which may be perceived as disrespectful with a disregard for a patient's dignity. She does not want to lose Joanna. What should she do?

ACTIVITY 15.15
TRAVELING THERAPISTS

Robin Blessing, rehabilitation manager at Moonlight Bay, has been promoted to area manager for six nursing homes in Manatino County. She discovers she has a completely new set of staffing issues. On one hand, she feels fortunate to have been able to establish a good relationship with USA Rehabilitation Travelers, and they have been providing a steady stream of competent therapists who typically work 6- or 13-week assignments in one of the nursing homes and then move out of the area.

She is reluctant to take them away from patient care to provide a solid, detailed orientation to the system (their patient skills are rarely an issue), but she finds that she is spending more time dealing with many daily issues that arise because of small misunderstandings about procedures or correcting their documentation and billing errors than she spends on anything else. She also feels like she is constantly in limbo because of this turnover. So does James Butler, the full-time physical therapist assistant in one of the centers who complains of constantly adjusting to new therapists for the 4 years he has been on staff. What should she do?

ACTIVITY 15.16
A CLINCAL AND FINANCIALCHALLENGE

Belinda Gentry, director of rehabilitation at Sea Shore Health and Rehabilitation Center, receives a call on Monday morning from the Executive Director, William Winters, requesting to meet with her today about a patient. When they meet, he asks Belinda if she had the opportunity to see the new patient Mr. Beasley, who was admitted over the weekend. Belinda reports that she had and that Mr. Beasley is a 66-year-old man, who has had a left total hip replacement. He was admitted on Saturday with orders for Physical Therapy and Occupational Therapy. Mr. Beasley was evaluated by a physical therapist on Saturday and an occupational therapist is in the process of completing her evaluation today.

William is pleased and asks Belinda for assurance that they will not miss the opportunity to capture the " reimbursement for Mr. Beasley at a RUG-level of Rehabilitation Ultrahigh. He has reviewed the monthly report and shares with Belinda the fact that utilization for the higher RUG levels of reimbursement has dropped by 25% and the average patient length of stay has declined by 4 days. He attributes these unfavorable numbers to the new therapy staff. He believes they are not seeking to treat patients aggressively enough, and they fail to strongly encourage patients to come to therapy. The bottom line, he tells Belinda, is that the therapy department is losing the nursing home money and he wants to know what she will do about it. How should Belinda respond? Does William have a valid concern? What action does Belinda need to take?

ACTIVITY 15.17
HELPING THE HELP

Keisha Williams has been a CNA at Sea Shore Health and Rehabilitation Center for about 1 year. She has been surprised at how much she enjoys her work and the people she is assigned to care for in the residential unit. She is very pleased that Belinda Gentry, the rehabilitation director has asked the director of nursing that she be assigned to the rehabilitation wing because she is so efficient and works so well with her patients.

Keisha tells Belinda that she is flattered and appreciates that her work has been recognized, but she is also concerned about the transfer. She feels her work will be harder physically and she doesn't know whether she likes the idea that there is so much patient turnover on the rehabilitation wing. What should Belinda do?

Chapter 16

Management Issues in Outpatient Centers

Learning Objectives

◆ Discuss components, characteristics, and types of contemporary outpatient care.
◆ Analyze key licensing, accreditation, and reimbursement requirements.
◆ Discuss contemporary outpatient practice issues (i.e., referrals, kickbacks, use of the term physical therapy, reimbursement limits, etc.).
◆ Analyze the work of physical therapists in outpatient centers.
◆ Determine the managerial roles and challenges to managerial responsibilities.
◆ Analyze managerial decision making in given outpatient situations.

Part 1
The Contemporary Setting

Overview of Outpatient Physical Therapy

Physical therapists have always provided care to persons in outpatient centers. Typically based in hospitals or physicians' offices in the early years of the profession, the emergence of nationwide rehabilitation corporations with the inception of the Medicare program in the 1960s and 1970s provided many additional outpatient employment opportunities for physical therapists. The advent of the Medicare program also led to another important outpatient development—private practices owned and managed by physical therapists as reimbursement policies made these opportunities attractive and lucrative.

Interest in outpatient physical therapy continues today. In the latest American Physical Therapy Association (APTA) practice survey of more than 45,000 physical therapists, 56% of them reported working in some type of outpatient setting.[1] In 2005, 11.9% of physical therapists who are APTA members identified themselves as full-time self-employed and 2.8% as part-time self-employed.[2] The private practice section of the APTA has about 4,000 members (about 5% of the total membership of the APTA).[3]

A shift from inpatient to outpatient care at all levels of health care also contributes to the self-employment of professionals. The more important factor, however, is that many physical therapists often find caring for outpatients with subacute and chronic musculoskeletal disorders more preferable than caring for patients with more acute, complex conditions found in all other practice settings. Currently, about three of every four patients in outpatient settings receive physical therapy services for musculoskeletal conditions.[2] This focus on outpatient care is supported by the fact that the 7,573 APTA-board–certified specialists are overwhelmingly certified in orthopedics (4,448), and sports (640).[4]

Medicare reimbursement policies also skew the patients to those with acute musculoskeletal problems or those who have had orthopedic surgery. Care for people with other diagnoses associated with chronic musculoskeletal or other complex medical conditions are less likely to receive outpatient services because of reimbursement policies. Therapists also may find it more difficult to develop goals for patients with chronic conditions if their potential for improvement is limited. These patients also tend to be sicker and find it less likely to make their way to an outpatient center on a regular basis.

Licensure, Certification, Regulation, and Accreditation

Regardless of the type of center, all outpatient physical therapy providers must be certified as individuals or as a group practice to be reimbursed for their services. Provider organizations are certified by agencies in each state to be either rehabilitation agencies or certified outpatient rehabilitation facilities (CORFs). These are complex certification processes. Simply stated, the difference between the two types of certification is in the services provided. A CORF must provide physician services, physical therapy, and psychological/vocational counseling. Typically, occupational therapy, and speech/language pathology also are included. A rehabilitation agency (or outpatient physical therapy facility) must provide services in an office, although it also may provide services in a patient's home. Minimum services required in a rehabilitation agency are physical therapy or speech/language pathology, and social or vocational counseling. Occupational therapy may be included.

The certification process involves an on-site survey and ongoing attention to recertification. In all cases, either the group or individuals also must seek approval of the appropriate Medicare carrier to obtain a provider number to bill Medicare for their services. See Sidebar 16.1.

> ### Sidebar 16.1
> #### Licensure
>
> See the State Operations Manual at http://www.cms.hhs.gov/manuals/downloads/som107ap_k_corf.pdf. Find the state agency responsible for certifications in your state and determine the requirements and process involved for both certified rehabilitation agencies and CORFs.

The Joint Commission on the Accreditation of Health Care Organizations (The Joint Commission) which accredits many types of health-care organizations, includes rehabilitation and outpatient physical therapy in its list of ambulatory care centers. The Commission on Accreditation of Rehabilitation Facilities (CARF) also accredits outpatient centers. Managers may be involved in preparations needed for unannounced on-site surveys by accrediting agencies as discussed in other chapters.

Contemporary Outpatient Issues

Turbulent changes in Medicare reimbursement policies have presented many hurdles for managers in all outpatient settings, and for independent practitioners in physical therapy in particular. These policies also influence the professional relationships between physical therapists and physicians. These relationships are generally and usually collaborative, ethical, and legal resulting in positive outcomes for many, many patients. However, three important issues may negatively affect this professional relationship. These are direct access of patients to the services of a physical therapist, physician self-referral, and kickbacks. Other issues related to reimbursement also are addressed in this chapter.

Direct Access

Efforts led by the American Physical Therapy Association (APTA) to influence state legislators to permit consumers direct access to physical therapists without physician referral through practice act rules have been very successful. However, it continues its lobbying efforts to convince members of Congress that Medicare payment for physical therapy services without physician referral should be allowed. Continued negotiations by the APTA with other private third-party payers about physician referral requirements for payment are equally difficult.

The inability of some patients to directly access physical therapy services without the referral from a physician may deny them the care they require to meet their functional needs. The need for a physician referral also places many independent outpatient practitioners at a competitive disadvantage with physician-based physical therapy services.

Without the resources available in large corporations, solo practitioners may also have more difficulty establishing referral relationships with physicians who are willing to refer patients to practices outside of their offices.

Practice Without Referral

Despite the legal ability to treat patients without physician referral, many physical therapists may not do so regardless of their work setting. One reason is reimbursement requirements discussed above. Another reason is their reluctance to give up the valued interactions they have with physicians in their clinical decision making. For instance, in a hospital-based outpatient practice, doctor-therapist interactions may be frequent and expected, because this communication is a strong part of an organizational culture that is physician-centered. Financial arrangements that hospitals have with physicians also may demand a referral relationship with its outpatient centers.

Identifying expectations for relationships with physicians on staff and developing strong relationships with physicians facilitates the transition of patients from one setting to the next within the hospital or health-care system. This communication responsibility is as important for hospital-based managers as developing a strong referral base is for managers in other outpatient settings.

Other outpatient therapists may feel that they lack the competence and skills for the independent decision making involved in the examination and evaluation of patients who have not seen a physician. Particularly when there is a need for diagnostic testing that is beyond physical therapists' scope of practice to order or interpret, there is some comfort in receiving physician referrals that include such important patient information. The ability to call a referring physician for more information is routine.

It is less routine for physical therapists to have relationships with physicians in the reverse. Patients with direct access to physical therapists may have suspicious findings discovered during their examinations that require further medical testing. It may be more difficult and time-consuming for physical therapists to make referrals to patients' physicians or to the most appropriate physician if a patient does not have a physician of record. Delays in the continuity of therapy services may result.

Self-Referral

Professional opposition to both referrals for profit and physician ownership of physical therapy services has been a long-standing legislative agenda item for the APTA. Such business relationships present a potential conflict of interest for physicians that may not be in the patient's best interest. They also may negatively affect the autonomy of physical therapists in their clinical decision making and in their fiduciary responsibilities to patients. Although the negative impact of self-referral on physical therapy autonomy and fiduciary responsibility may occur in *any* setting, the focus of the efforts of the APTA has been the provision of outpatient physical therapy Medicare services. The competitive disadvantage for physical therapists that results from self-referral, particularly for the independent practitioner, is difficult to overcome.

Physicians are in the position of "cherry-picking" patients who have the highest potential for the greatest reimbursement for their own practices. They also can exhaust a patient's benefits for outpatient rehabilitation services in their practices before referring them to another provider to continue service for patients to meet their therapeutic goals. Moreover, they may refer to other professionals only those patients who are the most difficult—financially or because of conditions that demand more treatment time. These financial and ethical issues fueled the development of federal legislation regarding self-referral.

Concern about the potential for the fraud and abuse inherent in self-referral, federal legislation, generally referred to as the "Stark Law," prohibits a physician from referring a Medicare patient to any organization for certain designated health services (i.e., laboratory services, radiology, physical therapy, etc.) if that physician holds a financial interest in that organization. See Sidebar 16.2. The Stark Law has been in effect in one phase or another for about 20 years with the inevitable development of exceptions to the prohibition of self-referral. The final Phase III of the Stark Law continues to refine this law to close loopholes and clarify financial relationship rules.

Probably the most important part of the complex and confusing Stark legislation for physical therapy managers has been the in-office ancillary services exceptions to self-referral. The resultant "rules" have evolved to include several conditions that must be

---

> ### Side Bar 16.2
> #### Physician Self-Referral
>
> Go to http://www.cms.hhs.gov/ Physician Self Referral/for more information on physician self-referral.

met for physicians to bill Medicare for physical therapy services provided in their offices. Essentially, the rule is that physicians are permitted to order and to provide physical therapy in their offices if it is ancillary to the medical services that they provide. Other criteria are that the services must be provided in the same building as the physicians' offices, and physicians no longer need to provide direct supervision of those services to be reimbursed.

To be paid, however, personnel who are identified by Medicare as providers of physical therapy must provide the services (i.e., physical therapists and physical therapists' assistants) and they must comply with state statutes regarding direction and supervision. Physicians may bill for these services under their Medicare provider numbers because they are ancillary services.

These employment arrangements raise several important concerns for physical therapy managers in physicians' offices. Establishing strong professional relationships with physicians in a practice is a key responsibility for a manager who must clarify and assure that the expertise of the physical therapists is respected. It is crucial so that the therapists' clinical decision making about specific patients is preserved. Simply following the specific, standard orders of the physicians must be avoided to assure autonomous decision making.

Because the physician's Medicare provider number and business office are used for processing physical therapy bills, physical therapy managers may have a higher responsibility for assuring the accuracy of claims submitted for reimbursement. Educating the business office staff about legal and ethical concerns that may override either contract agreements with Medicare carriers or office policies and procedures may be an ongoing primary managerial responsibility. Managers in this type of setting may need to be even more cautious about productivity goals and physician-established protocols for care that may be in the best interest of the practice rather than in the best interest of a particular patient.

Use of the Term *Physical Therapy*

It is possible that physicians may bill other non-Medicare health-care insurance companies for "physical therapy" that they either provide themselves, hire a physical therapist or physical therapist assistant to deliver, or direct nonlicensed staff to do. Because any health-care provider who is licensed to do so may bill Medicare using any current procedural terminology (CPT-4) code, they may treat patients using the interventions of heat, ultrasound, massage, exercise, etc. They often tell patients that they are receiving "physical therapy" although a physical therapist is not providing the care.

Using the term *physical therapy* exclusively to denote only those things that physical therapists do is another dilemma for the profession. Many of Medicare policies limiting access and reimbursement for outpatient services are linked to the high incidence of fraud and abuse in outpatient billing for the CPT codes most commonly used in treatment of musculoskeletal conditions—the 97000 series primarily. The problem continues to be that Medicare establishes the value of each CPT code in the Physician Fee Schedule but does not control or determine which health professionals bill for the services they provide using these codes. Medicare has assumed that all providers licensed to provide interventions that fall in the 97000 series are equally qualified to do so.

This means that physical therapists in private practice not only compete with other physical therapy outpatient providers in corporations and health-care systems, but they also compete with chiropractors, physicians, and any other provider who may directly bill for 97000 interventions. Sorting out which of these practitioners may be responsible for the fraud and abuse associated with the billing for CPT codes in the 97000 series remains elusive. The initiation of the National Provider Identification Standard may help to clarify this situation by identifying who is actually providing care billed for, and allow comparisons of different types of practitioners.[6] See Sidebar 16.2A.

Kickbacks

The Stark Law should not be confused with the Medicare and Medicaid Patient Protection Act of 1987, commonly called the "Anti-Kickback Statute," which was passed to address compensation arrangements that had the potential to adversely affect clinical decision making and lead to unfair competition. Simply put, this law prohibits the *offer or receipt* of any kickback, bribe, or rebate directly or indirectly in the form of cash or in kind for referrals by physicians (or their recommendations to purchase or lease supplies and services) of patients insured under Medicare and Medicaid.

Violation of the Anti-Kickback Statute is a criminal offense and it has been enforced to a greater degree than the Stark Law, a civil statute, which relies more on whistle blowing than criminal investigations to identify violators. Like the exceptions in the Stark Law, there are revisions of the Anti-Kickback Statute that identify safe harbors that exempt certain forms of kickbacks. See Sidebar 16.3. Managers seeking to widen their referral base must be careful to comply not only with these federal statutes related to Medicare and Medicaid patients but also antikickback statutes in their states, which may apply more generally to all types of patient referrals.

Despite these legislative solutions to serious problems, the current reimbursement system continues to support the positions that physicians hold in health-care decision making, and reflects their ability to lobby Congress for policies that favor their practices financially. Physicians also have the advantage of their positions of power and influence over patients. Although many people are more interested and skillful in gathering and analyzing information about their health-care choices, the impression is that most people continue to rely on and trust the recommendations of their physicians, although these recommendations may be influenced by other factors rather than the best interest of the patient.

Sidebar 16.2 A

National Provider Identification Standard

Go to http://www.cms.hhs.gov/nationalprovidentstand/for more information on this program.

Sidebar 16.3

Kickbacks

Go to http://oig.hhs.gov/fraud/safeharborregulations.html for information from the Office of the Inspector General on antikickback safe harbors.

Changing this patient dependence on physicians requires not only managerial strategies but also strategies for the physical therapy profession as a whole. Managers are faced with almost daily decisions about how much of their efforts should focus on "working the system" rather than changing it to achieve some of their most important business goals.

Reimbursement Limitations

Lobbying efforts also have been directed to reversing the implementation of an annual financial limitation (capitation) on Medicare Part B payments for physical and speech therapy combined and for occupational therapy. Hospital-based outpatient services have been exempt from this capitation to assure that access to therapy services is not denied to Medicare beneficiaries due to the limits imposed by this capitation. This ruling presents another potential disparity among physical therapy providers that is based on work setting alone. Outpatient managers must develop processes to assure that patients are not moving from one therapy provider to another within 1 year ("therapy hopping") to attempt to overcome these caps on the coverage of their outpatient rehabilitation services.

Identifying which patients may have already reached their annual capitation amount in one setting before initiating services in another setting can be time consuming. For example, a patient may receive physical therapy in a physician, chiropractor-based, or corporate practice setting and exhaust their allowable charges or reach their capitation amount. The patient's physician may make another referral and direct the patient to a private practice or hospital-based practice to continue therapy. Although hospital-based therapy is not capped for Medicare patients, the risk of denials of claims may be high if a patient's goals were documented as met in the prior setting. A private practitioner who continues any patient's care in this situation may risk denial of the claim for reimbursement if the annual cap has been reached in a nonhospital setting without his or her knowledge.

Authorizations

Managers also must be certain that approvals necessary to initiate and continue services are consistently and accurately followed by members of their professional and business office staff members for both Medicare and nonMedicare patients. The aim is to avoid denials of payment for services rendered because they were not preauthorized, or rules for continuing care were not followed. This required communication with insurers is another means of ensuring that payment for patient care is not intentionally, or unknowingly, denied.

Authorizations for the care of patients who receive services as part of their workers' compensation benefits or through personal injury insurance (auto accident insurance) is determined by state rather than federal statutes. Managers also must track these state statutes and rules for ongoing policy changes. Because many of the patients receiving workers' compensation benefits have been injured while working for large corporations, it is not unusual that attorneys also attempt to become involved in medical discussions as they champion benefits for their clients. Interactions with attorneys related to their client's rehabilitation can be time consuming for managers. See Sidebar 16.4.

Insurance Coverage for Rehabilitation Services

Congress continually acts to cut Medicare payments for rehabilitation services, regulate payment fees though annual adjustments of CPT code values, and adjust annual capitation on fees for rehabilitation services. This perpetual legislative activity keeps many outpatient physical therapy managers on an unpredictable course as they manage not only the current financing of physical therapy practice but attempt to predict growth of their organizations.

For private insurers, controlling costs often means limiting or eliminating coverage of "ancillary" health services, such as rehabilitation. It is no surprise that

Sidebar 16.4

Workers' Compensation

Find the WCRI Benchmarks Study at the Workers' Compensation Research Institute Web page. Analyze the results. Go to http://www.wcrinet.org/ benchmarks/benchmarks_06/benchmarks_ 06_tbl-B.html managers choose to narrow a practice to one form of reimbursement system and market to that population. Frequently, only organizations with extensive resources are able to support business offices prepared to deal effectively with Medicare, workers' compensation, personal injury, and other types of insurance concurrently. The complexity of any one of them can be overwhelming. On the other hand, it may be important to contract with different types of insurers because changes in any one of their policies may make one type of insurance more attractive than another at any point in time.

Alternative Income Sources

Physical therapists who wish to be truly autonomous, may decide not to contract with insurance payers at all and rely on a strictly cash business with patients who are able to directly access their services. The introduction of health savings accounts may allow more people to select and pay out of pocket for particular services they need. In any type of outpatient physical therapy settings, becoming the provider of choice becomes a major responsibility of the physical therapy manager.

Turf wars with chiropractors for patients with spinal disorders, with occupational therapists for patients with hand injuries, and with other providers who are on the fringes of formal health care (i.e., acupuncturists, Rolfers, massage therapists, etc.) often raise the concern of rehabilitation managers. Personal trainers are also eager to meet the needs of people who may have exhausted their insurance benefits and are willing to pay cash for individualized, private exercise sessions to continue their "therapy." Deciding when to align with other professionals to enhance a physical therapy practice, or when to clearly differentiate physical therapy from them is not an obvious decision.

A recent managerial response to declining reimbursement for rehabilitation services has been diversification of physical therapy practices. Efforts to provide related services such as spa services, health-club memberships, wellness programs, etc. that are paid for in cash rather than health insurance reimbursement are becoming more common. Managers of physical therapy practices may need to consider, however, the image these business decisions may project. It is their responsibility to clarify and solidify the role of the profession while promoting exclusivity of the use of the term physical therapy.

Unique Features of Physical Therapy Practice in Outpatient Settings

The focus of most physical therapy practices or rehabilitation outpatient centers is the care of people with musculoskeletal conditions, with sports-related injuries often identified as a special set of conditions treated within these centers. Outpatient practices also may care exclusively for children, or they may focus on particular conditions, such as the management of patients with lymphedema, women's health, or work-related injuries.

Sometimes, the specialization of a practice evolves from the specialty of the physicians who refer to that practice. For instance, if an orthopedic surgeon specializes in the treatment of shoulder impairments and refers the majority of his patients to one particular physical therapy center, that center will likely, by default, "specialize" in rehabilitation of disorders of the shoulder. Other centers establish themselves as a sports medicine center, for instance, and then build referrals to develop that specialty practice. The hiring of board-certified specialists also drives the specialization of a clinic. Again, it may be that the hiring of a specialist drives the practice, or the deliberate recruitment of specialists is a management strategy for developing a niche practice.

Types of Practices

Managers in any outpatient setting not only have variety in the clinical focus of a practice, but they also may have the opportunity to identify a preference for practice in a variety of health-care organizations shown in Figure 16.1 and discussed further in Sidebar 16.5 and the following sections.

Other Features of Hospital-Based Outpatient Services

Hospital-based outpatient rehabilitation services may address a wide range of specialty services. The range depends on the type and number of physician-owned or private practices in the community. For example, orthopedic surgeons who perform surgery in the hospital may refer those patients to their own practices or other outpatient centers rather than the hospital's

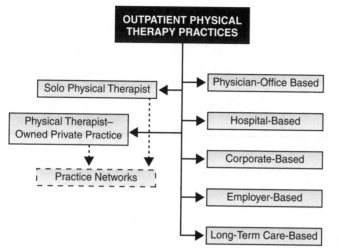

Figure 16.1 ✦ Types of outpatient practices.

Sidebar 16.5

Characteristics of Work in Outpatient Centers

Solo practices:

✦ Often are highly specialized.

✦ May be general practice meeting needs of patients across the life span.

✦ Provide the greatest opportunity for autonomy in clinical and business decisions.

✦ May find it difficult to negotiate contracts with third-party payers.

✦ Establishing a broad referral base may be difficult.

✦ May need to make special effort to avoid professional isolation.

✦ Need to remain current with both clinical evidence and reimbursement policies.

Private (independent) practice:

✦ Opportunity for unlimited business growth and the development of niche markets.

✦ May be interdisciplinary.

✦ Business responsibilities often override direct attention to patient care because the livelihoods of employees are based on responding to unpredictable reimbursement policies and contract negotiations.

✦ Cash flow and capital resources are common concerns.

Practice networks:

✦ Provide centralized support for contract negotiations and other aspects of billing, marketing, and quality care, etc.

✦ The independence of private practice is preserved.

✦ Flat fees that are paid to the network increase the cost of doing business.

Employer-based:

✦ There is a guaranteed population of employees who need services.

✦ Highly specialized practice.

✦ Location on the campuses of large corporations reduces space expenses.

✦ Convenient for employees.

✦ Opportunities for development of on-site prevention and wellness programs.

✦ Direct per capita reimbursement for services is often negotiated to avoid third-party payers.

✦ Boundary issues may arise if the practice is limited to employees with work-related conditions who also see other providers for nonwork related health problems.

Hospital or health-care system based:

✦ Opportunities for upward career mobility.

✦ Increased likelihood of strong continuity of care as patients' transition from one part of the system to another.

✦ Slowly changing bureaucracies.

✦ State-of-the-art facilities and equipment.

✦ General or specialty practice opportunities.

✦ Increased interaction among larger staffs.

Continued

Sidebar 16.5

Characteristics of Work in Outpatient Centers—cont'd

- ✦ Reimbursement issues less threatening.

Long-term care based:

- ✦ Strong continuity of care as patients move among units on a long-term campus.
- ✦ One management umbrella for both inpatient and outpatient services.
- ✦ Higher percentage of patients with complex, chronic medical conditions.
- ✦ Geriatric specialization opportunities.

Physicians' offices:

- ✦ Close working relationships with physicians.
- ✦ Typically large caseloads with high productivity demands.

- ✦ Potential limitations in autonomous clinical decision making that lead to ethical and financial conflicts.
- ✦ Opportunity for orthopedic specialization.

Corporate chain of centers:

- ✦ Upward career mobility opportunities in many locations.
- ✦ Central control of resources for development, marketing, staff recruitment, etc.
- ✦ Potential risk of focus on quantity rather than quality of care to please shareholders.
- ✦ High productivity demands.
- ✦ Stockholders are important stakeholders.

---

outpatient rehabilitation services. The hospital's specialization, therefore, may, by default, be anything other than postsurgical orthopedics. This self-referral leaves hospital-based outpatient centers dependent on referrals from other medical specialists. Hospitals are frequently the only provider of services to people who are underinsured or uninsured.

A recent trend for hospitals and health systems to develop outpatient centers separated from the hospital itself that are more conveniently located and accessible for patients is a response to the competition for outpatients. The more centers one organization has in an area, the fewer contracts a third-party payer requires to meet the needs of the people it insures. This is good for insurers who are able to reduce their administrative costs with fewer contracts, but it often presents difficulties for independent practitioners in those communities who also seek contracts with the same insurers.

Managers in hospital-based outpatient practices are part of a larger organization that meets a wider range of community needs. Their staffs may more likely be involved in staff meetings, clinical instruction, and institutional activities related to accreditation. Finding the means to address the needs of a broad patient base rather than a niche market may be a management responsibility that is not found in other settings.

Deciding how much to meld the inpatient and outpatient staffs into one unit may be an important decision in hospital-based practices, particularly if staff shortages are a major concern. Ideally, staff who are willing and able to float from inpatient to outpatient services and vice versa allows managers flexibility in staffing assignments. More often, the two staffs are either unwilling or unable to easily transition from one setting to the other as needed. The skill set, pace of work, and clinical specialties may be very different in these subgroups of therapists.

These factors contribute to a manager's decision to deliberately treat the two groups as separate entities, particularly when the inpatient and outpatient services are physically isolated from each other. Other managers may insist that staff maintain their skills in both areas. The ability of a physical therapist to remain a broad generalist to meet these job demands may only be possible in less complex hospital settings with a limited range of patient problems to be addressed.

Patient Outpatient Choices

Physician referrals for outpatient rehabilitation may be based on locations convenient for patients. They may be dependent on a center having a contract with a patient's insurer. Regardless of the preference of the physician to refer to a particular center, the third-party payer may limit where a person receives outpatient therapy to facilities that are within their provider network, with extra cost to the patient who chooses a center outside the network. The reality is that patients are most likely to do what their physicians recommend whenever possible, and physicians try to honor referrals to providers within patients' networks.

The most defining feature of outpatient physical therapy is that, unlike all other settings, the therapists do not have a captured audience. They are dependent on people voluntarily coming for treatment sessions, so managers must, above all, get patients in the door. An important first step in this responsibility is arranging as many contracts with insurance carriers as possible so that the organization is a potential provider for as many potential patients as possible. It is difficult for managers when people who seek to come to their centers cannot pass through the doors because they are "out of network." Many potential patients cannot afford the additional costs of going to a provider they prefer rather than one that is "in network."

Competition within a third-party-payer network, for the same patients, particularly for those deemed most desirable for a variety of reasons, becomes fierce. To be competitive and profitable, physical therapy managers in any outpatient practice setting must focus on the quality of services provided and payments for their services. Word of mouth about the successes and efforts of the staff in a practice may be the most valuable marketing tool a manager has. Perhaps the only way to tip the power and influence of physicians on patient choices about their physical therapy is to have more patients who are empowered to say that they prefer to go to a particular practice because of the reputation it has. At the same time, it is important for referring physicians to have confidence in the quality of the services that their patients receive. See Sidebar 16.6.

Quality of Care

Physical therapists who are considering management positions in different types of outpatient centers need to consider accountability expectations for assuring the quality of care as well as the profits. A discussion with potential employers about the amount of time a manager is expected to devote to these two broad categories of responsibilities may be revealing. The business side of these managerial responsibilities may be complemented or supplemented by other staff, but the professional ability to assure the quality of care cannot be delegated effectively to nonprofessionals, or even professionals from another discipline. The strength of a practice may lie with a quality emphasis, or approach, to management decisions.

Unlike other health-care settings in which Medicare has linked required electronic data collection on each patient to quality outcomes and costs, there is no standardized, formal documentation required of any outpatient rehabilitation setting from any payer. Although there are some systems available for purchase or those created by large organizations for their own use, it remains difficult to make comparisons of the quality of care and cost-effectiveness of outpatient organizations. Unlike nursing homes, this important information is not as available for public comparisons of centers.

Recent initiatives by the APTA may provide the ability of centers to participate in a national outpatient database.[6,7] Because there is no requirement to share data on the services they provide, outpatient centers may prefer to gather data for internal and marketing processes only, while intentionally avoiding comparisons with other centers. Since larger organizations may already have powerful internal mechanisms for quality and productivity measurements in place, efforts toward a national, standardized outpatient documentation and measurement system may require powerful planning and persuasion by the profession.

Patient Satisfaction

Surveys to determine patient satisfaction with physical therapy outcomes and care also may be useful in studying the quality of outpatient care, particularly because hands-on orthopedic treatments may be threatening or painful, and patients are expected to actively participate in their therapy.[8] One study of survey results suggests that outpatient satisfaction with physical therapy is most associated with a high-quality interaction with the therapist (e.g., time spent with patient, adequate explanations and instructions to patients, less use of supportive personnel) rather than environmental factors such as clinic location, parking, time spent waiting for the therapist, and type of equipment.[9]

Sidebar 16.6

Physician Quality Reporting Initiative

Go here for information on new physician quality reporting initiative, http://www.cms.hhs.gov/pqri/

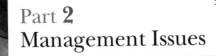

Part 2
Management Issues

Overview of Management in Outpatient Centers

Management opportunities in outpatient physical therapy are numerous and can be found in a variety of organizations and models that are attractive to entrepreneurs and employees who seek career ladders within large organizations. These managerial opportunities include:

- ✦ A solo practice, typically one office, in which the physical therapist provides all of the patient care and manages the practice with limited support personnel. This practice may also include provision of home care or contract services for other organizations.

- ✦ A large private physical therapy practice with either a single office that employs several other physical therapists and support staff, or multiple offices employing potentially large numbers of rehabilitation professionals and support staff.

- ✦ Solo or private practices that are part of physical therapy networks with centralized support for many aspects of the practices, which may be paid for either through flat payments or profit sharing with the network. Depending on the nature of the agreements, the practices in the network commonly operate with relative decision-making independence.

- ✦ Solo or private practices that lease space and pay for support services in a physician practice. This arrangement allows establishment of strong professional ties with physicians while clearly maintaining professional autonomy.

- ✦ Practices whose only business is a contract with a large employer(s) to provide all physical therapy services to employees, usually including job analysis and injury prevention services, and frequently on the campus of the employer's business.

- ✦ Outpatient services within hospitals or health-care systems that may range from supervisory responsibilities in one of several satellite offices to management of all rehabilitation services in all units of the hospital or the entire health-care system.

- ✦ Outpatient services provided in long-term care centers or communities. Outpatients may be residents in the center who are eligible for Medicare Part B outpatient rehabilitation, or patients who have been discharged from the facility and return to it as outpatients to continue their rehabilitation. Managers typically have responsibility for inpatient services in the same long-term care organization.

- ✦ Physician-owned (single or group) physical therapy services that are offered in-house to patients of that particular physician or physician group. The role of managers may be more limited because of physician interest in the practice.

- ✦ A national corporation that owns a chain of outpatient centers. Management responsibilities may range from one center to regional management of several centers or upper-level management positions.

Within any of these models, there may be board-certified specialists and niche target markets. Practices may focus on particular diagnoses or age groups, or they may be broad generalist practices that address a wide variety of patient needs. In any outpatient setting, managers assume similar responsibilities that are addressed in the following sections.

Managerial Responsibilities

Mission, Vision, and Goals

There may be more variation in mission, vision, and goals among outpatient settings than any other health-care settings because of the range of possibilities of ownership and size. Hospital-based outpatient units are linked to the larger organization's goals and outcomes to meet the mission and vision of the organization as a whole. Outpatient managers in those settings may contribute to the development of the hospital mission, vision, and goals; and will certainly be accountable for their unit's contributions to achieving them.

Managers in corporate-based outpatient centers also are likely to be handed the mission and vision of the corporation with minimal input into their development unless it is part of a special assignment to review or modify them. Private physical therapy practitioners have to consider the creation of a vision, mission, and goals as the starting point for setting their practices apart from others.

Managers in all types of outpatient settings work a little harder to differentiate themselves through their visions and missions because of competition for patients. For instance, home care is home care, and a general hospital's mission and vision is more like that of other general hospitals. Outpatient centers, on the other hand, may seek to have more differences than similarities to gain a competitive advantage.

Clearly differentiating the strengths of a practice through vision and mission statements may also be a powerful tool for recruitment of personnel and for development of a referral base, provided they are effectively communicated to stakeholders.

Policies and Procedures

Outpatient managers' responsibilities for policies and procedures also vary according to the size and type of organization. Managers may receive policy and procedures manuals developed at higher organizational levels for implementation, or they may assume total responsibility for development and implementation in independent practices or in physicians' offices. The larger and more complex the organization, the more complex policies and procedures become. In addition to the required policies and procedures that are needed to become a Medicare-certified provider organization, larger organizations may expand their policies and procedures to reflect the more complex interactions and management of resources that are the result of their size. Independent practitioners may feel less urgency for policies and procedures because the running of the business is more automatic and reflexive with less staff and simpler physical space.

Professional Courtesies

A policy and procedure that may be unique to outpatient settings is one that addresses extending the professional courtesy of free or discounted fees for treatment of physicians, other health professionals, and/or family members of employees. Although professional courtesy may be an effective marketing

strategy, there are inherent issues related to unfairness (unintentional or deliberate), or a potential violation of antikickback legislation. The Stark Law addresses professional courtesy only in hospitals but it provides "food for thought" for any setting. Their requirements for professional courtesy include:[10]

+ The policy for professional courtesy must be in writing and approved by the governing body responsible for the organization. It must not violate state or federal antikickback legislation.

+ The services offered are routine and typical and offered to all physicians regardless of the volume or value of their referrals.

+ The physician or family member cannot be a federal health beneficiary unless there is a financial need.

Establishing limits on the percent of the annual visits that can be devoted to professional courtesy may be necessary, particularly for the private practitioner. Determining the number of courtesy visits per physician and their extended families also may need to be set. Balancing professional courtesy and pro bono services may need to be considered in some practices.

Although managers cannot afford to give away their services, they also cannot afford to jeopardize the good will that may be accumulated through these actions. Establishing written guidelines for scheduling of these patients will avoid disruptions of services to clients who are paying for their services. Assuring all patients that they are receiving the same level of service whether they are paying for it or not may be a consideration in establishing this policy.

A similar policy may be necessary for the treatment of coworkers who require physical therapy services when there is an expectation that they also receive a professional courtesy. Professionals who treat family members may want to consider the ramifications of that decision. Managers should have a policy to address how professional courtesy extends to staff who treat family members directly and family members who are treated by other people on staff.

Pro Bono Services

Similar policy and procedures questions often arise in relation to the delivery of pro bono services. *Pro bono publico* is derived from the Latin and means "for the public good." It is used to describe professional services that are voluntarily provided without payment to people who are unable to afford them. With a basis in the legal profession, pro bono services commonly are offered by professionals in all fields. Some professions require their members to provide pro bono services to meet legal and ethical responsibilities, while others believe that pro bono is the voluntary choice of each individual.

Organizations do not have pro bono obligations, but they often incur bad debts because of providing services to people who are unable or unwilling to pay for them. To reduce these bad debt losses, managers are unlikely to encourage staff to provide pro bono services while working. However, they may establish guidelines for staff to engage in pro bono services on their own time in community-based organizations.

Typically, the use of its own facilities, even after hours, to provide pro bono services is discouraged because of liability concerns. Because professionals can often meet their pro bono responsibilities through a variety of means other than the direct provision of free services (e.g., financial donations to charitable groups), employers typically expect professional employees to meet their required or voluntary obligations on nonwork time.

Marketing

The managerial duties for marketing vary widely from one type of setting to another. Typically, large health-care organizations and corporations have full-time marketing staffs who generate materials and plans for implementation by managers among the units of the organization. Because of the expense involved, independent practitioners may be at a disadvantage in their marketing responsibilities. The time needed for inbound- and outbound-marketing activities intended to set a practice apart from others may be limited because the bulk of the manager's time is devoted to direct patient care and the management of finances. Moreover, the costs of a strong outbound-marketing program may be prohibitive, forcing these practitioners to rely on word of mouth to develop a strong, professional reputation for the services they provide.

A priority target of marketing efforts for the private practitioner may be managed care organizations. Overcoming their reluctance to enter into contracts with private practice physical therapists is a major managerial challenge. Although the prices set by private practices are commonly competitive, managed care organizations often are not interested in negotiating a contract for their services. Perhaps the reason for this lack of interest is that the business priority of managed care organizations is minimizing their administrative costs, which are typically fixed regardless of the size of an organization they contract with. If a managed care corporation already has a contract with a hospital in the community, it has little incentive to also contract with several small private practices. Each new provider that is added to their panel of providers increases their administrative costs.

Provider Networks

These third-party-payer contract difficulties led to the development of physical therapy provider networks that allow multiple private practices to negotiate collectively with managed care companies as a single entity. This model increases the possibility of gaining a contract that includes all centers because the network has enabled the insurance company to reduce their administrative costs. Their combined ability to develop a broader diversification of populations to be served, or to meet the unmet needs of particular populations also improves their ability to negotiate as a single entity with third-party payers.

The capability to present quality assurance, utilization review, and outcome studies across several practices also makes the idea of private practices more attractive to third-party payers, particularly if a group of practices can be flexible about the different types of reimbursement models insurers may offer. These network business opportunities also present professional opportunities for providers to share ideas and improve clinical practice. This may be an attractive opportunity for managers of solo practices willing to sacrifice some of their independence and control to continue operating a private practice.

Staffing

Because outpatient services are enticing and appealing to many physical therapists, managers may have a little less difficulty in recruiting staff than managers do in other health-care settings. However, they may face hurdles recruiting particular therapists with specialized skills for program development in niche markets. For instance, managers in different types of outpatient centers are more likely competing with each other than they are with other types of health-care settings in the recruitment of musculoskeletal specialists.

Salary and benefits are likely the big negotiating factors because of the number of outpatient opportunities in any location. Managers need to be insightful interviewers, who can spot an applicant who has the strong interpersonal skills requisite for establishing trusting relationships that lead to high levels of patient satisfaction with their care and for strong professional relationships with referring physicians.

Personnel decisions often are directed to the development of specialized services. Supporting specialist certification or advanced degrees in exchange for a long-term employment commitment to the organization is often good management strategy. Identifying both physical therapist and physical therapist assistant staff who have the potential to assume more administrative responsibilities also is important. Programs that nurture that potential have many advantages. Having the means to grow one's own staff with career ladder plans may be the most important decision about the utilization of human resources in outpatient practices.

Support Staff

Because services must meet the definition of "skilled" for Medicare reimbursement, the use of supportive personnel, other than physical therapist assistants, for direct patient care provided to Medicare recipients is typically not a management option. However, the use of other physical therapy extenders may be tempting, particularly in times of workforce shortages and reduced reimbursement. The direction and supervision of others who are not physical therapist assistants, and careful delineation of the duties that they may perform must receive the close attention of managers.

Even if these extenders (i.e., aides, technicians, etc.) are licensed in other disciplines, such as athletic training or massage therapy, or have education and credentials as exercise physiologists or personal trainers, they are not licensed to practice physical therapy. Although the skills they bring to a position in an outpatient practice may be very attractive, what

they can be legally assigned to do and whether the services they perform can be billed for must be weighed against the value of their contributions to patient care.

In some practices, there may be a reluctance even to hire physical therapist assistants. A practice that relies heavily on manual therapy is an example. The manager may decide that this staffing model is not conducive to a practice that is committed to consistent, one-on-one, high-touch therapy. Therapists directing others to deliver patient care is not part of this model. However, because staffing costs are so high, managers may have no choice but to hire physical therapist assistants. If not delivering direct patient care in this type of practice because it is so specialized, physical therapist assistants may be able to contribute effectively to other types of interventions and assume more administrative roles.

Supervision of Students

Small private outpatient practices, in particular, may show reluctance to engage in clinical education programs. Because outpatient practices have less difficulty recruiting staff, and their marketing commitment to provide patients with highly skilled specialists, they may hesitate to incorporate students into their practices. Other outpatient centers may be reluctant because of high productivity expectations that may not be met because of additional duties placed on clinical instructors. Conversely, other outpatient centers may be very eager to have students because of the extra hands that students bring to heavy caseloads with no additional personnel expenses.

Outpatient managers in *all types* of physical therapy practices have an obligation to ensure that the learning goals of students take precedence over maximizing billable units generated in those situations. Preparing staff to meet their important professional responsibilities as clinical faculty is key to meeting this obligation. Other managerial issues related to clinical education include:

✦ Integration of clinical education in the vision, mission, and goals of the organization.

✦ Criteria for establishing contracts with physical therapy and physical therapist assistant programs.

✦ Determination of which and how many staff are committed to the supervision of students at any time.

✦ Integration of clinical teaching into career ladders.

✦ Modification of staff assignments and productivity goals that reflect a commitment to students' learning goals.

✦ Evaluation of both teaching and clinical performance.

Patient Care

Managers must develop strong orientation sessions and establish monitoring systems (peer-review audits of documentation, for instance) to ensure not only the quality of services but compliance with the accurate and timely completion of documentation to meet legal and reimbursement requirements. There are challenges in meeting these requirements. For example, the goal-setting component of documentation for reimbursement of outpatient services demands a functional focus. This requires therapists to adjust their thinking about patients. Outpatients who require physical therapy must be well enough to get dressed and travel to therapy, which are high-level functional activities. Yet they must be "sick" enough to require the skilled services of physical therapists.

The premorbid functional level of many outpatients is often high. Pain or impairments rather than functional limitations are typically the basis of their need for physical therapy. Physical therapists must be diligent in linking their patients' concerns to functional goals. Other patients may have chronic conditions where improving long-standing functional limitations is not a reasonable goal, although therapy certainly may significantly influence their quality of life. It is often difficult to determine what is "reasonable and necessary" that "requires the skill of a physical therapist" for many of the patients with chronic conditions. Go to Sidebars 16.7 and 16.8.

Documentation

A primary patient/client management responsibility is that accurate documentation of the high-quality services that were provided comply with requirements for reimbursement established by Medicare and other insurance companies. Generally, for each insurer, managers should determine:

✦ Which staff members are recognized as certified providers responsible for clinical judgments and supervision of other personnel.

> **Sidebar 16.7**
> **Therapy Services and Medicare**
>
> Case examples of reimbursement issues can be found at *http://www.cms.hhs.gov/ TherapyServices/*

> **Sidebar 16.8**
> **Insurance Intermediaries and Carriers**
>
> Go to http://www.cms.hhs.gov/mcd/ index_lmrp_bystate.asp?from2=index_lmrp_bystate. asp& for more information on carriers for outpatient physical therapy services in each state.

✦ The level of care required for reimbursement as a skilled service.

✦ Documentation requirements (Level of skill? Justification for care? Goals? Patient response?)

✦ Content to be included in standardized forms to be submitted during the episode of care.

✦ Data needed for reauthorization or modification of plans of care.

✦ Required content in encounter (treatment) notes and progress notes.

✦ Discharge and discontinuance requirements.

An increased interest in medical necessity and outcomes is expected to be the federal government's next focus of Medicare rules about rehabilitation services. Pay for performance is expected to be the next major reimbursement initiative. Managers will need to evaluate the usefulness of new instruments and databases designed to address these issues, such as the Activity Measure-Post Acute Care Computer-based Format (AMPAC-CAT),[11] Focus On Therapeutic Outcomes (FOTO),[12] and the Outpatient Physical Therapy Improvement in Movement Assessment Log (OPTIMAL).[7]

Fiscal

A major financial concern, once contracts with insurers have been negotiated, is meeting the requirements for a clean claim (i.e., 100% complete, clear, no errors, no questions) that is reimbursable on its first submission. Being paid for services provided often seems to be based on capricious and arbitrary, if not silly, rules set by carriers. Outpatient managers must check that carriers are consistent with federal legislation regarding Medicare coverage policies. Keeping abreast of current decisions about reimbursement policies is also critical. Breaking the rules because they were unknown can have a very serious impact on cash flow and profits of an outpatient practice. See Sidebar 16.9.

It has become commonplace for employers to encourage employee enrollment in health insurance plans with high deductibles and co-payments. Employers are thus able to reduce their costs for this benefit and employees' payroll contributions for their insurance are decreased. However, these higher deductibles and co-pays may deter many people from choosing to attend physical therapy sessions at all, or to reduce their attendance (i.e., no-shows and cancellations) to levels that they can afford. These insurance plans may be ideal for major, catastrophic illnesses or injuries, but they may have a negative effect on services like physical therapy that have a co-payment due at the time of each treatment session. The Medicare co-payment for outpatient services also may be prohibitive for many senior citizens on limited retirement incomes.

Managers need to be prepared to have frank discussions with patients about their ability to pay and the potential negative effects of ignoring problems that may be relieved with physical therapy intervention. Payment plans and other creative strategies may be necessary within the scope of what is legal and permissible. Offering certain discounts and waiving fees may be illegal.

Legal, Ethical, and Risk

A broad ethical issue for the profession is the potential disparity in patients who are able to access services. A recent study summarized some factors that determine utilization of physical therapy services. Generally, people were more likely to receive physical therapy if they have more than one musculoskeletal condition, have some limitation in function, have seven or more diagnostic codes, have a college degree, and reside in an urban area. People who were not as likely to receive physical therapy were older than 65, had no high school degree, were of Hispanic ethnicity or African American, had public or no insurance, and were living anywhere except the Northeast United States. Patients with musculoskeletal disorders were more likely to be referred by an orthopedic surgeon or an osteopathic physician than primary care physicians, and particularly if they also had workers' compensation insurance.[13]

Although overutilization of services is the focus of third-party payers, this study suggests that outpatient managers may find an urgent need to address underutilization. To do so, managers may develop business goals that address social and cultural norms along with programs to educate groups about physical therapy.

Overcoming language barriers may be a powerful way to counteract underutilization. Many patients with the need for physical therapy and the insurance to pay for it may not seek it because of these communication barriers. Other patients may face cultural barriers because their physicians have been educated in other countries and lack an understanding of contemporary physical therapy practice in this country. Managers also need to advocate for patients who need rehabilitation in Medicaid programs that may be very restrictive and vary from state to state. See Sidebar 16.10.

The salient legal and ethical issues in outpatient settings lie with fraud and abuse in Medicare billing. See definitions in Sidebar 16.11. Federal investigations through the Operation Restore Trust and analysis of Medicare Part B Extract Summary System

---

Sidebar 16.9

Medicare Coverage Database

Go to *http://www.cms.hhs.gov/mcd/search.asp? from2=search1.asp&*. Explore this resource by finding the local coverage in a state, then select a topic in physical therapy or a CPT code.

Sidebar 16.10

Office of the Inspector General

Go to *http://oig.hhs.gov/publications/docs/ workplan/2008/Work_Plan_FY_2008.pdf* and identify which upcoming activities of the Inspector General are important to physical therapy managers.

(BESS) data, the Comprehensive Error Rate Testing (CERT) Program, and activities of the Office of Inspector General have resulted in much attention to fraud and abuse in the Medicare system with physical therapy (or more accurately, the use of physical medicine CPT codes) at the heart of this investigation.

These investigative programs to reduce fraud and abuse also have provided the means for federal and state agencies to cooperate. They also enable public citizens to use hotlines to directly report suspected Medicare fraud and abuse to the proper authorities. These initiatives have been very successful in recovering millions of dollars and have resulted in the prosecution of many health-care providers. Some examples of fraud and abuse are fraudulent diagnoses, billing for services that were not provided, duplicate billing, and claims for medically unnecessary services.

Monitoring efforts that include the statistical analysis of claims and on-site reviews of Medicare providers with high reimbursement rates continue to reduce inappropriate payment of Medicare claims. Utilization management programs assure that payments are made only when it is clear that beneficiaries actually received the services that were billed. Incomplete or inaccurate documentation about patients' diagnoses and conditions, extent of services provided, and lack of medical necessity underlie suspicions of fraud and abuse. Managers can expect continued initiatives to address Medicare payments, which forces them to be diligent about documentation requirements and the skills of therapists to meet them.

Many of the problems with the reimbursement of rehabilitation services relate to the fact that data on a particular diagnosis is more difficult to pinpoint when the need for therapy is often the result of multiple diagnoses. It is also difficult for outsiders to understand why there is a wide range in the length of time the same condition may be treated. The wide variation in the quality and outcomes of those services does not seem to be in direct relationship to the amount of therapy received. Defining the amount or mix of services needed for specific patients or categories of patients remains elusive. Without a standard way to determine the ability to perform the activities of daily living and the specific needs for therapy derived from such a determination, a needs-based payment system cannot be easily established.

All of these initiatives make it important for managers to be aware of their organization's inclusion in these data collection and analysis efforts by federal agencies, and to remain current about actions taken in response to these analyses. It is also beneficial that staff clearly and consistently understand that coding the services provided is determined by what the physical therapist is doing rather than by what the patient is doing.

Communication

Outpatient physical therapists rely on phone and fax in their communications with physicians regarding the care of particular patients. The opportunities to communicate about patient data or problems may be most important in outpatient centers because the source of information is often limited to what a patient reports. Access to diagnostic test reports and other information from a medical record is not always available. Each communication with a physician also becomes important as an opportunity to strengthen a referral base and establish good will and professional relationships.

Managers need to constantly remind staff of the importance of these communications. Calls to physicians for clarifications of referrals or additional diagnostic information also are opportunities to demonstrate the knowledge and expertise of staff, and to determine the preferences and needs of the referring physicians.

Establishing strong communication patterns with the staff members in a physician's office alleviates the need for repeated attempts to speak directly to a physician. Developing a rapport with the person who answers the phone so that they know that the physical therapist would not be calling unless it was something that demands attention is a critical skill for managers to instill in physical therapists and support staff.

Physician Certifications of Plans of Care

Medicare documentation requirements add an additional burden for timely completion of physicians' approvals of established plans of care and their revision that often involves follow-up calls to physicians to remind and encourage them to complete the paperwork. Specifically, Medicare's conditions of coverage state that Part B outpatient rehabilitation services are paid for only if:[14]

+ A physician certifies that a plan for outpatient rehabilitation services was necessary when it is established or soon after. Physicians (i.e., doctor of medicine, osteopathy, or podiatric medicine), physical therapists, occupational therapists, or speech pathologists may establish plans of care and if these plans not established by a physician they must be reviewed and certified by a physician.

+ The services are or were furnished while the patient was under the care of a physician.

+ The services are or were reasonable and necessary to the treatment of the patient's condition.

+ The physician provides written recertification for the need for services under the same plan of care at least once every 90 days.

Insurance companies that contract as Medicare carriers may determine if these certification and recertification requirements are met in any format they choose. Documentation must be filed and submitted with reimbursement requests. Failure to do so results in denial of payment.

Verbal Orders

Managers need to assure that all requirements are being met for receiving verbal orders from physicians or physician extenders. State statutes or third-party payer rules may determine who may refer a patient to physical therapy. For instance, in an exchange of phone calls about modifying a patient's plan of care, the result may be that a physician

assistant returns the call to the physical therapy clinic approving the change requested. The only person available to accept the call is a physical therapist assistant who may or may not be involved in that patient's care.

Whether or not the phone conversation between the physician assistant and physical therapist assistant is acceptable may depend on several factors. For instance, whether the physician assistant is speaking for the physician who is engaged in other activities at a particular moment, or whether the physician assistant is independently making the decision on the revised plan of care must be made clear if physical therapy statutes specify from whom physical therapists may accept orders or referrals.

At the same time, it may be acceptable in some jurisdictions for the physical therapist assistant to take the call while the physical therapist is engaged in other activities as long as it is not perceived as the physical therapist assistant is modifying the plan of care rather than simply taking a message. Documentation of all of these communications must be clear and detailed to reduce legal and reimbursement risks. Managers should encourage their staffs to avoid assumptions and blanket rules about these communications related to patient care decisions.

Peer Support

The outpatient setting is conducive to opportunities for professional interaction and mentoring in all but the solo practitioner setting. This may be another factor that makes the setting attractive for many physical therapists. Interdisciplinary teamwork is not a driver of most outpatient practices, but interactions among therapists of the same discipline in larger centers is much higher than other practice settings where they may be more isolated in their daily work.

There is more opportunity for professionals to consult with each other and share their expertise because the more open, common "gym" area in outpatient centers permits more ongoing interaction among staff. Managers have more opportunity to observe work performance as well. This strengthens communication about clinical decision making, which may contribute to improving the quality of care. Outpatient managers may more easily identify common clinical issues that can be addressed in staff meeting or journal clubs because of the large number of patients with similar conditions.

Caseload Models

Managers in larger outpatient settings also need to consider the impact of their caseload model. Does the same therapist follow their assigned patients from admission to discharge? Are daily patient assignments made based on a generated master schedule, which means that any available therapist or physical therapist assistant may see a patient at any point? As an efficiency issue, managers may prefer that each therapist's schedule is filled regardless of who initially treated the patient. From a patient satisfaction perspective, there may be a risk in frequently changing the providers who see the patient. If this is the case, however, establishing timely, written documentation requirements may be necessary to avoid the need for staff to make and take time to discuss patients with the providers who saw them at the last visit. These models also require managers to assure the patients' rights to confidentiality and privacy. The more people involved in a patient's care, the greater the risk of inadvertently violating these rights.

Direction

Perhaps more than any other setting, outpatient clinics also provide the best opportunity for unquestionable direction and supervision of physical therapist assistants and other supportive staff, again, because of the open, yet contained environment that facilitates interaction among the staff. Communication about patients may become an issue depending on the ratio of physical therapists to physical therapist assistants. Situations in which there are many physical therapist assistants and one physical therapist may require managers to identify communication methods that are very different from those required when there are many physical therapists and one physical therapist assistant.

Conclusion

The long history of outpatient physical therapy suggests that its future is secure. As new technology, new health-care business models, and new opportunities for specialized practice continue to develop in a system shifting to outpatient care, managers will find, and create, many opportunities. As the most popular work setting of physical therapists, outpatient physical therapy services provide many professional opportunities for managers who are willing to carefully attend to the complexities of billing and payment for the services provided. Managing professionals who are often specialized and highly skilled can be very rewarding. Activities 16.1 to 16.16 address many of the decisions facing managers in outpatient settings.

ACTIVITY 16.1
PATIENTS OR CLIENTS

Are the people who receive rehabilitation services in outpatient centers more like patients or clients as defined by the American Physical Therapy Association? Defend your answer in a group discussion. What difference does it make?

ACTIVITY 16.2
DIVERSIFYING OUTPATIENT SERVICES

Patrick Peterson is manager of the 5th Avenue Physical Therapy Center that is one of 123 centers owned by U.S. Rehabilitation Corporation. At the last regional meeting, all eight managers in his region were assigned to devise a plan for expanding services in their centers. Role-play the planning meeting in which eight managers develop their plans for incorporating cash business in their centers. All of these centers are solo practitioner centers with limited floor space.

ACTIVITY 16.3
PERSONNEL RECRUITMENT

Jack Steuben is manager of outpatient services for the Great Plains Health Care System. His responsibilities include staffing the six outpatient centers that are 30 to 40 miles from each other in the rural area around the county seat. Currently, he has an open position in each center because of population growth in the county and marketing efforts that have increased the visibility of rehabilitation services in the system. He has asked for another meeting with Linda Lopez who is his contact in the Great Plains Human Resources Department. Although there have been three applications from physical therapists submitted over the last few months, Jack has been reluctant to hire any of them because they are board-certified specialists who want to limit their assignments to their specialty areas. He wants Linda to regroup and come up with some new ideas because staff vacancies are now resulting in a waiting list for physical therapy appointments in all of the centers. Role-play this meeting.

ACTIVITY 16.4
EXPANSION OF A PRACTICE

Michael Moriarity has been a successful solo practice physical therapist for 7 years in Greendale, a suburban community. He feels that he is ready to take on more responsibilities. Recently he has been approached by U.S. Rehabilitation Services who is interested in buying his practice and having him stay on as the manager of his clinic and two others. He has also identified a possible new location for opening another office in his practice, in Whitehurst, another suburb, which is growing rapidly. Finally, Westshore Village, the largest retirement community in the area, has approached him with a contract to provide rehabilitation services in their nursing home and outpatient center. How should Michael decide which professional opportunity is most attractive?

ACTIVITY 16.5
STAFF RETENTION

Joslyn Robertson has owned and managed Robertson and Associates, Physical Therapists for 10 years and currently has a staff of three physical therapists and three physical therapist assistants. Her most senior therapist, Annabelle Walsh, tells Joclyn that she has been offered another position with U.S. Rehabilitation Services that is opening a clinic about 3 miles away. Although she likes her current position, the opportunity to move up within the U.S. Rehabilitation Services is very attractive. Annabelle feels she will never be more than a staff PT if she remains in her current position. What should Joslyn do?

ACTIVITY 16.6
NONLICENSED PERSONNEL

Tony Massino is the new manager of Citywide Rehabilitation. Although he knew when he accepted the position that there were two athletic trainers and a massage therapist on staff, it was not until he got into the position that he became concerned. The athletic trainers and the massage therapist have been assuming a great deal of responsibility for patient care. They even have their own caseloads and they complete charge slips for the patients that they treat. When he asks the other physical therapists about this, they report that they turn patients over to them once they have stabilized. They are not sure why he is concerned. Should he be?

ACTIVITY 16.7
PHYSICIAN RELATIONSHIP

Dr. Ramirez has called Susan Wishart, Manager of Rehab Action to voice his concerns. He has been receiving complaints from his patients in the last few months about the therapy they have been receiving at Rehab Action. The complaints include patients who say they are ignored for long periods, another who says the therapy made her worse, and others who have asked if they can go somewhere else for their therapy because the clinic is so busy.

He wants Susan to resolve her problems or he will call Americare, the primary insurance carrier for these patients to find another provider. Susan is very upset because she had no idea patients were so unhappy. She has relied on Dr. Ramirez as her primary referral source for the past several years and her business is at financial risk without his patients. What should she do?

ACTIVITY 16.8
A BILLING ISSUE

Daniel Devereau is one of the six staff physical therapists who work in the physical therapy department of Northern Orthopedic Associates. He tells Polly Alberts, Rehabilitation Manager, that he believes the billing department is not posting charges as he has submitted them. Although he and the other therapists are not involved with billing, he happened to see a former patient at the market last night who was very upset with him because the bill she received for therapy did not match the therapy she received. Daniel was embarrassed and promised to look into it and get back to her. What should Polly do?

ACTIVITY 16.9
DOCUMENTATION

Despite the several warnings that Burt Duncan, the manager of the outpatient rehabilitation services at St. Anthony's Hospital, has given Tamara Berkman, she has gotten several days behind on her patient documentation again. Although she is a very effective physical therapist who is admired by her patients and coworkers, she just seems unable to manage the paperwork. When pushed, she stays after hours to catch up but reverts to her old patterns very easily. What should Burt Duncan do?

ACTIVITY 16.10
GIFTS

Getting signatures on the plans of care from the physicians in Northern Orthopedic Associates has been very difficult and frustrating for Karen Larson, the manager of a small private practice. About 20% of her patients are referred from Northern Orthopedic yet she seems to spend 80% of her time resolving issues with them. At a meeting with her staff, they brainstorm some ideas to solve their issues with Northern Orthopedic. One of the staff suggests that they offer an in-service on rehabilitation of the shoulder to the physicians and provide a nice dinner to encourage them to come. Another therapist says that is a kickback and its illegal to do that. Is she right? What are other ideas for Karen to consider?

ACTIVITY 16.11
SCHEDULING

Marla McCormick has been the receptionist and scheduler in the Sandy Shores Physical Therapy practice for several years. She really likes her job but feels overwhelmed with the recent expansion that includes four physical therapists. She seems to make one of the physical therapists angry every day because of some scheduling decision that she made. Discussing these problems with them makes her very nervous. She tells them that she is just trying to accommodate the patients, no matter what. This has been what she has always done with scheduling, and has been encouraged to do by Burt Evans, the owner of Sandy Shores. What needs to be done?

ACTIVITY 16.12
WORKERS' COMPENSATION

Cynthia McLean, the manager of the Rehabilitation Care at Southside, overhears one of her staff therapists, Kitty Salmonson, on the phone. Kitty is discussing a patient's care and condition in detail. When Cynthia asks Kitty whom she is speaking with, she says it is Mr. Caan's workers' compensation attorney. What should Cynthia do?

ACTIVITY 16.13
SERVICE EXPANSION

Eleanor Prentiss is the new regional manager for U.S. Rehabilitation Services. She has been asked to develop a clinic in a predominantly Hispanic, middle-class neighborhood where most of the people are employed by a nearby assembly plant. This is the first effort of U.S. Rehabilitation Services to break into this underserved market. What are the factors that Eleanor needs to address to make this a successful venture?

ACTIVITY 16.14
SURVEY RESULTS

Tonya Montes is very surprised. She has reviewed the results of the patient satisfaction surveys completed in the last 3 months and 30% of the patients rated their experience in her outpatient clinic as "somewhat dissatisfied" or "very dissatisfied." The only thing that has changed is that she hired two physical therapist assistants about 4 months ago, but they seemed to be doing very well and handle their assigned caseloads without difficulty. What does Tonya need to investigate?

ACTIVITY 16.15
OUTCOMES

Jerome Fielding is the manager of a private practice, All County Physical Therapy, that has grown to include three outpatient centers. He feels the timing is right to begin to explore some software to capture outcomes of the patients treated in his centers. What should he look for in these products?

Jerome also has been invited to join the National Physical Therapist Network. What does he need to consider to make the right decision? What are other networks that are possibilities?

REFERENCES

1. American Physical Therapy Association. PT demographics: Type of facility. 2007. Available at: http://ww.apte.org/AM/Template.cfm:Section=Demographics&CONTENTID=41549&TEMPLATE=CM/ContentDisplay.cfm. Accessed October 24, 2007.

2. American Physical Therapy Association. Physical therapist member demographic profile 1999–2005. Available at: http://www.apta.org/AM/Template.cfm?Section=Demographics&Template=/MembersOnly.cfm&ContentID=38175. Accessed November 14, 2007.

3. American Physical Therapy Association. Private Practice Section. Available at: http://www.apta.org/AM/Template.cfm? Section=Chapters&template=/aptaapps/componentsonline/componentsonline.cfm&processForm=1&componentType=Sections&specChoice=E&convertList2Form=yes. Accessed November 14, 2007.

4. American Physical Therapy Association. Profile of a certified specialist. Available at: http://www.apta.org/AM/Template. cfm? Section=Certification2&Template=/

5. Centers for Medicare and Medicaid Services. National provider identifier standard. Available at: http://www.cms.hhs.gov/NationalProvIdentStand/. Accessed December 14, 2007.

6. American Physical Therapy Association. Get connected with APTA CONNECT! Available at: http://www.apta.org/AM/Template.cfm?Section=Info_for_Clinicians&CONTENTID= 43616&TEMPLATE=/CM/ContentDisplay.cfm. Accessed November 21, 2007.

7. Guccione AA, Mielenz TJ, DeVellis RF, et al. Development and testing of a self-report instrument to measure actions: Outpatient physical therapy improvement in movement assessment log (OPTIMAL). *Physical Therapy.* 2005;85:515.

8. Monnin D, Perneger TV. Scale to measure patient satisfaction with physical therapy. *Physical Therapy.* 2002;82: 682–691.

9. Beattie PF, Pinto MB, Nelson MK, et al. Patient satisfaction with outpatient physical therapy: Instrument validation. *Physical Therapy.* 2002;82:557–565.

10. Centers for Medicare and Medicaid Services. Professional courtesy §411.350 scope of subpart. Available at: http://www.cms.hhs.gov/PhysicianSelfReferral/Downloads/Unofficial_Redlined_411_350.pdf. Accessed December 14, 2007.

11. Jette AM, Haley SM, Tao W, et al. Prospective evaluation of the AMPAC-CAT in outpatient rehabilitation settings. *Physical Therapy.* 2007;87:385–398.

12. Resnik L, Hart DL. Using clinical outcomes to identify expert physical therapists. *Physical Therapy.* 2003;83:990–1002.

13. Carter SK, Rizzo JA. Use of outpatient physical therapy services by people with musculoskeletal conditions. *Physical Therapy.* 2007;87:497–512.

14. American Physical Therapy Association. MED-MANUAL, §270. Available at: http://www.apta.org/AM/Template.cfm?Section=Private_Practice1&TEMPLATE=/CM/ContentDisplay.cfm&CONTENTID=18881. Accessed December 14, 2007.

TaggedPage/ TaggedPageDisplay.cfm&TPLID=206&ContentID=25738. Accessed November 20, 2007.

Chapter 17

Management Issues in School-Based Services

Learning Objectives

- ✦ Discuss the characteristics of contemporary school-based services.
- ✦ Analyze key legislation impacting the delivery of school-based services.
- ✦ Discuss contemporary school-based practice issues.
- ✦ Analyze the work of physical therapists in public schools.
- ✦ Determine the managerial roles and challenges to managerial responsibilities.
- ✦ Analyze managerial decision making in given school-based situations.

Part 1
The Contemporary Setting

Overview of School-Based Rehabilitation Services

Although school systems are not part of the health-care system, many of the 6.7 million people ages 3 to 21 in special (sometimes labeled *exceptional*) education receive interdisciplinary-related services, including physical therapy, in the schools they attend.[1] In addition, almost 300,000 infants from birth through age 2 receive early intervention services through local school systems or other approved agencies to improve their opportunity for success when they enter school.[2] These special education and related services are provided by each state through federal legislation mandates, primarily Individuals with Disabilities Act (IDEA).

IDEA and IDEIA

Initiated in 1975 with subsequent revisions—IDEA was reenacted and revised in 2004 as the Individuals with Disabilities Education Improvement Act (IDEIA). Part B of IDEA defines children with disabilities as individuals between the ages of 3 and 21 who have one or more of the following conditions that adversely affects their educational performance:[3]

+ Mental retardation
+ Hearing impairment (including deafness)
+ Speech or language impairment
+ Visual impairment (including blindness)
+ Serious emotional disturbance
+ Orthopedic impairment
+ Autism
+ Traumatic brain injury
+ Specific learning disability
+ Attention-deficit disorder (ADD)
+ Attention-deficit hyperactivity disorder (ADHD)
+ Other health impairment

Although not clearly defined, school systems are required to provide a *free and appropriate* education and the support or related services necessary for each student to achieve his or her educational goals. These related services include:[4]

+ Speech-language pathology and audiology services
+ Psychological services
+ Physical and occupational therapy
+ Recreation, including therapeutic recreation
+ Social work services
+ Orientation and mobility services
+ Medical services for diagnostic and evaluation purposes
+ Interpreting services
+ Psychotherapy
+ One-to-one instructional aide
+ Transportation
+ Art therapy
+ Technological devices
+ School nurse services

Least Restrictive Environment

A key element of IDEA is that the special students receive an education in the least restrictive environment. The legislation reveals a preference for mainstreaming a student into regular classrooms with the assignment of aides to assist the student, the provision of other supplemental services, and the use of assistive technology. However, IDEA recognizes that a more restricted environment may be the only one possible for some students, and that it must be provided. Although mainstreaming is preferred (about 90% of children with special needs are mainstreamed to some degree[5]), the reality is that for a student with complex problems requiring a very specialized curriculum and many related services, the need for an appropriate education may trump the right to be mainstreamed into a general classroom.

At the least, students with disabilities are expected to attend schools as close to their homes as possible, in classes with peers near the same age. Support and services are to be taken to the students, and general and special educators are expected to collaborate to maximize opportunities for interaction between students with and without disabilities, and to assure that their education is as close as possible to the general curriculum.

As a result, school districts provide a menu of possible placements for students with special needs that range from support in the regular curriculum, to a mix of regular and special education classes in regular schools, to separate special schools, residential programs, home instruction, or even hospital placement for students who are medically unstable. During their K–12 experience, some students may require different placements as their learning needs change, while other students may qualify for the same level of support throughout their educational experiences.

The Individualized Education Plans

The determination of a free and appropriate education in the least restrictive learning environment is a detailed process made by interdisciplinary teams of professionals, the parents, or guardians of the student, and the older student, through the establishment of individualized education plans (IEPs). Not only must school districts assure that an IEP is established for every student identified with special needs, they also are responsible for assuring that every student with special needs is identified and evaluated through Child Find, which is another program mandated by IDEA.

Each student's IEP must be reviewed annually. Typically, a meeting is held to discuss the proposed IEP with parents (legal guardians and others who assume the roles of parents) as equal partners in the planning who have the right to accept or reject the IEP. Unique to students in special education, also because of the IDEA legislation, school districts are responsible for assuring that each child's right to an evaluation of learning needs, an appropriate education in the least restrictive environment, an IEP, and notice of changes in the IEP are met and documented as part of the formal school record. Students, through their parents, may dispute that schools have met their responsibilities for assuring these rights. These disputes may be resolved through mediation or formal administrative hearing processes that each school district must have in place.

An initial eligibility IEP determines a student's placement in special education for the first time. After which, every annual program IEP specifies a student's current status, and the educational goals for the next year. The school district and parents must agree upon an IEP for each student before the beginning of each school year. The IEP is essentially a binding agreement that the school district will provide what is in the IEP. Because they are typically completed toward the end of the school year, any necessary changes in an IEP because of unanticipated changes in the student over the summer, or as the school year progresses, must be agreed upon in writing. IEPs include descriptions of:[6]

+ Specific educational goals for the next school year.
+ The effect of a student's disability on involvement and progress in the goals for the general curriculum used in the regular classroom.
+ The means for meeting the student's need to be involved in general curriculum.
+ The special education and related services that will help a student reach his or her annual educational goals (involvement in general curriculum, extracurricular, and nonacademic activities; and participation with students with and without disabilities).
+ Related services to meet the developmental, corrective, and other needs for the student to meet individualized educational goals. The frequency, duration, and length of treatment sessions, provider qualifications, and ratio of providers to students are included.
+ Necessary program modifications or support for school personnel.
+ Plans to regularly inform parents of a student's progress.
+ The student's participation in any district or statewide assessment of student achievement used for the general education population and required modifications or accommodations that will be necessary.

Other Components of IDEA

Physical therapists and other members of the rehabilitation team also may be involved in state-approved early intervention programs through a variety of organizations that operate under IDEA's Program for Infants and Toddlers. The program guidelines encourage the most natural environment possible for interventions. There is much less consistency from state to state in these programs than there is in the implementation of Part B of IDEA. For instance, in some states these programs may fall under the U.S. Department of Health rather than the U.S. Department of Education. A lead state agency typically coordinates and supports the services of all early intervention providers.

The target population of the Program for Infants and Toddlers are children who already have, or who are at risk for, developmental delays that may impede their education. In some states, this Part C of IDEA (birth through 2 years) may be extended to age 6. Parents have to decide to waive their right to Part B of IDEA to continue to receive Part C services at this age. These early interventions may decrease referrals to special education because they assist a wider range of students who are struggling with language or learning, but a major goal is successful *transition* of the young child into the less restrictive school environment.

The required Part C Individualized Family Service Plan (IFSP), which is comparable with the IEP required in Part B, reflects the mandate that Part C is family-focused rather than child focused. Recognizing the emphasis on providing care in the context of the family system requires the physical therapist to develop strong collaboration skills and to develop more respect for the priorities of the family than might be expected in health-care settings.

At the other end of the educational spectrum is another transition point. Beginning at age 16, IDEA demands that IEPs address a transition plan for how the student will proceed after high school. Whether it is the development of skills to live independently as an adult or preparation for college or a training program, the plan must have measurable postsecondary education goals and a plan to meet them.

Assistive Technology

IDEA has set other regulations related to the provision of assistive technology and the associated services related to these assistive devices and equipment. Assistive technology may range from eyeglasses to complex, specially designed communication systems. The IEP team determines that assistive technology is necessary to support the right to access to the general curriculum, special education, or related services. The equipment may be used at home if it supports education but it is the property of the school. For many students assistive technology may be the only way for them to access a general curriculum.

Some school systems may collaborate with community agencies to exchange, recycle, and refurbish assistive equipment that students no longer need or have outgrown. Payment for assistive technology may come from a variety of resources beyond the funds in the school system's budget, such as grants, third-party payers, and donations. It is not unusual for school districts to have centralized assistive technology services that coordinate the provision of equipment and devices recommended by the IEP teams throughout the system.

Other Legislation Affecting Special Education

Several other pieces of legislation are related to the rights of people with disabilities. Those most important to schools, include the Americans with Disabilities Act (ADA), Section 504 of the Rehabilitation Act, and the more recently enacted, No Child Left Behind (NCLB) education legislation, which resulted in revisions of IDEA.[7]

The ADA Title II addresses *all* activities of state and local governments and requires that people with disabilities receive an equal opportunity to benefit from all of their programs and services, which include public education. Accomplishment of this equal opportunity may take two forms. Specific architectural standards in the new construction and alteration of buildings must be met or programs may need to be relocated to more accessible locations. Standards include alternative means of communicating to people with hearing, vision, or speech disabilities so that they may maneuver within the buildings (i.e., floor announcements in elevators, and Braille signage). The other component of ADA requirements is for reasonable modifications to policies, practices, and procedures where necessary to avoid discrimination of people with disabilities.

Related legislation that applies specifically to any program or agency that receives any federal funding is Section 504 of the Rehabilitation Act. ADA is a broader application of this older Rehabilitation Act, and they are similar but not the same. Section 504 requires that those funded entities do not discriminate against, or deny benefits to qualified individuals with a disability. Each federal department and agency has its own set of Section 504 regulations that applies to its own programs, but they all include the requirement that reasonable accommodations are to be made, which are similar to those required in ADA. Because Section 504 does not come with funding to meet its requirements like IDEA, school systems may find it more difficult to comply with these regulations.[8] Children receiving services under Section 504 are required to have a plan in place similar to the IEP required for IDEA.

Section 504 is broader in scope than IDEA, which addresses only the rights of children with specific diagnoses. Section 504 requires the elimination of any barriers for *anyone* with a physical or mental impairment that substantially limits one or more major life activity. The ability to learn in school is considered a life activity. This of course includes all students eligible for IDEA services, but also children who may have temporary or intermittent disabilities, such as asthmatic episodes or self-limiting infectious diseases, for example. To compare another way, IDEA is often considered an affirmative action rather than an antidiscrimination act because children who qualify for IDEA receive additional services and protections, which go beyond the equal protection assured by Section 504.[8]

The newer NCLB Act imposed standards for teacher qualifications and core academic subjects that were included in the amendments to IDEA in 2004. States imposed educational standards for reading and math, demanding school districts show annual improvements in scores. Corrective actions and opportunities for students to transfer from schools that are not meeting the standards or to seek supplemental services to meet standards are part of this act. Although too soon to tell, the potential negative financial impact on special education as funding is directed to meeting standards for all students is a possible concern. Sidebar 17.1 leads to more information on these topics.

Sidebar 17.1

More Legislative Information

Other data about IDEA and special education can be found at the U.S. Department of Education's Web page at https://www.ideadata.org/index.html and Wrightslaw is a Web page that provides tools for parents to advocate for their children at http://www.wrightslaw.com/.

Unique Features of School-Based Physical Therapy Practice

The most obvious feature of school-based physical therapy is that services are provided in schools rather than in a health-care setting. Collaboration may be the best word to describe the effort required by physical therapists to work with other members of the related services team and with general and special education teachers to evaluate, plan, and support instruction. Without an understanding of instruction and curriculum, physical therapists may find it difficult to contribute to decisions about the least restrictive environment for students.

For the students with gross motor deficits, the physical therapists' collaboration with adaptive physical education teachers becomes very important in the development and implementation of IEPs. Adaptive physical education is part of the federal special education mandate so it must be provided to all students. If physical therapy is no longer needed for a student to benefit from instruction, adaptive physical education may be a powerful means to continue to work on goals related to movement and physical activity, and for physical therapy and adaptive physical education programs to complement each other when resources are limited.

The needs of students during a school year, and their needs as they advance in grade levels make school-based positions the only positions in which physical therapists establish such long-term relationships with patients (students). Although it may not be typical, it is possible that a school-based physical therapist could work with the same child from ages 3 to 21. Participating in IEP meetings and the other less formal contact with parents over the years leads to establishing lasting professional relationships with families that are unknown in health-care settings. These collaborations place parents on equal footing with teachers and related services providers in the care of their children.

Funding Resources

Like health-care systems, school systems face many financial challenges. Despite the authorization that Congress contribute 40% to the costs of implementing IDEA, its funding is discretionary rather than mandatory, which has resulted in a huge financial shortfall, with federal funds actually contributing less than 20% of that funding.[9] School districts must find the rest of their funding from state and local taxes that may fluctuate widely from year to year. Managers made need to make a point of following federal and legislative action closely as a result.

Some states permit Medicaid reimbursement to school systems for children who are eligible and require related services. The shifting of state and local resources from education to other public demands is common and expectations to do more with less continues to be an educational management challenge, particularly in terms of salaries, which are often established through collective bargaining negotiations.

Salaries

Teachers are represented by National Education Association's bargaining units in each state. Although physical therapists may not be members of these units, they may be bound by the pay scales and merit raises negotiated for teachers. These pay structures may make it difficult to recruit physical therapists because school-based salaries often are not competitive with the health-care sector. Some school districts may choose to contract for related services through community-based organizations that provide pediatric rehabilitation services. They can offer higher salaries to their employees because these are practices that receive reimbursement from other sources in addition to school system contracts.

This contracting of services may solve the need for more competitive salaries, but it presents challenges for physical therapists who may already be perceived as "related to" rather than strongly integrated into some schools. If they also are perceived as not even employed by the school system, overcoming the perceived or actual distances between teachers and therapists may be challenging.

Collective bargaining may also lead to strict rules about teaching assignments and the time devoted to specific assignments. Because school systems tend to be tightly regulated bureaucracies anyway, these two factors may make the integration of related services challenging. The daily scheduling of classes, lunch breaks, transportation, and other activities may be made down to one-half minute intervals with very little room for deviation. Physical therapists who are more accustomed to the freedom of scheduling their own patients and control of their workdays, may find schools very restrictive as they seek to ensure that the goals to be met by related services are addressed in students' daily schedules.

Concurrent Community Services

Another challenge for physical therapists new to school systems may be limiting goals for children to those only related to their accomplishment of educational goals in the least restrictive environment. The hours in school, after all, are a small proportion of the entire time that children with disabilities face challenges. For instance, bed-to-chair transfers or environmental barriers in the home may need to be addressed although they are not related to the ability to function in school. As a result, some students may concurrently receive community-based therapy services. If so, school-based physical therapists may need to extend their collaboration networks to include other professionals who are providing services to students outside of school.

Responsibilities for assistive technology may be higher for school-based therapists who may rely on a special centralized countywide team for acquisition of any item, equipment, or system needed to improve the functional abilities of students. The technology may be purchased, fabricated, or leased; and the responsibility for fitting, repairing, and maintaining the devices or technology lies with the rehabilitation team whose primary responsibility is to train the student and others in its use. Remaining current in new technology becomes an important professional responsibility for school-based therapists and their colleagues in community-based private and public practices, and pediatric hospitals.

Sidebar 17.2 summarizes the factors that managers may present as components of the fulfilling and rewarding world of school-based physical therapy. As a member of the education team, physical therapists have an important role in assuring the achievement of educational goals of children.

Sidebar 17.2

Characteristics of School-Based Physical Therapy

✦ Establish long-term relationships with students, families, and transdisciplinary education team.

✦ Services are integrated into a tightly controlled schedule.

✦ Need for creative approaches to focus only on the educational needs of students rather than more typical patient goals.

✦ Detailed collaboration with education professionals and other members of the rehabilitation team.

✦ The role of physical therapy may be poorly understood by education professionals.

✦ Coordination and collaboration with community-based providers offering concurrent care.

✦ Highly individualized planning for meeting yearly education goals.

✦ Outcomes of therapeutic efforts may be long-term rather than immediate, and more difficult to determine.

✦ Shift of focus of care on educational rather than therapeutic goals for students.

✦ Competition for limited resources (often including space) available to school systems leading to financial and administrative constraints on services.

✦ Shorter workdays because of public school schedules, and potential for extended summers.

✦ Isolated from other physical therapists because of distances among schools in a system.

Part 2
Overview of Management in Public Schools

Management of School-Based Physical Therapy

Each school district may have a central coordinator of special education services who is based at the county's board of education. There may or may not be another person who coordinates the related services in special education for the entire district. Depending on the number of students in special education and the need for related services, supervisors for each of the related disciplines may be assigned to regions within a district. This makes school-based management a field operation similar to management of rehabilitation services in home care.

Because most IEPs are completed on each child before the beginning of the school year, district-wide needs for related services can be somewhat predicted. Because the needs of each child may vary from year to year, new students transfer into the system, and others graduate, the assignment of therapists among schools each school year remains a major challenge.

Depending on the number of students in each level of educational placement, physical therapy staff may be assigned:

✦ To one special school where there are many students with multiple disabilities and many related needs. They may provide actual, direct physical therapy interventions in therapy rooms in the schools and devote more attention to assistive technology in special education classes.

✦ To travel among several schools at all levels of education where students may be in both general education and special education classes. Their role may be more consultative (indirect) and intermittent to assure inclusion in these least restrictive environments.

✦ To programs for infants and toddlers who are at risk. Physical therapists may provide direct services with an emphasis on family education in early intervention centers.

✦ To some combination of the above models.

School district coordinators meet these needs by hiring therapists who are employees of the school district or by contracting the services of private companies or independently practicing physical therapists. Assuring that these contracts allow time for participation as an active team member beyond the provision of direct services is important so that contracting physical therapists are prepared to meet all of the responsibilities of school-based therapists.

The needs of students in special education cover a broad range of diagnoses and levels of disabilities, and a particular child's needs change over time. Physical therapists must have a broad range of skills to address a wide variety of conditions complemented by a strong understand understanding of teaching and learning for these special populations. Coordinators of related services in larger school districts may assign physical therapists the responsibility for interdisciplinary rehabilitation teams providing services in a cluster of schools in a particular location.

Management Responsibilities

Mission, Vision, and Goals

Perhaps the most important challenge to the mission, vision, and goals is orienting new staff as they make a major shift to a commitment to the philosophy and mission of IDEA and to an educational rather than health-care approach to the provision of services. Managers may need to clarify each particular school's philosophy and commitment to the "idea" of IDEA and compliance with its rules and regulations. Although the interdisciplinary focus may be secondary nature to many physical therapists, the heightened role of parents and teachers in decision making may be something that managers need to convey to the people they supervise. Limiting goals to those related to education in the least restrictive environment may be another important component of orientation for new employees.

Policies and Procedures

Broad policies and procedures are developed in the offices of the school board and distributed throughout school districts for implementation. Managers are unlikely to have responsibility for policies and procedures unless they are temporarily assigned to review them.

Clarification of the roles of the members of the IEP team may be the most important policy and procedure. Perhaps more than any other practice setting, the integration of services to avoid their overlap and to identify gaps in services, is critical in providing school-based services. Resources often are inadequate and must be managed conscientiously and carefully to eliminate waste and duplication.

In addition to IEP mandates, policies and procedures may need to be in place to clarify the responsibilities of members of the team and to establish stopgap measures in the provision of services. For instance, it may be helpful to develop a list of assessments, interventions, etc. commonly used by physical and occupational therapists, and then create a chart to delineate which discipline is primarily responsible for which ones. A similar clarification of the roles of supportive personnel in the related services and instructional paraeducators becomes important to ensure compliance with professional regulations and to establish clear lines of responsibility and communication.

Managers also may be responsible for determining which standardized developmental and functional scales should be used across the district and which should be used at the discretion of individual therapists. Investigating evidence to support these decisions may be a new role for managers as their accountability for the outcomes of services provided becomes dependent on standardized measurements.

Unlike health-care decisions, physicians may never be involved in actual IEP processes and decisions. Whether or not school-based therapists must have physicians' orders to "treat" children in school systems may vary from state to state. Managers may have to assure that policies and procedures address the expected relationships with physicians and compliance with legal requirements for the provision of service, particularly if Medicaid funding of services is a consideration. Assisting staff in a major shift of responsibility for clinical decisions without the medical support that is more common in health-care settings is another role of managers.

Marketing

Because related services in special education are so dependent on federal and state legislation, new programs may be limited to those that are mandated with little opportunity for creating other new programs. However, some managers may have the opportunity to identify funding sources and prepare grant proposals for alternative funding from other public and private sources. The support services available for preparation of proposals may vary widely from one school district to another so grant writing workshops and in-services may be valuable to managers who either are assigned or take the initiative to pursue outside funding.

Networking may be a more appropriate function than marketing for school-based managers. Due to IDEA requirements for referral of students to identify their potential need for related services, managers may not need to internally market related services in most schools. Internal networking may be more important to managers to identify and establish working relationships with all of the key players in each school. Beginning with the principal and continuing with teachers and other service providers, it may be critical for managers to clarify the roles of the physical therapists and other members of the rehabilitation team and to confirm that the goals for services are incorporated in the plans and mission for each school on an ongoing basis.

Formal and informal community networking is also important for the identification of support groups for caregivers and other community resources important to special education in general, and to meet the goals of specific IEPs. For example, managers may need to take the initiative to establish professional relationships with durable medical equipment suppliers, orthotists, and prosthetists.

Getting to know the family physicians, orthopedic surgeons, and other doctors who care for children receiving related services may be critical. Their understanding of the services provided in schools may be limited. Managers may make opportunities to educate physicians in face to face encounters to broaden the service network that supports the requirements of children with special needs while opening doors for better interdisciplinary communication between school-based and community-based providers of care.

Perhaps most importantly, managers need to be the face and voice of the school-based team to other providers of pediatric rehabilitation services. Not only are these services important as potential sources of providers in the school, but managers may need to open these doors so that school-based staff are able to coordinate effectively all of the care a child receives.

Staffing

Determination of a full-time caseload presents challenges to school-based managers. Three major factors to be considered in school-based caseloads have been identified:[10]

- ✦ The students to be served: type and amount of services provided to each student, geographic area to be covered, number of schools, and distances between them.
- ✦ The therapists' other responsibilities: documentation, meetings, consultation with teachers and parents, outcomes studies, and supervision of support personnel.
- ✦ Other factors: consultation with classroom staff and parents, support available, number of one-on-one sessions, community contacts required, and continuing education requirements.

Taking these identified tasks, managers may analyze staff caseloads by creating a log to determine the percentage of time in a 37.5-hour week that each full-time equivalent (FTE) employee devotes to various activities. Possible activities in a time log may include, direct student contact, paperwork, IEP and other meetings, travel time, assessments, consultation, lunchtime, and other union contract work conditions (e.g., breaks, preparation time).[10] Managers may ask staff members to complete the time logs consistently or they may select certain weeks for data collection with time logs. Data analysis may assist managers to adjust work assignments on an ongoing basis, redistribute staff, compare the work of full-time and part-time staff, or establish productivity goals for each staff member.

Recruitment

Recruitment of full-time staff to be employees of the school board may be challenging because salaries tend to be less than competitive with those offered in other work settings. Juggling the needs of students in all schools with the needs and preferences of contract service providers, or independent per diem contractors, and aligning them with the expectations of full-time school board employees makes assignment decisions and scheduling, particularly in large school districts (i.e., either population or geographically large) very time consuming.

For instance, contracting with a community-based pediatric practice may mean it provides services to the school district only on Tuesdays and Thursdays because they have outpatient visits in their offices scheduled on other days although IEPs call for related services to be delivered 3 times per week. Independent contractors only may work in one particular school that is convenient for them, or choose not to work into extended year programs during the summers. Full-time employees may become resentful if they are always representing other per diem or contract therapists in IEP meetings because the full-time therapists are more available.

School-based managers may face more pressure than managers in health-care settings to avoid staff turnover because the services provided in schools are long-term and complex. The time required for new people to establish rapport with children may delay or interfere with the progress toward goals. Consistency of personnel is more likely to result in better collaboration among members of the IEP team as well, particularly in field operations where a physical therapist may be a part of numerous teams in several schools.

Like other field operations, employees of the school district who travel among schools may spend as much time commuting between schools as they do delivering services. Often the staff are available but unevenly distributed because some locations are more desirable than others. This preference presents another management challenge if there are no resources to offer incentives for less attractive assignments. Hiring physical therapist assistants at lower pay scales may be one management solution, particularly if more assistants than therapists are available for hire. Because physical therapist assistants may be more tightly tied to a particular community, turnover of staff may be reduced, but managers should be cautious about other potential problems that may arise.

Physical Therapist Assistants

The roles of physical therapist assistants may be limited to the provision of direct care and providing instructions to teachers and support staff because consultation and the development of IEPs may be beyond their scope of practice. Evaluation, treatment planning, and supervision of others are typically the responsibilities of physical therapists that cannot be delegated to assistants. This delineation of roles further limits the distribution of the potential workforce. Utilization and supervision of physical therapist assistants is determined by state statutes, which may mean that physical therapists do not need to provide direct or on-site supervision to physical therapist assistants in schools. Depending on those practice rules, supervision of assistants by the physical therapist of record may mean that the therapist has supervisory responsibility for several assistants who are assigned to different schools. When a physical therapist assistant is assigned to only one school serviced by an itinerant physical therapist, managers may need to pay particular attention to assure compliance with practice acts.

For instance, if the physical therapist assistant is more readily available in a particular school than the physical therapist is, care needs to be taken that practice acts are not violated. There may be unintentional, well-meaning decision making and problem-solving by the physical therapist assistant that occurs because of the day-to-day questions that arise about the care of a child, which are actually the responsibility of the physical therapist. Managers may find it necessary to spend more efforts distinguishing the legal responsibilities of physical therapists and physical therapist assistants for parents and education professionals. Orientation of therapists and assistants in school-based practices may need to include communication strategies for dealing with these potential issues about decision making to avoid potential practice act violations.

Patient Care

Even for physical therapists with pediatric experience in other settings, distinguishing only those goals that are related to the achievement of school-based goals may require a careful analysis of a child's ability to function. Moving from a "medically necessary" model of thinking to a "learning relevant" model may not be as easy as it sounds for some therapists, particularly if the therapists are also working in community-based pediatric services where the emphasis is one-on-one interventions. Shifting gears may not happen without effort.

Managers' monitoring of this critical component of school-based services and their assurance of staff expertise to address a wide range of diagnoses and learning needs may be their primary roles in the actual delivery of services. Managers should not be hesitant to hire therapists who seek new opportunities in school systems even though their prior work experience may be with adults. It may, however, be somewhat easier to start with a clean pediatric slate than it is to modify strong, long-held opinions about the care of children with disabilities.

Classroom Integration

Making certain that the determination of providing direct interventions *only* when necessary and consulting (indirect) services *always* when necessary may be another management concern. Deciding when to shift services from isolated therapy rooms to integrated services in the classrooms remains controversial as therapists balance the child's need for practice to learn new skills with the need to function in the most natural environment—the classroom. It follows that determining the frequency of treatment interventions also becomes challenging because the effectiveness of interventions is muddied by many external factors—positive and negative, including the actual implementation of recommendations made to teachers and caregivers.[11]

Managers may need to encourage their staffs to be creative in identifying resources and in collaborating to meet the needs of students. Increased collaboration may require having the tools to resolve potential conflicts among the rehabilitation team, teachers, and family members. School-based managers may need to offer more assistance to their staffs in reaching more compromises than are expected in health care. Teachers become vested in students that they have known for years, and parents' opinions are taken very seriously.

The negotiation skills of managers also may be more important in school-based practice because resolving conflicts at one level of management may create additional problems at others. For instance, if upper-level district managers of special education and related services do not come from the same professional disciplines as the people they supervise, or if members of one IEP team report to different supervisors in a district, additional management issues can arise. School districts are complex, bureaucratic organizations in which the chains of command are not always clear, particularly as limited resources demand frequent organizational changes.

Performance Evaluation

Because school-based services are a field operation, evaluation of performance of staff may be difficult.

There may be only one annual opportunity to observe treatment sessions to determine the therapist's clinical expertise and ability to manage the behavior of children. Managers often rely on input from other members of the IEP team, including parents and students to complement these direct observations. Tweezing out the contribution of each discipline in student outcomes may not always be straightforward nor clear, and the outcomes of education are often long-term with many intervening variables along the way. Having staff self-report on their activities and their contributions to IEPs may be an important management tool. For instance, in addition to the direct provision of services, evaluation of performance may include:

✦ Compliance with the IDEA, Section 504, and ADA
✦ Knowledge of the general education curriculum as it relates to therapy
✦ Effective use and analysis of assessment tools
✦ Consultation and collaboration skills

Fiscal

Although managers in health-care settings may face many budgeting and cash-flow challenges, they seem to be compounded in school systems. Through complex federal and state funding, which is typically driven by legislative budgeting processes, school-based managers may have a minimal role in any financial decision making, but a great deal of accountability for controlling costs.

School districts may enroll as providers of Medicaid services, which allow them to be reimbursed for services provided under IDEA Parts B and C to students whom are eligible for Medicaid. This Medicaid Certified School Match Program includes reimbursement for direct services, such as all of the rehabilitation services, counseling, nursing, and transportation. Administrative activities, such as referrals to determine Medicaid eligibility and for the coordination of services, also are reimbursed.

The intent of these Medicaid match programs is to improve students' access to medical care and to promote a better understanding of care available to families, which will improve students' health. It is also a source of income for school districts that helps to meet their costs for delivery of these mandated services, with some remaining funds available to reinvest in the expansion of services and to purchase supplies and equipment for special education programs. Managers may need to develop the means to prevent duplication of Medicaid services when children are concurrently receiving therapy in community-based agencies.

Legal, Ethical, and Risk

Because special education is so tightly linked to legislation, failure to meet these mandates presents potential legal issues. There are numerous legal cases surrounding special education and IDEA, which have been taken to the U.S. Supreme Court. For instance, courts have been asked to determine what is a related service versus a medical service. The determination of the adequacy of physical therapy services for a particular child also has been addressed by the courts.[10]

Role Release

In addition to the legal issues surrounding the supervision and direction of physical therapist assistants, the delegation of care to paraeducators (also called paraprofessionals or instructional aides), teachers, and parents may be equally risky, although necessary. These professional decisions about who does what are about directing and instructing rather than delegation. They require careful consideration because it is more the rule than the exception that physical therapists and other health professionals in the related services "release" their roles to others in the schools and to parents for students to meet their goals.[10]

Therapists are often less available for the daily carry through of interventions that students need to practice because they are spread thin among schools to meet the demands for services when workforce and other resources are limited. It is important that physical therapists understand that role release does not mean abdication of responsibility. Documentation of the training of others to perform assigned tasks and supervising that performance with a particular student is critical especially in this transdisciplinary, educational model of care.[10]

These role-release decisions are even more complex because IEPs are discipline neutral. This transdisciplinary nature of therapeutic services in schools may cause physical therapists to struggle with reinforcing what is and what is not physical therapy.

Because physical therapy is defined as only what a physical therapist does or directs a physical therapist assistant to do, it may be helpful to clarify that others who are following the instructions of the physical therapist in the classroom or at home, are not, legally "doing physical therapy."

Managers also must understand their legal responsibility for patient/client instruction and the education of other caregivers are also professional responsibilities. They may take on greater significance in complex school settings in which many people are involved in students' IEPs, particularly when the therapist is intermittently on the premises. Assuring that all care providers are adequately trained for their global responsibilities and for particular tasks assigned for each student, must be confirmed and documented by the physical therapist and other providers of related services.

Confidentiality

Another legal and ethical concern is maintaining the confidentiality of student records, which is as important as maintaining the confidentiality of medical records. Therapists may need to be reminded that all statutes regulating practice, professional codes of ethics, and standards of practice apply to health-care and school-based settings.

Like health care, a lack of resources often leads to ethical dilemmas. Pressure from principals or school-board members to standardize policies and procedures about the frequency and duration of related services for children with particular diagnoses, or to establish productivity goals that negatively impact IEP outcomes, requires managers to be prepared to present the legal and ethical dilemmas that such actions place on therapists.

Communication

Managers of any field operations often take a variety of means to communicate with staffs that are scattered over a large geographic area following different work schedules. E-mail, phone conferences, cell phones, access to electronic databases, and other forms of communication have facilitated efforts to communicate and track services provided. School-based managers may find the need to spend much time in the field to determine the effectiveness of services provided under their supervision in each school.

Managers may need to confirm that physical therapists who supervise physical therapist assistants have established the importance of scheduling ongoing communication and supervisory sessions. Physical therapist assistants must have accurate contact information so that the physical therapist is readily available should student emergencies arise. Whether or not the level and frequency of supervision of supportive personnel in school-based practice are defined in state statutes, supervisory responsibility and the documentation of communication is essential. This is particularly important if the physical therapist and the assistant are not in the same place at the same time—which may be a more common staffing model in school-based practice than it is in health care.

Similarly, instructions to, and follow-up of care provided by, nonlicensed school aides and paraeducators under the direction of physical therapists or assistants must be clearly documented. Managers may need to determine training needs and prepare programs for them accordingly. Physical therapists need to be prepared, or need to assign physical therapist assistants, to provide one-on-one instructions to non–health-care professionals to meet the needs of particular students.

Informal Communication

The informal communication among related service providers and all of the teachers involved in a particular student's IEP has been facilitated by the availability of e-mail. Because the therapists may move among several schools, there may be little downtime in a particular school for informal, face-to-face interactions. Therefore, to enhance communication, managers must assure that there is time for staff to represent rehabilitation services at formally scheduled meetings of the special education team. Emphasizing the importance of accurate documentation of the services provided and filing that documentation in a centralized location for timely access by all members of the IEP team also is critical for communication among the team.

Conclusion

The management of school-based physical therapy services offers unique challenges and rewards. It provides the satisfaction that comes from being a respected, indispensable part of a transdisciplinary special education program, and someone who is responsible for staff who must be effective team players, communicators, and documenters throughout a school system.

Because there is a higher legal standard of care expected when people are less able to take care of themselves, managers must be vigilant in addressing the legal and ethical issues confronting physical therapists who care for children. The rewards of establishing long-term professional relationships with children and their families often more than balances all of the system requirements that must be addressed. The financial support of special education programs, personnel shortages, and government mandates may demand as much of the attention of managers as their responsibility for the quality of care provided through the related services.

The team approach to solving complex problems helps to focus on the big picture of least-restrictive learning environments. School-based practice presents many opportunities to take pride in contributing to the accomplishments of many children who might otherwise not have a chance if not for the combined efforts of many health and education professionals. Activities 17.1 to 17.14 provide the opportunity to address school-based management decision making.

ACTIVITY 17.1
SCHOOL-BASED MANAGERS AND STUDENTS

Are students who receive related services in schools more like patients or clients as defined by the American Physical Therapy Association? Defend your answer in a group discussion. What difference does it make?

ACTIVITY 17.2
THE BIG PICTURE

In addition to her responsibilities for all rehabilitation services in the K–12 schools in Hamilton County, Marsha Miller is assigned to a task force to address the rise in obesity among all students and to identify potential grant-funding opportunities. She has to determine the potential role of the rehabilitation team in program development and implementation. What should she recommend? What other concerns about school-aged children have been identified by the APTA?

ACTIVITY 17.3
COMMUNITY RESOURCES

Larry Eubanks has moved to Uniontown to become the Coordinator of Rehabilitation Services for Union County Schools. He wants to develop a link on the school-board's Web page for community resources that parents, students, and staff alike may access. He wants the list of resources to be comprehensive and relevant, leaving no stone unturned. How should he go about implementing this idea?

ACTIVITY 17.4
UNSATISFACTORY PERFORMANCE

Larry Eubanks spent one day in the last year, unannounced, in each school to observe clinical performance and interactions of his staff with school personnel. He was impressed with everyone's efforts and felt confident that he had inherited a good team doing a good job. He was surprised by a call from Fred Fielding, the teacher who is the orthopedic program coordinator at Jackson Middle School. Fred is demanding that Sonja Sammons, the physical therapist, not return to the school because of her disruptive behavior, and expects Larry to replace her as soon as possible. Fred reports that Sonja spends more time socializing and provoking student conflicts than doing her job. Larry's observations of her clinical interventions with three students were acceptable. What should Larry do?

ACTIVITY 17.5
SCHOOL-BASED VERSUS COMMUNITY-BASED

Larry Eubanks has been working closely with Total Therapy Care to coordinate the care of several students with disabilities in Union County Schools over the past year. He negotiated a contract between Union County and Total Therapy Care to provide services in one of the county's special education centers. That contract has been working well with no issues. However, Larry has received calls from two different parents of children who are being treated by Tanya Vargas, a full-time physical therapist employed by the school board for K–12 schools in the northern half of the county. The parents report that they are very concerned because their children also receive therapy 3 times/week at Total Therapy Care, and the physical therapist there tells them that what Tanya is doing is undermining what they are trying to do with their children. What should Larry do?

ACTIVITY 17.6
CASE STUDY STAFF SHORTAGE

The good news is that Union County is the fastest growing county in the state. The bad news is that the school board is having difficulty meeting the educational demands of the additional students who have moved to the area. Larry Eubanks has been rehabilitation coordinator for Union County Schools for 5 years now. He received a memo from the Sarah Chiles, County Director for Special Education requesting a meeting next week. She asked that Larry be prepared to identify at least three ways to control costs other than staffing and three strategies for recruiting staff to meet the needs of 120 new special education students next year. What are some ideas that Larry may present?

ACTIVITY 17.7
CLINICAL EDUCATION IN SPECIAL EDUCATION

One of the recruitment strategies that Larry Eubanks suggested during his meeting with Sarah (see Activity 17.6) was to establish clinical education agreements with the local university's physical therapy program and the community college's physical therapist assistant program. This also may relieve his personnel shortage to have professional students helping with care. He reported to Sarah that the program coordinators have approached him in the past but he did not feel that his staff was ready. What are the issues that Larry and Sarah need to consider before they meet with the coordinators of clinical education from the university and community college?

ACTIVITY 17.8
CASE STUDY: ADAPTIVE PHYSICAL EDUCATION

Larry Eubanks has received his third message from Melissa Quintos, one of the adaptive physical education teachers in Union County. She has been insistent in her requests for him to devise a countywide plan to integrate therapy more effectively into adaptive physical education. He has been avoiding her because he does not feel prepared to address the issues. What does Larry need to do before meeting with her?

ACTIVITY 17.9
CASE STUDY: SUPERVISION OF PT ASSISTANT

Clarice Montiago, Charlie's mother, has called Larry Eubanks to say that she no longer wants Sally Simmons, the physical therapist assistant, to work with Charlie. She just learned that Sally is not a licensed physical therapist. Clarice states that she knows her son's rights and he must be treated by a physical therapist. What should Larry do?

ACTIVITY 17.10
CASE STUDY: TO WALK OR NOT TO WALK

There is only one item on the agenda for the Fall physical therapy staff meeting. Larry Eubanks has sent a memo stating the meeting will be a workshop to develop recommendations for policies and procedures about determining which children are to incorporate walking during school hours as part of their IEPs. This issue has been a source of contention between the therapists, who strongly feel that students who can walk, should walk, and teachers and administrators who insist that only students who can perform within the demands of schedules should be walking between classes and to and from activities. Their argument is that it is disruptive for students to be excused early or to be late for every class and lunch because of the extra time they need to walk. What literature is available on this issue? What should the policy and procedure state?

ACTIVITY 17.11
MAINSTREAMING VERSUS INCLUSION

Larry Eubanks just realized that the communication problem that he has been having with some of his staff is because of a difference of opinion about least-restrictive environment. Some of his therapists believe that their job is to adapt the child to the school as much as possible and that they should only be in classes and activities in which they can succeed. Other staff members believe that the school should make all efforts to adapt classrooms, and the school as a whole, to meet the needs of all the children. Which view is right? What difference does it make? What should Larry do?

ACTIVITY 17.12
PARENTAL DEMANDS

Joe and Anne Lee have asked for a meeting with Larry Eubanks, rehabilitation coordinator for Union County Schools and Joyce McCullen, Principal at Pretty Lake Elementary School. They are very unhappy with the decision made at the last IEP meeting that their daughter Lulu will not be receiving physical therapy in school. Lulu had been receiving physical therapy 2 times/week at Kids-R-Great Rehab in town, but the Lee's health insurance no longer covers these services. They believe that she has not reached a plateau and only can improve with more physical therapy. Although they attended the IEP meeting and heard that all accommodations have been made for Lulu to meet her learning goals, they are not satisfied. The Lee's have advised Mrs. McCullen that they have contacted a lawyer and know their rights. Role-play this meeting.

ACTIVITY 17.13
DIRECTION AND SUPERVISION

Terri Edmundson, physical therapist at Pretty Lake Elementary School, has established the method that Timmy Fletcher is to use to ascend and descend the school-bus steps. She has directed Jake Ortiz, the physical therapist assistant to have Timmy practice on the steps 3 or 4 more times in the next week. Terri also tells Jake that when he is satisfied that Timmy can perform the stairclimb, he is to instruct Debra, the orthopedic aide assigned to Timmy, to meet him at the bus everyday to supervise him getting on and off the bus until further notice. Timmy's mother calls Larry Eubanks, rehabilitation coordinator, at the end of the week to ask if she should be helping Timmy on and off the bus at home everyday since he is doing it at school, or if he should continue to use the wheelchair lift on the bus at the home end? What questions should Larry ask of whom? What other concerns should Larry have?

ACTIVITY 17.14
PRODUCTIVITY

Based on the analysis of time logs submitted for 4 random weeks by 12 physical therapists Larry Eubanks is faced with the following results based on 37.5 hours/week of work:

ACTIVITY	MEAN PERCENTAGE OF TIME SPENT BY PTs TRAVELING AMONG SCHOOLS	MEAN PERCENTAGE OF TIME SPENT BY PTs ASSIGNED TO ONE SCHOOL
Student contact	44%	46%
Paperwork	19%	20%
Meetings. including IEPs	16%	28%
Lunch	6%	6%
Travel	15%	0%

What should Larry conclude about the work of his staff? Should the percentages for the distribution of work of physical therapist assistants be the same?

REFERENCES

1. U.S. Department of Education, Office of Special Education Programs. Children and students served under IDEA, part B, by age group and state: Fall 2005. Available at: https://www. ideadata.org/tables29th/ar 1-1.htm. Accessed September 21, 2007.

2. U.S. Department of Education, Office of Special Education Programs. Table 6-1. Infants and toddlers receiving early intervention services under IDEA, Part C, by age. Available at: https://www.ideadata.org/tables29th/ar_6-1.htm. Accessed September 21, 2007.

3. United States Congress. Individuals with Disabilities Education Improvement Act 2004. Sec 101, Part AA, Subpart 4, Sec 602 (3)(A) Definitions. Available at: http://thomas.loc.gov/cgi-bin/query/D?c108:5:./temp/~mdbsfV1ryh::. Accessed April 5, 2009.

4. United States Congress. *Related services in IDEIA 2005.* Sec 101, Part A, Subpart 4, Sec 02 (26)(A). Available from: http://thomas.loc.gov/cgi-bin/query/F?c108:1:./temp/~c10864HVJj:e761:.

5. Osgood RL. *The History of Inclusion in the United States.* Washington, DC: Gallaudet University Press, 2005.

6. Siegel LM. *The Complete IEP Guide: How to Advocate for Your Special Ed Child.* 4th ed. Berkeley, CA: Nolo, 2005.

7. United States Department of Justice. *A Guide to Disability Rights Laws.* September 2005. Available at: http://www.usdoj.gov/crt/ada/cguide.pdf. Accessed September 21, 2007.

8. Rosenfeld SJ. *Section 504 and IDEA: Basic Similarities and Differences.* Available at: http://www.wrightslaw.com/advoc/articles/504 IDEA Rosenfled.html. Accessed September 21, 2007.

9. IDEA Funding Coalition. IDEA funding: Time for congress to live up to the commitment mandatory funding proposal. Available at: http://www.nea.org/lac/idea/images/mandatory 2006.pdf. Accessed September 21, 2007.

10. McEwen I, ed. *Providing Physical Therapy Services Under Parts B & C of the Individuals with Disabilities Education Act (IDEA).* Alexandria, VA: Section on Pediatrics, American Physical Therapy Association, 2000.

11. Kaminker MK, Chiarello LA, O'Neil ME, et al. Decision making for physical therapy service delivery in schools: A nationwide survey of pediatric physical therapists. *Physical Therapy.* 2004;84:919–933.

Chapter 18

Management Issues in Home Care Organizations

Learning Objectives

✦ Discuss the characteristics of the range of contemporary home care services and hospice.
✦ Analyze licensure, certification, and accreditation demands in home care.
✦ Discuss contemporary home care practice issues.
✦ Analyze the work of physical therapists in home care settings.
✦ Determine the managerial roles and challenges to managerial responsibilities.
✦ Analyze managerial decision making in given home care situations.

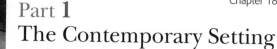

Part 1
The Contemporary Setting

Overview of Home Care

Home care is that broad array of professional and paraprofessional services, postacute and long-term care, with medical and social services provided in nonmedical, residential settings that include two broad parallel and inter-related functions: [1]

- ✦ Social and supportive services. Their purpose is to keep the person in the home and as functional as possible by providing personal care. This type of home care is often uncompensated care by family and friends. If additional supportive assistance is needed, it is more often than not paid for out of pocket. These paid services do not require a high level of skill. Contrary to popular impressions, it may be more expensive than institutional care if it is needed 24/7 and the client is severely dependent.

- ✦ Postacute services. These may be episodes of care of intermediate or intensive length, which include intermittent, short-term visits by health professionals. They are professional, skilled services; therefore, reimbursement by Medicare, Medicaid, and other health insurance policies applies.

Society has a long history of the care of the sick and elderly in the home. Only recently has that care become an important part of the business of health care. People of all ages who have a wide range of physical and mental impairments receive home care. Children and working age adults, commonly receiving Medicaid benefits, comprise 40% of home care patients. People over the age of 85 are the smallest age group (16%) who receive home care services, but they use a disproportionate amount of it. Home care payment is 48.7% Medicare funded, 24.2% Medicaid, 3.8% other insurance, and 22.8% out of pocket. [1] About 20% of these payments go to approximately 20,000 provider organizations, which deliver home care services to 7.6 million people in the United States. These organizations supplement rather than replace the informal, unpaid care that families, neighbors, and friends provide in the home. Family and other unpaid providers provide *all* of the care for 74% of the dependent elderly in the community. [2]

The purpose of home care is to maximize health and functioning in people with long-term needs so that they may remain in the community in the least restrictive environment, while supporting the families who care for them. The goal of health-care policy has been to prevent unnecessary use of more costly inpatient health-care services. Changes in hospital reimbursement have resulted in earlier hospital discharges made possible by new portable technologies. Services, such as intravenous nutrition, chemotherapy, respiratory therapy, dialysis care, fetal monitoring, telemonitoring, and other high-tech therapies have moved into the home setting. The resultant rapid growth in home care services has become a major issue in the provision of health care. [3]

These technological advances have skewed the home care population to clients who are frailer and more medically compromised, yet who seek to remain safely in their homes. Meeting the needs of this population involves creative and complex discharge planning from hospitals and long-term care organizations. After all, the return to home is a time-honored goal of hospitalization, and an important stage of rehabilitation. Shifting from the dependency of inpatient care to independence at home requires the serious planning of many people. It must be taken seriously because the control of one's environment is the major criterion for a person's independence. The unique circumstances of each patient make it difficult to anticipate every potential problem related to the return to home after an episode of inpatient care. At the least, the discharge plan needs to include the determination of: [4]

- ✦ Safety and accessibility of the home environment.
- ✦ Willingness of the patient to receive home services.
- ✦ Availability of willing and able family or caregiver to assist the patient in activities of daily living (ADLs) and instrumental activities of daily living (IADLs).
- ✦ Additional resources available to supplement family caregiving.

See Sidebars 18.1 and 18.2.

Sidebar 18.1

Contemporary Home Care Issues

Other data about contemporary home care and current policy issues can be found at the Web pages of the National Association for Home Care & Hospice. http://www.nahc.org/.

Sidebar 18.2

Terminology

Terms used to name and discuss the care provided in the home may be used inconsistently and result in confusion. Assumptions should not be made about the legal or certification status of a business based on its name. For instance, home health and home care may be used interchangeably, or home health may refer to nursing services with home care reserved for the broader context of all services, or home health may mean Medicare certification of an agency and home care refers to private pay services.

Types of Home Care

Table 18.1 summarizes the differences among the three broad types of home care and the role of physical therapy services in each. Any of these services may exist as part of an integrated health-care delivery system, a franchise (unit of a national company), a joint venture, or a freestanding, privately owned organization. Only 25% are hospital-based organizations.[1]

The Family and Home Care

For many people with acute and chronic conditions living at home, assistance from family, benevolent volunteers or paid caregivers is generally required (although not always available). These needs for assistance and issues related to them transcend class, race, ethnicity, age, gender, place, and time. For example, family members often fear the patient's failure to die or to get well. Uncertainty about the length of time their support will be needed is a common concern for many families involved in the care of loved ones at home. This uncertainty influences their willingness to begin to engage in the care of a person. More importantly, the growth in single-parent homes and blended families complicates the provision of unpaid home care. These new kinship roles have changed the traditional family model and tend to erode the informal caregiving required to keep the ill and elderly in their homes.[6]

Family members assume four roles when involved in home care regardless of the type of disability the loved one has, the funding source for care, and the amount or the types of services required:[7]

+ Providers of direct care. Most family members believe that this care is their responsibility or obligation. They may be reluctant to have "outsiders" in their homes, but must agree to outside help because they lack specialized skills to care for the very sick.

+ Task sharers. Family members perform special tasks that are unique to meeting the particular needs of an individual that only family members can meet. Family sharing of these responsibilities requires clarification of normal household duties. Meeting these patient needs supplements and complements rather than substitutes for outside services that are provided.

+ Brokers. Arranging home care services for a patient among the myriad of fragmented services, eligibility requirements, and funding requires family members to develop organization and coordination skills to meet this role.

+ Monitors. Determining the quality of the task-related skills and the interpersonal relationships of health-care workers with the patient becomes a family responsibility. It is a critical component of assessing the effectiveness of care often provided by several people.

Even if family members are comfortable assuming these roles, the advantages of home care—convenience, more independence and control for the patient, and personalized attention—must be weighed against the disruption to the order of the home as it moves from a place of refuge and privacy to becoming a health-care setting. For informal caregivers, who are predominantly spouses and female adult children, "caring" remains inconvenient, challenging, and disruptive to the daily patterns of living and working. In U.S culture, the demands of home care are grossly undervalued and codified

TABLE 18.1 Characteristics of home health agencies, hospices, and home care aide agencies and the role of physical therapy in each

TYPE OF HOME CARE	PURPOSE	PATIENT ELIGIBILITY REQUIREMENTS	ROLE OF PHYSICAL THERAPY
Home Health (Care) Agencies	Skilled intermittent care that includes disease state management	Typically certified as Medicare agency. To be eligible for home care as a Medicare beneficiary: Must be homebound, MD certification of need, require skilled intermittent or part-time care. Must be medically necessary. Continues until outcomes reached or maintenance program established and can be turned over to less technical provider (custodial care).[1]	Integral component of an integrated, interdisciplinary approach to skilled care
Hospices	Professional (medical) and volunteer (social) services for those at the end of life (77% of hospice patients die at home)	Certified as Medicare agency. To be eligible for hospice services, need documented proof of only 6 months to live but can live longer and continue to receive care. Agree to palliative rather than curative or life-prolonging care.[5]	May range from a more consultative role with a focus on assisting caregivers as a patient's condition declines, to a strong interdisciplinary team approach to palliative care at the end of life.
Home Care Aide Agencies	Homemaker, personal care services to assist with activities of daily living	No certification requirements because it is not a covered skilled service. Licensure rules vary from state to state.[2]	May have consultative or teaching role in the agency in preparing home care aides for their duties with complex, dependent patients. The coordination of skilled services with home care aides occurs when both skilled services and home health aides are provided concurrently.

Note: Organizations that provide private duty nursing, home medical equipment, infusion therapy, and home pharmacy may be included in an "other" category.

as housework, family obligation, or perhaps a voluntary charitable responsibility.[3] Although policy makers see care provided in the home as a potentially less expensive care setting, patients and their families often are simply relying on home care services for relief—as caregivers, paying consumers, and managers of care.

Home Care and Public Policy

Home care is full of dichotomies for health-care policy makers. For instance, home care is both formal professional services provided by paid staff and unpaid assistance furnished by such informal supporters as families and neighbors. It is both acute and long-term care with medical and/or social components. It is a service with merits of its own while also valued in terms of reductions in institutional care. Depending on which lens is being used, the determination of the goals and components of home care and its place in the continuum of health care can be complex.

Because of these complexities, policy makers revisit the costs and benefits of home care constantly. Professional providers of home care are continually adapting and adjusting case mixes and patterns of care to match available reimbursement without reducing the home services needed or desired by the sick and vulnerable. Because of the uncertainty and complexity of the system, it is no surprise that home care is not always the hoped for thrifty substitute for costly institutional care that policy makers desire.

Some tough political questions are yet to be addressed effectively, such as:[3]

✦ Is caring for the sick at home a private family obligation or a responsibility shared with a caring society?

- ✦ Should home care be provided only under the most restrictive of circumstances, or whenever it can help?
- ✦ When will the fundamental question of how to determine the appropriate recipients and payers of home care be resolved?
- ✦ How can the unwillingness to pay for home care because of lack of trust of services provided privately in a person's home be overcome?

Licensure, Certification, Regulation, and Accreditation

Generally, all home care organizations are licensed in accordance with state statutes. Requirements for licensure may include assurance of financial stability and liability insurance, lease agreements, compliance with background screening checks of employees, qualifications of the administrator and director of nursing, corporation documents, etc.

To provide services to patients insured by Medicare and Medicaid, a home care organization is required to be certified by the Centers for Medicare and Medicaid Services (CMMS). Accreditation of the organization is a voluntary process that federal, state, and other reimbursement models are dependent upon in their certifications of providers of home care.

The Community Health Accreditation Program (CHAP) of the National League for Nursing is one of the accrediting bodies for home health organizations. Since 1965, CHAP has taken a lead in developing mechanisms for recognizing excellence in community health. CMMS granted CHAP deeming authority for home health and hospice organizations, which means that CHAP, not state agencies, may have responsibility for surveys of these organizations to determine that an organization meets Medicare's conditions of participation for reimbursement of the services they provide.[8]

The CHAP accreditation process is based on standards of excellence for management, quality, client outcomes, adequate resources, and long-term viability. The goal of this process is to assist all types of community-based health-care organizations to do the following:[9]

- ✦ Strengthen internal operations
- ✦ Promote continuous quality improvement
- ✦ Promote consumer satisfaction

- ✦ Promote positive client outcomes
- ✦ Meet community health needs in a cost-effective and efficient manner
- ✦ Maintain the viability of community health practice nationwide
- ✦ Assure public trust in community-based services and products

CHAP, like most accrediting bodies, provides guidance and criteria to be met as evidence of efforts to accomplish these goals. Their criteria are based on four key underlying principles that drive their standards:[9]

- ✦ The organization's structure and function consistently supports its consumer-oriented philosophy, mission, and purpose.
- ✦ The organization consistently provides high-quality services and products.
- ✦ The organization has adequate human, financial, and physical resources to accomplish its stated mission and purpose.
- ✦ The organization is positioned for long-term viability.

Another, more recent, home care organization accrediting body is The Joint Commission of Accreditation of Health Care Organizations, which began as the accrediting body for hospitals. Now called simply The Joint Commission, its seal of approval is nationally recognized as an indication that an organization meets certain quality standards. Unlike CHAP, The Joint Commission accredits a wide range of health-care organizations. They also administer Disease Specific Care Certification to health plans, disease management service companies, hospitals, and other care delivery settings that provide disease management and chronic care services. The positioning statement of The Joint Commission is "helping health-care organizations help patients."[10]

The Joint Commission's standards for each type of organization are organized around the important functions of patient safety, patient care, and management, which are framed as performance objectives based on continuous quality improvement concepts. Oryx is The Joint Commission initiative for the collection of standardized data on these performance objectives that is not fully developed for home care organizations. Instead, in its home care accreditation decisions, The

Joint Commission uses data generated through Medicare's Outcome and Assessment Information Set (OASIS). OASIS is the documentation/reimbursement system required by Medicare to assess outcomes in home care organizations. Like CHAP, The Joint Commission surveys can be approved as a substitute for federal and state agency surveys of home care organizations for certification or licensure.[11]

Hospice and Rehabilitation

Management of physical therapy and other rehabilitation services in hospice requires a broader view of quality of life to address the dignity of people in death and dying. Managers need to begin the orientation of staff to their roles in hospice with the concept that hospice is an environment and attitude of care rather than a place.

For many people, dying is a lingering process of difficulties with each stage resulting in a little more loss of the capacity to bounce back. It has been called rehabilitation in reverse because the role of the rehabilitation members of the team is to address the deteriorating rather than the improving changes in the patient's condition. Optimizing function at each stage must be discussed with the patient and family so that expectations are not threatening.[12]

Using the same skills that they bring to all settings, therapists in hospice care may need to deal with their own feelings about death and dying. Accepting the following classic premises underlying hospice helps to address new adaptations or skills required to maximize function and safety for the patient and family:[13]

- ✦ Basic regard for the recipient of care.
- ✦ Acceptance of death as a natural part of living.
- ✦ Consideration of the entire family as the unit of care.
- ✦ Maintenance of the patient at home for as long as possible.
- ✦ Assistance for the patient attempting to assume control over his or her own life.
- ✦ Instructions for patient self-care.
- ✦ Reduction or removal of pain and other distressing symptoms.
- ✦ Comprehensive provision of services by an interdisciplinary team.
- ✦ Total, not fragmented care.

Although every Medicare-certified hospice is mandated to have an occupational, physical, and speech therapist contracted, the use of those services is not mandated. Managers responsible for rehabilitation staff in hospice may need to develop strategies for educating other members of the hospice team about the role of the rehabilitation team, particularly if there is concern that receiving rehabilitation may raise false hopes of recovery. The care provided in hospice tends to be more holistic and the roles of members of the team become blurred and overlap as a result. As the predominant health professional, the nurse often determines the involvement of other professionals on an as-needed basis.[12] Sidebar 18.3 contains additional information on hospice.

Unique Features of Physical Therapy Practice in Home Care

Although physical therapists may work in any type of home care agency (see Table 18.1), they are most likely to be employed by, or contract their services with, home care agencies that provide skilled services to people across the life span. Home care also may be a part of their responsibilities although their primary work occurs in inpatient or outpatient settings. The following list includes examples of potential models of organizations in which physical therapists may manage home care services:

- ✦ Pediatric private practice that provides services to children in the home and office.
- ✦ Home care agency providing pediatric services only.
- ✦ Private, nationwide home care corporation with many locations.

Sidebar 18.3

Hospice Sources

For additional information on hospice go to the American Academy of Hospice and Palliative Medicine at http://www.aahpm.org/sites/index.html and the Hospice Foundation of America at http://www.hospicefoundation.org/.

✦ Skilled nursing facility that has rehabilitation staff who provide home care services within the retirement community of which it is a part.

✦ Home care agency that contracts with an adult congregate living facility to provide all home care services in the community.

✦ Home care unit whose staff is employed by a hospital organization and who provide services only to patients discharged from that hospital.

✦ Freestanding home care agency that forms a legal relationship with a hospital that then becomes a unit of service in that health-care system.

✦ Physical therapy company that provides per diem staff to several home care agencies.

✦ Registry of health-care professionals that provides staff either locally or as travelers typically through short-term contracts with agencies.

✦ Physical therapist who is an independent contractor accepting cases from a variety of home care organizations. NOTE: Medicare patients requiring more than one home care service must receive those services through a Medicare-certified home care agency rather than from individual providers.

✦ Hospice programs.

The work of home care physical therapists seems to present the same universal challenges and rewards of work found in any other setting. The unique aspects are just because the care is provided in the home. Coke[14] has identified some characteristics of work in home care that are presented in Sidebar 18.4.

Sidebar 18.4

Characteristics of Work in Home Care Settings

✦ Patient-focused care for approximately 45 minutes with one patient (and his or her family) at a time who is typically highly motivated to participate.

✦ Excessive paperwork.

✦ Difficulty scheduling visits because of the patient's own commitments, such as physician appointments, coordinating the presence of the caregiver for teaching, and the visiting schedules of other members of the care team.

✦ Involvement with comprehensive care in an interdisciplinary team.

✦ Driving in various weather conditions.

✦ Entering unfamiliar neighborhoods.

✦ Unkempt homes that are less than ideal circumstances for treatment and comfort.

✦ Creative and professional challenge to devise relevant care plans and obtain measurable clinical outcomes.

✦ Professional rewards of patient appreciation for individualized, personalized caring.

✦ Independence in structuring therapist work time based upon client needs.

✦ Travel breaks that allow "breathing time" rather than continuous patient care.

✦ Focus on mastering activities of daily living, assessing and instructing in the use of durable medical equipment, and provision of caregiver training. These factors often determine the patient's ability to remain at home.

✦ Addressing safety concerns is a top priority. Layout of a home is often more confining and requires more maneuvering. Fear can certainly be a barrier to improving function and a limiting factor in the patient's recovery process when there is no one to depend on for assistance.

✦ Patients must be true partners and follow through on instructions on their own. They may have cooperated in the hospital to be discharged, but may need encouragement to sustain motivation when at home and other activities compete more for a patient's time.

✦ A shift from a focus on strengthening specific muscle groups that are important for a particular functional activity to performing functional activities as exercise. Exercise is uniquely tailored and highly individualized to meet specific patient needs and address unique functional deficits.

Particularly for therapists who transition to home care from other health-care settings, work in home care presents additional factors for consideration, such as:

✦ Productivity goals that are affected by factors beyond one's control, such as traffic congestion, road conditions, or weather conditions.

✦ Greater responsibility for detailed and extensive documentation to meet reimbursement and accreditation requirements.

✦ The potential for long work hours due to schedule changes, unpredictable circumstances during travel or in the homes of patients, and difficulty coordinating schedules with other members of the team.

✦ Limited opportunities for face-to-face communication and interaction with other team members for patient care discussions and peer support because of the short time spent in the office of the organization.

✦ Decreased control of therapy because patients are on their own turf.

✦ A shift to a more collaborative role with emphasis on problem-solving *with* the patient.

✦ A shift in perceptions about the functional ability of the very ill.

✦ A shift in the focus of goals to the relevant, immediate function needed to achieve maximum level of independence in the home environment.

✦ Increased responsibility for patient safety 24/7 rather than only during the treatment visit.

✦ Increased need for understanding of comorbidities and the interaction of multiple medications.

✦ Need for a more comprehensive view of the patient and his or her environment.

✦ Less than ideal treatment areas because of the physical layout of homes and/or the size and type of furniture present.

Home care physical therapists and other professionals often need to encourage patients to set aside the enjoyment of secondary gains, such as being cared for, having reduced family responsibilities, or simply taking pleasure in the attention they receive in their new situations. To achieve their full potential at home, the rehabilitation team needs to get patients and their families on the same page about their home care plans and goals. This often requires a delicate balancing of the eccentricities of all the parties, which may include extended family members, household staff (e.g., housekeeper, personal chef, or handyperson), home care aides, or private duty nurses. At the other extreme are the challenges presented by less fortunate patients with limited, unreliable, or unpredictable support systems who insist upon staying in their homes even if the risks to their safety and well-being are very high.

Physical therapists in home care settings also must make a shift in their plans of care and goals to reflect the importance of social and cultural influences in home care. Unlike other settings, where these factors are considered in terms of adaptations to the culture of the organization, home care physical therapists find themselves enmeshed in the culture and psychosocial dynamics of *each* family they work with. A broader understanding of all of the factors affecting the outcomes of rehabilitation at home is required. Because these influences are more pronounced and hard to avoid when on the patient's turf, physical therapists may need to develop a series of questions to be better prepared to identify, at least, the cultural influences that are important to the patient. Some suggestions for questions to ask are provided in Sidebar 18.5.

Sidebar 18.5

Questions to Determine Possible Cultural Influences on Patient Outcomes.[15]

How would you describe yourself?
Tell me about your cultural heritage or background (i.e., ethnicity, racial identification, language). How important is this to you?
What was your religious upbringing? How important is this to you?

What was your family's social economic status growing up? How did this affect you?
Do you have any experience with disability or being a caregiver?
What did it mean to grow up as a girl (boy) in your culture/family?

Part 2
Managing in Home Care

Overview of Management in Home Care

Managers in home care may assume a wide range of responsibilities depending primarily on the structure of the home care organization. The following list includes some examples of potential managerial roles in home care:

+ The director of nursing or some other assigned person in a small, developing home care agency assumes responsibility for the hiring and assignments of physical therapists.

+ Regional managers of physical therapy in a large national chain of home care agencies recruit, orient, and supervise the overall care provided by physical therapists in several different locations in their assigned region. As part of the management team, they contribute to decisions related to the organization as a whole and interpretation of outcomes and other data. Each office in the region may have a person who assigns patients and supervises other patient-related care duties of the physical therapists.

+ The director or supervisor of rehabilitation in a freestanding or hospital-based home care agency supervises all members of the rehabilitation team regardless of their disciplines.

+ The director of rehabilitation in a large teaching hospital handles all aspects of physical therapy services provided in various inpatient, outpatient, and home care units. The larger the organization the more likely that unit supervisors manage the day-to-day operations of these units. They may have some flexibility in shifting staff among units as staffing needs demand.

+ Owner of a private practice, particularly pediatric practice, coordinates assignments of physical therapists that are a mix of outpatient and home care patients.

+ Managers of contract therapy companies negotiate contracts for assignment of physical therapists in any of the above home care settings.

In all of these scenarios, managers face the same challenges in the delivery of high-quality physical therapy services in home care. These managers are presented with the same management challenges found in other health-care settings, but they are compounded by the fact that home care is a field operation. The "field" that is managed in home care may encompass several counties or a large metropolitan area. This offsite arrangement may make face-to-face contact with other staff at a central home office impractical on a daily basis because of distances that they must travel and productivity goals they must meet.

Management Responsibilities

Mission, Vision, and Goals

Gathering support from the staff in the field to carry out the mission, vision, and goals of a home care organization may be difficult to structure because interactions with coworkers and supervisors are limited. Opportunities to convey the big picture of home care may not easily present themselves. Because this incohesiveness may contribute to staff turnover, managers may need to identify a variety of means for transforming the mission and vision into action, and for demonstrating the link between the goals of the organization and their day-to-day responsibilities. For instance, expecting *all* providers of care in the organization to participate in regularly scheduled staff meetings is a strategy to reinforce the vision and mission and update everyone on the big picture of the organization.

At the same time, managers need to participate in the creation, or regular review, of the mission and vision of a home care organization so that they reflect the role of contemporary rehabilitation practice. As health-care policy changes, opportunities for identifying and clarifying the role of rehabilitation in the goals of home care agencies lie with managers.

Policies and Procedures

Federal and state regulatory demands dictate many of the policies and procedures in home care because of the long lists of "musts" that are in their regulations. Managers are responsible for the review of these regulations, and for their coordination with the goals and performance of the staff they supervise. They may prepare a mini rehabilitation version of the policy and procedure manual to accomplish this review of the key policies and procedures and to update information that may assist staff in the performance of their duties. For instance, specific application of ethical principles and legal responsibilities in home care may need to be included. Clinical guidelines, either adopted or created by the home care agency staff, may be coordinated with policies and procedures. The more useful and user-friendly it is, the more likely a modified version of policies and procedures is likely to be adopted by staff.

Marketing

As in other large health-care settings, managers in large, national home care corporations are more likely to be presented with the tools for organization-wide program development and marketing plans for implementation than they are to be responsible for their development. On the other hand, managers in freestanding agencies may have more input into this overall planning for an agency, or they may be assigned to program development for physical therapy or interdisciplinary rehabilitation services. The trend toward niche markets and disease management programs presents opportunities for the inclusion of physical therapy in marketing plans.

Managers need to be diligent in championing physical therapy in home care organizations that are historically dominated by nursing care–driven goals and programs. Because nurses are typically the designated case managers of patients in home care, physical therapists have been dependent upon the nurses for referrals to physical therapy. Recently, a shift to a rehabilitation model in home care because of changes in Medicare-reimbursement expectations has helped to increase the utilization of physical therapy services. Encouraging nurses to have broader perspectives of the role of rehabilitation in hospice, and of patients who have acute and chronic conditions of multisystems, is an important managerial role. Having nurses ride along with physical therapists also may be helpful in improving the understanding of the role of the physical therapist, distinguishing it from the role of the physical therapist assistant. These are opportunities for physical

therapists to learn more about nurses and their home care roles.

Staffing

Because most jurisdictions require it, and home care agencies prefer it, physical therapists who work in home care generally have experience in other clinical settings. Because home care is a field operation involving complex clinical decision making, managers prefer people who have already demonstrated skill and confidence in settings that permit interaction with other professions on a regular basis for at least 2 or 3 years. Guiding the successful transition of physical therapists to the world of home care may require careful selection of employees. A formal, structured orientation is essential because home care is an atypical setting with a shift in the patient/therapist relationship that may be difficult or uncomfortable for some therapists.

Therapists who have previous acute hospital experience are used to heavy caseloads and short treatment sessions. These therapists may need guidance to adjust to the slower pace of home care and longer one-on-one treatment sessions with patients. On the other hand, home care physical therapists who also have worked in outpatient settings may be reluctant to set high goals for patients who appear very ill compared to the level of function observed in outpatients. Addressing the characteristics of home care listed earlier and anticipating needs of therapists as they transition to home care work, are management priorities.

Ride-Alongs

Managers should not underestimate the need for ride-alongs—making visits with other staff—as part of the orientation process. Typically, the clinical expertise needed for direct patient care is not problematic for therapists new to home care. Rather it is learning the formal regulation requirements of a home care system, planning a daily schedule, and finding strategies for care within the limited space and minimal resources of a person's home that must be addressed. These issues may be included during ride-along orientation sessions, which also identify commonly used neighborhood shortcuts and other time-saving strategies. Managers who implement such orientations help new employees develop a sense of *esprit de corps* in their new positions.

Managers in home care face the same issues as managers in other settings in managing a mix of physical therapists who are full-time employees with those who work part-time or on a per diem, or as-needed basis. Per diem positions in home care may be more desirable than in other settings for people who seek less than full-time work. Home care is probably the setting that offers the most flexibility for work schedules that accommodate personal needs.

Although not considered good management practice for staff assignments, some managers may allow per diem employees to accept or reject new assignments, limit their service area, or schedule vacations with short notice. Because they are paid a flat fee per visit, allowing them to "cherry-pick" is often seen as a way to encourage them to accept more patients. This practice may be good for per diem staff but often leads to resentment among full-time staff who may not be at liberty to refuse assignments because they have productivity expectations to meet. Allowing unfair practices may create further problems if full-time salaried employees become dissatisfied and leave because they perceive that they are at a disadvantage when expected to care for more patients, those that are most difficult, or those farthest away.

Avoiding a sense of unfairness among full-time employees who see per diem staff as being at an advantage, while concurrently encouraging per diem staff to "belong," is a compounded problem in home care because it is a field operation. Careful control of these factors can require intricate balancing because a manager's need to supplement full-time staff with per diem workers may fluctuate. Without much notice, managers may eliminate or significantly reduce the number of assignments to a per diem pool of therapists because of reduced referrals for physical therapy. Just as quickly, the demand for services may increase. In order to shift from one circumstance to the other, establishment and enforcement of consistent policies and procedures for *all* employees becomes critical.

The flexibility and freedom in home care work that makes it attractive for therapists makes it a major challenge for managers. For instance, if an agency seeks to development interdisciplinary teams in certain geographic areas or for disease management programs, it may be difficult to get staff to commit non–patient-care time to program development and implementation efforts. This development work is perceived as unpaid labor, particularly if physical therapists' productivity is based on the number of visits they make, and upper management discourages any activity that is nonrevenue generating.

Physical Therapist Assistants

Statutes that control licensure rules in each state may determine whether physical therapist assistants are employed in home care agencies. Should physical therapist assistants be permitted to practice in home care, managers need to determine their role and the supervisory role of the physical therapists with whom they work.

As the complexity and acuity of patients in home care continues to increase, managers need to question whether physical therapist assistants are prepared for making immediate clinical decisions for *every* patient. After all, many patients present serious, unexpected decision-making challenges, even for the physical therapists who care for them.

It is critical that managers avoid making blanket policies and procedures regarding the roles of physical therapists and physical therapist assistants, and the assignment of patients to assistants. The ability of physical therapists to make individual judgments about directions to a physical therapist assistant about *each* patient's care must be preserved by managers to deter potential legal and ethical issues.

A physical therapist must weigh the condition and needs of the patients against the experience and skills of assistants, who may require different levels of direction and supervision for each patient, and for the same patient over time. A necessary starting point for managers is to clearly define these professional supervisory relationships and responsibilities for patient care. Verbal and written communication and formal reporting expectations must be specific and followed.

Patient Care

Medicare's OASIS is a group of data elements that drive the clinical work of home care across all disciplines. The data generated forms the basis for measurement of outcome-based quality improvement (OBQI). Its use is part of Medicare's Conditions of Participation for Medicare certification—in other words, it is not an option. In addition to sociodemographic data, health and functional status data are emphasized. Although designed for aggregate outcome measures, OASIS data also are used for patient assessment and care planning for individuals. At the agency level data are used for case-mix reports including patient status at the start of care and the identification of areas for improvement within the agency. The expectation is that documentation of care integrates OASIS terminology and concepts.[16] See Sidebar 18.6.

The orientation of physical therapists to their responsibilities in the generation of OASIS data must include the importance of this information. An agency's management decisions about who gets how much care is critical in the delivery of effective, and cost-effective, patient care that is consistent with evidence-based practice and professional duty. A systematic approach to comparing key factors at the start of care, at 60-days, and upon discharge[17] provides opportunities for analysis of physical therapy effectiveness at a variety of levels. Physical therapy managers in home care may look at OASIS outcomes to answer questions, such as:

✦ What was the change in a particular patient's status from admission to discharge?

✦ What was the value of physical therapy for an individual?

✦ Was physical therapy included appropriately (not underutilized and not overutilized) for patients in a selected diagnostic or case-mix group?

✦ How do physical therapists compare with each other in their care of similar patients?

✦ In the aggregate scores, what can physical therapists do to improve patient outcomes across the board?

This system, although time-consuming and detailed, may serve as an important management tool to answer questions that go beyond required reporting. It provides an advantage over outcome studies in other settings, which do not have similar conditions of participation for reimbursement. See Sidebar 18.7.

Managers in agencies that provide services to patients with private insurance policies need to consider adoption of similar, relevant outcome measures for these patients. If the home care agency is in a state that participates in a Medicaid Comprehensive Assessment and Review for Long-Term Care Services (CARES) program (determines the least restrictive setting appropriate for adults), or the similar Children's Multidisciplinary Assessment Team (CMAT) program for children, managers may identify opportunities for analysis of their data related to physical therapy and other rehabilitation disciplines.

Durable Medical Equipment

Physical therapy managers also may play an important decision-making role in home care involving the provision of durable medical equipment and the incorporation of new technology into patient care and patients' homes. Identifying and informing physical therapists of the impact of medical devices and communication technology available to monitor or improve the functional ability of patients is an important role for home care managers.

Physical therapists need to be prepared to understand and instruct patients in new technology from ergonomic devices for safety to medical devices for monitoring physiological status. Preparing home care physical therapists for teaching and persuading

---

Sidebar 18.6

OASIS

Go to http://www.cms.hhs.gov/OASIS/ 02_Background.asp#TopOfPage and http://www. cms.hhs.gov/HomeHealthQualityInits/12_HHQ IOASISDataSet.asp#TopOfPage for more detailed information on the components of OASIS.

Sidebar 18.7

OASIS Quality Outcomes

Go to the Web page for Medicare's COMPARE program, which is based on OASIS data at http://www.medicare.gov/HHCompare/Home.asp? version=default&browser=IE%7C7%7CWinXP& language=English&defaultstatus=0&pagelist= Home&CookiesEnabledStatus=True. Identify home care agencies in your area. Which one has the best outcomes? What else do you want to know about them? Should there be a similar program for all health-care organizations?

patients and their families to handle new technology may be more important in home care than any other setting. Managerial support to assure the comfort level of the staff with technology may be necessary if they are expected to make clinical decisions about selection and funding.

Fiscal

Although rehabilitation services have always played an important role in home care, the introduction of the Medicare prospective payment system for rehabilitation benefits in home care has directed even more attention to its management. Payment for a home care episode of care can be significantly increased if the number of therapy visits that are medically necessary is increased to a level that justifies categorizing a patient in the high-therapy case-mix group. This potential for increased reimbursement and the shift to the rehabilitation rather than the medical model for the determination of outcomes of care have resulted in a greater demand for physical therapy services in the last few years.

Fiscal responsibilities of middle managers in home care agencies typically include the need for:

✦ Understanding Medicare and Medicaid reimbursement and monitoring changes in rules.

✦ Educating the staff assigned to them regarding accurate patient assessment, clinical decision making, case management, and documentation in compliance with the regulations within these payment systems.

✦ Advising upper management of the effect of their administrative decisions on the professional standards of care, legal rules, and ethical obligations of their staffs.

Because they are in the middle, managers of therapy services are in a pivotal position to decrease the potential for misuse of physical therapy services while contributing to the profitability of agency. It may be dependent on incentives to the home care agencies for using these services. Correcting agency policies (formal or "understood") that may undermine the professional responsibilities of their staff is as important as the generation of revenue. Physical therapists should be able to turn to their managers for guidance and for advocacy with upper management when conflicts between agency expectations and professional duties occur.

Physical therapy managers may have other fiscal responsibilities that commonly arise during strategic planning and budgeting cycles. At the least, their contributions into these processes are important to the identification of, and commitment to, the resources required to provide physical therapy and other rehabilitation services in a home care agency. Accountability for utilization of resources and achievement of budgeted revenue expectations lie with these managers.

One certainty in today's unpredictable health-care environment is that managers will continue to do more with less. Controlling costs becomes a focus of managerial energy as a result. Often the expense of technology compared to its contribution to increased communication and efficiency of work and, additionally, to the quality of care often requires convincing arguments. The responsibility of managers to identify potential resources and to justify their requests may be intensive. Persuading physical therapists who are reluctant to change or to learn new technology may be another hurdle. Perhaps looking at field operations in other businesses such as UPS or FedEx, may identify existing means for addressing communication, scheduling, training, and quality issues.[18]

Legal, Ethical, and Risk

Assisting physical therapists in resolving legal and ethical issues in home care may present unique managerial challenges because the settings are patients' homes. Each home is the private domain of the patient who invites, or permits, the health-care team to enter as an agent of the home care agency. As such, the agency is answerable for all the actions of those employees within the scope of their work, and for all foreseeable consequences of that work.

Supervision

Home care managers have a responsibility for finding a reasonable means to supervise the actions of employees although they occur over a wide geographic range. Supervising strategies include follow-up calls to patients to ask how therapy is going, some random scheduling of reporting by the therapists to the manager, or unannounced on-site visits. What is reasonable supervision depends on the risks each of the physical therapists presents. Experienced physical therapists with unsolicited positive compliments from their patients may require less supervision than physical therapists who are new to home care, or about whom patient or coworker complaints have been made.

Moreover, supervision is important because home care is a high-risk environment for physical therapists. They have less control of the treatment setting and less authority in the home setting. At the same time, they have direct observation not only of a patient's clinical status, but also their social and family situation. It becomes more difficult for therapists to distinguish their job responsibilities from professional responsibilities and their moral duty. Managers may provide guidance on, or at least discussion of, these important issues and their influence on decision making in home-based care.

Safety

It is difficult for any home care provider to avoid action concerning unsafe or abusive conditions because they are direct observers of the situation. If they are unable to effect change directly, reporting and seeking help are critical actions. Attending only to physical therapy goals and interventions is much more difficult in home care. Environmental, socioeconomic, cultural, and family relationship issues often overshadow the immediacy of the patient's therapy needs. The one-on-one interactions and real-life problem-solving that make home care so attractive to many people is also what increases its complexity and its risks.

Because of these risks, managers must demand careful documentation as a paramount responsibility. Regardless of OASIS requirements, documentation of home care also must specifically address risks identified and action taken. Because patients may decline to accept the advice or comply with the suggested action, especially in their homes, documentation of what is said and done is obligatory.

Fraud

Like all health-care settings, the potential for fraud exists, but due to the nature of the field operation of home care, managers have a more difficult job of monitoring the potential for and the occurrence of fraud, which includes:[19]

- ✦ The provision of unnecessary services
- ✦ Billing for services not provided

- ✦ Overcharging
- ✦ Forgery
- ✦ Negative charting (only document the problems, excluding improvements)
- ✦ Substitution of lesser qualified providers
- ✦ Double billing
- ✦ Kickbacks

Managers may find themselves responsible for protecting their staff from fraud committed by higher management and for protecting higher management from fraud committed by their staffs. The nature of home care may require managers to exert a higher level of diligence to prevent and expose fraud.

Underuse

Underuse of care presents another risk for managers to monitor. If patients do not receive the amount of care they need, particularly to live safely at home, managers have to investigate the reasons and take action accordingly. Underutilization also is a factor if therapists prematurely discharge a patient who may be difficult or unpleasant or whose home situation makes the physical therapist uncomfortable. Managers need to be alert for discharge trends that may be an indication of this "dumping" of patients.

The delegation of skilled care to family members and other nonskilled paid helpers may also lead to potential underutilization of skilled services. Although teaching caregivers is a critical intervention in home care because skilled visits are intermittent, reductions in visits should reflect the accomplishment of patient goals rather than the increased availability of caregivers. Managers need to develop a strategy to avoid the latter.

Admissions and Discharge

Risks to patient safety in home care are increased because "discharge to the community" is a quality indicator for hospitals. To achieve their quality goals, a hospital's decision to send patients to their homes rather than to long-term care facilities may inadvertently place the patient in unsafe conditions once at home.[20]

Home care managers need to prepare their staffs for the effects of these hospital decisions on their plans of care for patients who may be medically unstable because they may have been discharged too soon. Given a choice, patients usually choose discharge to home, without a full understanding of the efforts that will be necessary to accomplish their goals. Once they are home, it becomes more difficult to persuade them that an alternative placement may have been more appropriate. Hospital readmissions become another indicator for managers to analyze as they develop strategies to address this issue.

Communication

Having all staff in the same building at the same time may be an infrequent occurrence in home care. The manager's interaction with staff is more often one-on-one, which may become burdensome for the manager unless electronic modes of communication become routine and interactive. In smaller organizations, managers may get to know staff members better because of these individual interactions, but in larger organizations, it may be impossible to know the staff whom they supervise because of the limited contact time with each person on a regular basis. It may be that a manager meets with new employees for orientation and rarely sees them after that unless accreditation standards demand formal, systematic review of performance and competency.

Communication limitations also affect the availability of managers to troubleshoot specific clinical decision making and other practice problems that may be more urgent and complex in a patient's home. The ability to handle broad problems across several staff is compounded by the fact that each staff member is working in isolation. If formal efforts to develop professional and social interactions among staff, beyond the required patient conferencing, are not made successfully, the manager may be a home care physical therapist's only formal connection to the agency and the only source of one-on-one professional advice.

Should the manager of rehabilitation in a home care agency not be of the same discipline as a therapist, the importance of establishing a networking and mentoring program increases dramatically. The sharing of experiences, identification of similar practice problems, and informal socialization may contribute to the improvement of quality services. The ability of managers to provide these opportunities, perhaps at

monthly staff meetings, in field organizations is an important responsibility.

In addition to informal feedback, formal evaluation of work performance by managers may include written data from patient satisfaction surveys, employee self-assessments, and outcome reports combined with direct observation of performance. Regardless of accreditation requirements, without mechanisms for feedback and evaluation, managers only assume what the level of work performance is. Satisfactory often means no complaints, but it also may mean substandard care provided by physical therapists who may not meet competency expectations.

Conclusion

The management of home care physical therapy requires a very different set of skills from management in other health-care settings. The skills that make managers effective in another health-care organization do not necessarily transfer to home care. Attention to the unique aspects of field operations and the special work of caring for people who are often very sick in their homes requires additional preparation.

Because the home care environment poses greater risks and the performance of employees is commonly unknown and unsupervised, managers in home care must have a high level of trust in the people they hire. Careful screening of the credentials and attitudes of potential employees, and detailed orientation to the home setting is critical to success.

Managers must develop therapists with strong patient skills to work with complex patients with minimal resources. They must prepare staff for the greater influence that cultural and social factors have on care in the home. Managers must develop skills that lead to positive experiences so that patient *and* employee dissatisfaction is diminished. Activities 18.1 to 18.20 provide the opportunity to address home care management issues.

ACTIVITY 18.1
PATIENTS OR CLIENTS?

Are the people who receive home care services more like patients or clients as defined by the American Physical Therapy Association? Defend your answer in a group discussion.

ACTIVITY 18.2
THE BIG PICTURE

Pleasant Valley Regional Home Health Services has all three components of home care in its organization—Pleasant Valley Home Care Agency (a provider of skilled care), Pleasant Valley Hospice, and Pleasant Valley Home Care Aides (a provider of private care). The role of physical therapy in the hospice and home care aide organizations is very informal. Occasionally, a particular patient's needs or problems arise and the physical therapy manager is called upon to address them.

The Board of Directors of Pleasant Valley Regional Home Health Services has asked the physical therapy manager to investigate the need for a more formal rehabilitation presence in their hospice and home care aide businesses. What should the manager's report to the Board be?

ACTIVITY 18.3
HOME CARE AGENCIES IN YOUR STATE

Find the requirements for licensure of the three types of home care organizations in your state. Are there any qualifications for physical therapy?

ACTIVITY 18.4
CERTIFICATION OF HOME CARE AGENCIES

Find the requirements for certification of home care agencies and hospices at the CMS Web page. http://www.cms.hhs.gov/default.asp? Are there any qualifications for physical therapy?

ACTIVITY 18.5
COMPARISON OF CHAP AND THE JOINT COMMISSION

Review the information on the Web pages of these organizations. If given the opportunity, which accrediting body would the team of a home care agency prefer? Why?

ACTIVITY 18.6
ORIENTATION TO HOME CARE PHYSICAL THERAPY

Jackie Mankowitz is a new manager of rehabilitation for Glenn County Home Care. She is developing a fact sheet (brochure) to present to potential employees to summarize the unique challenges and expectations for physical therapists working in home care. What should she say?

ACTIVITY 18.7
A STAFF SHORTAGE

Adam Anderson has been the manager of rehabilitation services at No Place Like Home, a Medicare home care agency for 3 years. For the first time, the administrator of the agency, Sally Simmons, has demanded that Adam begin direct patient care duties full-time because recruitment efforts have been unsuccessful in filling the two open physical therapy positions. The agency is at risk of losing referrals because of limited therapy services, and the nurses are becoming angry that the shortage of therapists is affecting their outcomes. Adam reluctantly agrees and voices his concern about losing ground on the great progress he has made on program development, boosting staff morale, and improving quality outcome scores, which he was hired to do. Sally agrees with him but insists more patients need to be seen. She asks for suggestions to maintain his positive work efforts while meeting patient care demands. If you were Adam, what would you suggest?

ACTIVITY 18.8
A PATIENT CALLS

Rose Rodriquez, physical therapy manager at We Come to You Home Care, receives a call from the Maude Morgan, the daughter of Frank Fabrizi, because a physical therapist has not made a visit to Frank in more than a week. She is wondering why therapy suddenly stopped. When Rose investigates, she finds Frank's signature on four treatment slips for the days in question and reports it to Maude. When Maude insists that this cannot be so, Rose and Guy Trujack, the administrator of the agency, go to the Fabrizi home to show Frank the signed treatment slips. They become convinced that the physical therapist, Ruthie Myers, forged Frank's signature and did not provide treatment on those 4 days. What should happen next?

ACTIVITY 18.9
HIRING A PT ASSISTANT

Although permitted by statute, Comfort Home Care has not hired physical therapist assistants to provide care. The three new positions for physical therapists because of the growth of the agency have not been filled for more than 6 months. Delilah Deavon, the manager of rehabilitation, receives an application from Jonathan Wiley, a physical therapist assistant with 20 years of experience including 3 years most recently in home care in another state. She has mixed feelings—excited to finally have an applicant and disappointed that it not from a physical therapist. What should Delilah do next?

ACTIVITY 18.10
A NEW OPPORTUNITY

Barbara Bradley has been the rehabilitation manager for a home care agency for adults for 2 years. She has been approached by a new agency, Kids at Home, to become their rehabilitation manager in developing programs for home care services to children and young adults who are homebound. What questions should Barbara ask Kids at Home? What should she ask herself?

ACTIVITY 18.11
THE JOINT COMMISSION REPORTING

The Joint Commission has just published its new manual for upcoming surveys in home care. They have added a new section to the patient safety goals regarding the risk for falls. It requires additional documentation for each visit by the physical therapist. Failure to demonstrate 12 months of compliance with the new requirement can result in a scoring deficiency during the survey, which is expected to occur in approximately 18 months.

Jody Wilson, the rehabilitation manager, realizes that this news will add to her staff's already detailed charting requirements. How should she present this new requirement to staff to minimize their feelings of being overloaded? Can you recommend a particular method for her to use in developing the additional part of documentation to assure that staff follow the new guideline?

ACTIVITY 18.12
ROLE OF REHABILITATION IN HOSPICE

Dr. Brooks just received a request from the nurse to have a physical therapist evaluate his patient in hospice, Mr. Clark. She told him that Mr. Clark is still ambulatory but spending more time in bed and his ability to use the bedside commode is declining. The doctor questions how a physical therapist can help in what is the expected declining progression of Mr. Clark's disease and functional abilities. The director of nursing asks Sam Solomon, PT to call the doctor to explain the role of the physical therapist in this case, and in hospice in general. What should Sam include in his discussions with Dr. Brooks? Prepare a brochure that nurses may share with other physicians in the future.

ACTIVITY 18.13
MANAGING PERFORMANCE

Sam Solomon, director of rehabilitation in a home care agency, is concerned about Leslie McDonald, one of the staff physical therapists who continues to have significant overtime on most days. Her caseload is no heavier than the other therapists and her driving miles are not excessive. She appears to remain in each home a long time yet does not complete her documentation in that time. These extended visits and completion of her documentation at the end of the day are adding to her hours. The agency encourages staff to document at the point of care. What should Sam do? What suggestions might Sam have for Leslie? He is considering a field visit or ride-along with Leslie. Is that a good decision? At what point should Sam start formal disciplinary action?

ACTIVITY 18.14
SAFETY OF STAFF

Barbara Bronski, the director of rehabilitation at National Home Care Services at Sunset Lake has been appointed to a corporate task force to develop policies and procedures to guide managers in decisions about assignments that may place employees at risk in patients' homes. Particularly, three recent issues need to be addressed:

- Overt presence of weapons and/or illegal drugs in a patient's home.
- Entering homes where patients are smoking when oxygen is in use.
- Assistance with obese patients.

Working in teams, develop policies and procedures regarding the safety of employees of National Home Care Services for these and other employee safety issues the team may identify.

ACTIVITY 18.15
A MEETING OF THE MINDS

Joanna Gilbert, the director of home care rehabilitation, has had minimal contact with three other rehabilitation managers in the same health-care system, two of whom are in the general hospital and one is in the rehabilitation hospital. She must ask for a meeting to discuss some issues. Her home care staff's concerns about the transitioning of discharged patients from the hospitals to home continue to grow. She is starting the meeting with her two top agenda items:

- Inappropriate therapist recommendations for equipment to be delivered to the patients' homes.
- Inpatient documentation that the family has been instructed in exercise or transfers when the family reports that they only observed and were not really trained.

Role-play the four people attending the meeting to address these problems.

ACTIVITY 18.16
DOWNSIZING

Carl Cutbertson's position as the home health rehabilitation coordinator has been eliminated as part of the downsizing of staff that occurred with the merger of two health-care systems. It has been decided that the nursing supervisor of each district in the reorganized home health division will be responsible for the rehabilitation services in each district, which includes assigning therapists to patients and evaluation of their performance. Carl is not surprised at yet another decision to decentralize therapy services throughout the system. His staff has asked to meet with him before he leaves his position to help them strategize what they need to do to continue to provide quality services in this new model. What should Carl recommend?

ACTIVITY 18.17
SCHEDULING

Sally Sanchez has asked to be with Joanna Gilbert, the new rehabilitation manager of the home care agency where she has worked for the last 4 years. Sally is very upset to learn that her vacation request for 2 weeks during the holidays has been denied. She thought the policy was that staff rotated every other year for holiday coverage and this is her off-year. She and her family have already made reservations for their holiday trip. Joanna apologizes but says she had no choice because there is no one to replace her. The temporary pool (on-call staff) has been eliminated because of budget cuts and the three per diem staff members have told her they also are taking their vacations at that time. What are their choices for the next step?

ACTIVITY 18.18
SUPERVISION OF PT ASSISTANTS

Wanda Roman, the nurse who manages rehabilitation services in Winding River Home Care, believes in following the rules, often literally. The practice rules that control physical therapy practice in her state say that the physical therapist must make at least every fifth visit to a patient who is being treated by a physical therapist assistant. Physical therapists in the agency, up to now, have made independent decisions about which patients physical therapist assistants would work with and when they would make supervisory visits within these rules.

They have received a memo from Wanda stating that under the new policy, all patients will be turned over to a physical therapist assistant after the initial evaluation has been completed and that supervisory visits will be made only on the fifth, 10th, and 15th visits unless she gives prior approval to do differently. Has Wanda made a good management decision?

ACTIVITY 18.19
A PT ASSISTANT DILEMMA

Jack Blair, the rehabilitation manager for a home care agency, is excited because of his success in finally filling one of his positions in physical therapy. He has hired an experienced physical therapist assistant (PTA). At the staff meeting the following day, he announces that the assistant will begin the first of the month, and asks the three physical therapists to identify patients who can be transferred to the PTA. He is shocked when two of them state that they will not work with a PTA because it increases their work. They also say that they like providing treatments themselves so they will not hand their patients over to someone else. The other therapist has worked with a PTA briefly in the past and did not like it, but is willing to try again. What is Jack to do?

REFERENCES

1. Cox DM, Ory MG. The changing health and social environments of home care. In: Binstock RH, Cluff LE, eds. *Home Care Advances: Essential Research and Policy Issues.* New York, NY: Springer Publishing; 2000.
2. Basic Statistics About Home Care. Available at: http://www.nahc.org. Accessed August 28, 2007.

ACTIVITY 18.20
A RISKY SITUATION

Betsy Petersen, rehabilitation manager for Best Home Care, receives a call from Charlotte Goldman, who is one of her full-time staff therapists. Charlotte reports that she has just left a patient's home and is too afraid to go back. She asks Betsy to reassign the patient to another therapist and suggests a male therapist may be a good idea.

When Betsy asked for details, Charlotte reported that although the home is in one of the better neighborhoods with expensive furnishings, it was in shambles. Except for the bedroom where the patient was, the house was cluttered and there was foul-smelling garbage. More importantly, however, the patient had a gun on the table next to the hospital bed and she suspects that he may have been under the influence of drugs. He appeared anxious when Charlotte asked him about family members who might be able to help him. He told her she should not worry about the gun, because he has to have some way to protect himself when he is alone in the house. The patient is unable to leave his bed without assistance and he requires intensive nursing care and rehabilitation to improve his functional status. She also is concerned about the other members of the team currently assigned to him. What should Betsy do?

ACTIVITY 18.21
PERSONNEL DIFFERENCES

John Anderson is director of rehabilitation for Central Home Health. He has received an application for one of his full-time therapist positions from Judith Marquez. Judith came to the United States from the Philippines through a recruitment agency that arranges placement of health professionals trained in other countries. She was assigned to work in several nursing homes during her 5 year contract, which has now expired. Her references are excellent.

John's experience with another foreign-trained physical therapist was negative. That person was shy, has a heavy accent, and required assistance because of her small size. He is also concerned that the patients treated through Central Home Health might make staff from other countries uncomfortable or even resist care from them. What should John consider in his interview with Juidth? Should be hire her? What may be that most important things in the orientation?

3. Buhler-Wilkerson K. *No Place Like Home: A History of Nursing and Home Care in the United States.* Baltimore, MD: John Hopkins University Press; 2001.

4. Crossen-Sills J, Bilton W, Bickford M, et al. Home care today: Showcasing interdisciplinary management in home care. *Home Health Nurse.* 2007;25:245–252.

5. Moore PC, McCollough RH. Hospice: End-of-life care at home. In: Binstock RH, Cluff LE, eds. *Home Care Advances: Essential Research and Policy Issues.* New York, NY: Springer Publishing; 2000.

6. Binstock RH, Cluff LE. Issues and challenges in home care. In: Binstock RH, Cluff LE, eds. *Home Care Advances: Essential Research and Policy Issues.* New York, NY: Springer Publishing; 2000.

7. Miller B. Families and paid workers: The complexities of home care roles. In: Binstock RH, Cluff LE, eds. *Home Care Advances: Essential Research and Policy Issues.* New York, NY: Springer Publishing; 2000.

8. Community health accreditation program—history. Available at: http://www.chapinc.org/chap-info.htm. Accessed August 27, 2007.

9. Community health accreditation program CHAP standards. Available at: http://www.chapinc.org/chap-soe.htm. Accessed August 27, 2007.

10. Facts about The Joint Commission. Available at: http://www. jointcommission.org/AboutUs/joint_commission_facts.htm. Accessed August 27, 2007.

11. Understanding Joint Commission home care accreditation 2007. Available at: http://www.jointcommission. org/NR/rdonlyres/BA6AEFA4-BC7B-4385-816E-D62EE667F9CC/0/07_OME_SAP.pdf. Accessed August 27, 2007.

12. Pizzi MA, Briggs R. Occupational and physical therapy in hospice: The facilitation of meaning, quality of life, and well-being. *Topics in Geriatric Rehabilitation.* 2004;20:120–130.

13. Koff T, ed. *Hospice: A Caring Community.* Cambridge, MA: Winthrop; 1980.

14. Coke T, Alday R, Biala K, et al. The new role of physical therapy in home care. *Home Healthcare Nurse.* 2005;23:594–599.

15. Hays PA. Addressing the complexities of culture and gender in counseling. *Journal of Counseling and Development.* 1996;74:332–338.

16. CMS. OASIS main components. Available at: http://www.cms.hhs.gov/OASIS/Downloads/maincomponentsandgeneralapplication.pdf. Accessed August 28, 2007.

17. CMS. OASIS data set. Available at: http://www.cms.hhs.gov/OASIS/046_DataSet.asp#TopOfPage. Accessed August 28, 2007.

18. Cluff LE, Brennan PF. The use of technology in home care. In: Binstock RH, Cluff LE, eds. *Home Care Advances: Essential Research and Policy Issues.* New York, NY: Springer Publishing; 2000.

19. Payne BK. *Crime in the Home Health Care Field: Workplace Violence, Fraud, and Abuse.* Springfield, IL: Charles C Thomas; 2003.

20. Polzien G. Promoting safety and security at home. *Home Healthcare Nurse.* 2007;25:218–222.

Chapter 19

Management Issues in Inpatient Hospitals and Health Systems

Learning Objectives

- Discuss the characteristics of the types of contemporary hospitals.
- Analyze licensure, certification, and accreditation demands in hospitals.
- Discuss contemporary hospital practice issues.
- Analyze the work of physical therapists in hospitals.
- Determine the managerial roles and challenges to managerial responsibilities.
- Analyze managerial decision making in given hospital situations.

Part 1
The Contemporary Setting

Brief Overview of Hospitals and Health Systems

In the last 25 years, the organizational changes that have occurred in hospitals may have had more of an effect on the actual practice of physical therapy than any other factor in any other setting. Rehabilitation services in acute care moved from major revenue generating centers in the fee-for-service model of reimbursement in the early years of Medicare to a cost center in the current prospective payment system of Medicare. The focus of management has become reducing the cost of care per patient. This organization change presented a difficult transition for many physical therapists. Their roles changed from providing as much rehabilitation care as patients needed in acute care before discharge to home, to a focus on specific, limited functional goals to prepare patients for discharge as soon as possible.

Once the gold standard of physical therapy practice, and often the preferred work setting of many physical therapists, new graduates were encouraged to take their first jobs in large acute care hospitals because it was perceived to be the foundation for all other practice settings. Most physical therapists sought to work in acute care at the beginning of their careers because that was where the majority of patients were cared for the majority of the time they needed rehabilitation services. The variety of clinical experiences presented by patients with a wide range of diagnoses in acute care settings, opportunities to follow patients for extended periods in the early stages of their recovery, and the availability of experienced mentors were perceived as important to professional development of novice physical therapists.

Many of these factors continue to affect the career choices of physical therapists. The current high patient turnover in hospitals provides therapists with a large variety of patient experiences, many that are often unique or at least rarely seen. Mentors often are available in hospital systems with large staffs, and novice therapists remain challenged by complex, on-the-spot clinical decision making required in hospital-based practices. The following facts gathered by the American Hospital Association in their 2005 survey of hospitals[1] may be useful in understanding some of these organizational changes that have had an impact on the practice of hospital-based physical therapy:

+ Of the 5,756 hospitals in the United States, almost 2,716 are in a health system (a corporate body that may own or manage health-provider facilities or subsidiaries) and 1,455 are part of health networks.

+ 51 deals involving 88 hospitals in 2005 were added to the 59 mergers and acquisitions involving 236 hospitals in 2004.

+ 946,997 hospital beds were staffed.

+ 47% of outpatient surgery was done in hospital-owned facilities with the rest performed in freestanding surgery centers or physician offices.

+ 60% of hospital systems also offer home health services, 60% offer hospice services, and 45% have skilled nursing facilities.

+ The average hospital length of stay decreased from 7.6 days in 1981 to 5.6 days.

+ Outpatient visits to hospitals tripled to 600 million in 2005 from 200 million in 1981.

+ 60% of all surgeries were performed as outpatient surgeries.

+ Payment-to-cost ratios for private insurance were 130%, for Medicare 95%, and for Medicaid 86%.

+ Costs of employment in hospitals increased 4% in a year.

+ 39% of hospital costs are related to care of patients with Medicare, 37% to patients with private insurance, and 6% of hospital costs are uncompensated.

+ Hospitals employed 4 million full-time equivalent (FTE) employees.

+ 60% of the costs of hospitals were wages and benefits.

+ 11% of hospitals had fully integrated electronic health records and 57% had partially implemented systems in 2005. Hospitals with more than 500 beds in urban settings that were part of systems were furthest ahead in implementation of electronic health records.

Given this information, it is no surprise that the focus of hospital and health-care systems is financial management so they survive and grow to provide health services to the community. They accomplish this by:[2]

+ Generating of a reasonable net income (revenue-expenses)
+ Making sound investments in assets that work for the organization.
+ Adequately and appropriately responding to governmental regulations and accreditation requirements.
+ Facilitating strong relationships with third-party payers as customers to be satisfied.
+ Influencing the method and amount of payment by closely monitoring capitation and prospective payment systems.
+ Monitoring the orders of physicians who account for 32.3% of health-care spending as the source of procedures conducted, medications prescribed, possible negligence in care provided, etc.
+ Protecting their tax-exempt status, which is under judicial and public scrutiny.
+ Assessing and improving quality as it becomes the major competitive factor (lower prices that often become equalized in a community are often a less important factor).

Selected Issues in Inpatient Hospital Care

As these trends suggest, freestanding community hospitals may soon be outdated if mergers and acquisitions continue on their current course. This section is directed to selected contemporary issues among general hospitals and health-care systems, academic health centers, specialty hospitals, and subacute care centers (which may occur in a variety of organizations) that may demand the attention of mid-level managers in each setting.

Growth of Hospitals

Another trend of importance to inpatient managers is that, despite all of the concerns about lack of funding and increased regulations, constant growth appears to be the actual state of the hospital industry. Hospitals seem to be constantly under construction or renovating. This expansion suggests that health care continues to be insulated from actual market forces that negatively affect the growth of other large businesses, such as the retail sales, construction, and manufacturing. Health-care systems do not seem to lack the assets needed to back these large projects. Mergers have contributed to this growth because they have allowed hospitals to shed redundancy and eliminate waste while building on the strengths of several organizations to enrich a single bottom-line.[3]

Managers who embrace the challenges of growth organizations as they continue to evolve find many unexpected upward career opportunities. This may involve an ever-increasing separation from the roles of a health-care professional to the new roles as a management professional. Because these positions in hospitals do not require licensure, it only takes desire and determination to begin to climb managerial career ladders in hospital systems.

Health-Care Systems and Hospitalists

One of the emerging trends important to acute care managers is the role of hospitalists in acute care medical practice. Although inpatient medicine specialists have been common in hospitals in other countries, hospitalists are a relatively new branch of medicine in the United States. The term was first introduced in 1996 to identify physicians who serve as the physicians-of-record for inpatients, returning them back to the care of their primary care providers at the time of hospital discharge.[4] They are immediately available to respond quickly to the daily demands of inpatients so that they positively influence decisions to shorten lengths of stay. Decreased costs through this increased efficiency results.[4]

Because the concept and their roles are so new, it is difficult to determine the effectiveness of hospitalists. Measurement of changes in patient and primary care physician satisfaction, lengths of stay, hospital costs, mortality, and readmissions are suggested determinants.[5]

Patients admitted to a hospital who do not have primary care physicians may be assigned to a hospitalist without a choice in the matter. Patients with primary care physicians may continue to receive care directly from them, or they may be cared for by a hospitalist with little notification or explanation from their primary care physician. Because it is a new specialty in medicine, many patients may not even know the role of the hospitalist in their care, or even care about that role, particularly when they also are under the care of one or more surgeons or other medical specialists. For other patients with chronic, complex medical conditions, beginning all over with a new physician with each hospital admission may be frustrating. Patients may be unhappy or fearful, if the continuity of care that their primary care physician had provided is lost.

Initially driven by hospitals and managed care groups to cut costs and improve the quality of care, primary care physicians were resistant to this new model of care and reluctant to transfer the care of their patients to hospitalists. As reimbursement rates continued to drop, however, they discovered that hospitalists save them both time and money. Interrupting their office practices for quick visits to attend to their patients in the hospital were no longer needed, and frequent phone call interruptions during patient visits in their offices from hospital nurses seeking orders decreased.

For hospital managers, the immediate availability of hospitalists has the potential to improve communication and decision making about direct patient care issues as they arise. Communication with the broader cadre of primary care physicians often resulted in delays in communication and miscommunication because discussions were not always face-to-face. As hospitalists, physicians may play a more consistent and central role as members of frontline care teams.

The dependence of hospitals on admissions by primary care physicians also may change as managed care organizations or hospital-sponsored physician networks take an expanded role in admission and inpatient care plan decisions. The rise of hospitalists may lead to even more of a distinction between health-care providers who are inpatient providers and those who are outpatient providers as inpatient care becomes a specialty unto itself. It may be that medical students will be making earlier career choices about whether their careers will be inpatient- or outpatient-based.

Academic Health Centers

The Institute of Medicine has identified the unique role and challenges that academic health centers (AHCs) face in health care. They concurrently train health professionals, conduct research that advances health, and provide care—often to the most ill and poorest populations. Their integration of these three responsibilities produce the knowledge and evidence that are the foundations for treating illness and improving health.[6]

AHCs are degree-granting institutions with a medical school and at least one other health professional academic program that owns, or has an affiliation with, a teaching hospital, health system, or other organized health-care providers. They may be private or public organizations. Some are based in universities while others are freestanding institutions. Either they are organized as an integrated model with teaching, research, and patient care the responsibility of one board of directors, or they are a split model. In the split model, typically, there is a chief executive officer for teaching and research who reports to a board in an academic institution. Another chief executive officer is responsible for patient care in an affiliating health-care system that reports to a different board of directors. Variations of these models, or AHCs that move among models as local factors and politics affect their organizations, are not uncommon.[7]

In any model, AHCs are complex business enterprises that continue to move toward corporate models of integrated operations to more effectively encompass all three of their roles than was possible in more traditional academic models. Upper-management positions have been transformed to reflect these organizational changes with increased accountability and broader responsibility for resource allocation, often among competing priorities. They are often at the mercy of state legislatures or city and county boards for funding.

AHC managers must balance these new corporate paradigms with traditional academic models that emphasize creativity and academic freedom. They accomplish all of this without losing sight of their greater responsibility for their societal missions that cannot be overshadowed by the business of research, teaching, and patient care.[7]

AHCs play a unique role in the community. They often provide services that are not available in other health-care organizations for the care of patients with complex medical conditions and severe trauma. While competing with other health-care organizations, they must also cooperate with them so that patients who require specialized care are referred to the AHC, and patients are referred appropriately to other health-care settings upon discharge from an AHC.

Like other health-care organizations, academic health centers face the same legislative and market pressures that other health-care organizations face in surviving economic upheavals. They must:[8]

✦ Focus on the competition. Increase awareness of the effect of other health-care organizations on the number of patients and visits to academic health-care centers. AHCs must recognize the competition's strengths and weaknesses and develop strategies to prevail.

✦ Improve their leverage in negotiations with third-party payers. Because payers have the upper hand, AHCs must leverage their strengths—superior physicians and outcomes, creating services for special populations, etc.

✦ Develop facilities in other markets. AHCs may need to develop centers in underserved markets rather than compete in heavily saturated markets.

✦ Consolidate supply. The alternative to new market development is to decrease the competition with mergers and acquisitions.

Managers in academic health centers are faced with even more complexity in their assigned roles because internal competition for resources is spread over teaching, research, and patient care. Particularly for managers who aspire to academic roles, these settings may offer attractive career opportunities.

Because they are in teaching hospitals, there may be more pressure for managers to include clinical educational opportunities for students in all rehabilitation disciplines than there is in nonacademic health centers. Accommodating the request of universities for student placements may be considered an important recruitment tool that has to be balanced against productivity goals and available staff with experience and willingness to be clinical instructors.

Specialty Hospitals

Specialty hospital is an umbrella term that includes a wide range of nonprofit or for profit, public or private organizations whose purpose is to provide either short-term or long-term care for particular populations such as people who:

✦ Need alcohol and drug abuse rehabilitation
✦ Need physical rehabilitation

✦ Have tuberculosis
✦ Have cancer
✦ Are women (and their infants)
✦ Are children
✦ Are veterans or military personnel
✦ Have ear, nose, and throat impairments
✦ Have cardiac disease
✦ Require orthopedic surgery
✦ Have other chronic diseases (e.g., respiratory)

Although some of these specialty hospitals have had a long history, such as those for children and veterans, maternity or tuberculosis hospitals, and rehabilitation centers; a recent surge in the number and different types of specialty hospitals has raised some concerns. In certain areas of the country, collaborations between specialty hospitals and physician groups have raised suspicions about the financial arrangements they have made with each other. These arrangements have been perceived to have a negative effect on funding for neighboring general hospitals.

Supporters of specialty hospitals see them as providing financial incentives for hospitals and for physicians to produce higher quality outcomes more efficiently. Because they are smaller with more focused patient-centered care, they argue that they spur on other hospitals to innovate and improve. Detractors believe that physicians compete unfairly by referring patients to their own specialty hospitals, and that these hospitals focus only on the most lucrative procedures for the healthiest and best-insured patients.

The counter argument is that many general hospitals have policies that demand physicians refer patients only to their hospitals. They often purchase physician practices and direct those physicians to refer to that hospital exclusively, and they operate health plans that include network referral requirements. They may really be no different from specialty hospitals in terms of their dependency on relationships with physicians.

The effect of physician-owned cardiac, orthopedic, and surgical specialty hospitals on the Medicare program lead to a report to Congress in 2005. Highlights of that report, based on analysis of only a few hospitals with the data available at the time, included the following facts:[9]

✦ In physician-owned specialty hospitals, costs for Medicare patients are not lower but their patients have shorter lengths of stay.

✦ They do treat patients who are generally less severe cases (with expectations for more profits) and they concentrate on particular diagnosis-related groups (DRGs), some of which are relatively more profitable.

✦ They tend to have a lower share of Medicaid patients than community hospitals.

✦ The financial effect on community hospitals in the same markets has been limited.

✦ Many of the differences in profitability across and within DRGs that create these financial incentives for patient selection can be reduced by improving Medicare's inpatient prospective payment system for all acute care hospitals.

✦ The hospitals are established to gain greater control over how the hospital is run, to increase their productivity, and to provide greater satisfaction for them and their patients.

✦ Physicians also may be motivated by the financial rewards, some of which derive from inaccuracies in the Medicare payment system. (The report makes recommendations for remedying these problems with DRG values and outliers.)

In a more recent study of Medicare data on 10,478 patients who underwent total hip replacement and 15,312 patients who had total knee replacements from 1999–2003, they determined that fewer Medicare reimbursed surgeries and more private insured surgeries were conducted in physician-owned specialty hospitals than in nonphysician owned. The patients in the physician-owned hospitals had lower rates of the common comorbid conditions of obesity and heart failure and fewer of the patients were African American although they were situated in neighborhoods with a higher proportion of African American residents.[10] Controversy surrounding these physician-ownership issues is expected to continue.

Rehabilitation Hospitals

Other specialty hospitals that are not physician-owned also may face challenges. Of particular interest to physical therapists are inpatient rehabilitation hospitals, which also are in the midst of dramatic reimbursement changes as they adjust to a new Medicare prospective system that became effective in 2002. The system is based on a patient assessment instrument similar to that used in skilled nursing facilities and home care agencies for data

collection. Medicare defines a rehabilitation hospital as one in which a certain percentage of patients (the 75% rule) require intensive rehabilitation with diagnoses that fall into this recently revised list of 13 diagnostic groups: [11]

✦ Stroke

✦ Spinal cord injury

✦ Congenital deformity

✦ Amputation

✦ Major multiple trauma

✦ Fracture of femur (hip fracture)

✦ Brain injury

✦ Neurological disorders, including multiple sclerosis, motor neuron diseases, polyneuropathy, muscular dystrophy, and Parkinson disease

✦ Burns

✦ Active polyarticular rheumatoid arthritis, psoriatic arthritis, and seronegative arthropathies

✦ Systemic vasculitides with joint inflammation

✦ Severe/advanced osteoarthritis

✦ Joint replacements (if bilateral, or patient is extremely obese, or frail and elderly)

The major struggles with Medicare reimbursement for inpatient rehabilitation managers have been the steady and dramatic decline in patient volume attributed to these policy changes, and the related concern of limiting patient access to inpatient rehabilitation services.[12] Another ongoing issue is related to the patients' ability to participate in intensive rehabilitation. Because patients are discharged sicker and quicker from acute care settings, they may not be able to meet the requirement of participating in 3 hours of therapy a day. Others may not need 3 hours of therapy to meet their goals. Failure to predict patient outcomes may have negative financial consequences.

Lack of, or limited, coverage for both inpatient and outpatient rehabilitation in many new models of health insurance also contributes to a decline in inpatient rehabilitation volume for patients who are not Medicare recipients. As these policy and reimbursement issues continue to be addressed, managers in rehabilitation hospitals can continue to expect organizational adjustments.

Another management responsibility in inpatient rehabilitation is the admissions committee. Among the Medicare requirements for admission to an inpatient rehabilitation hospital is that patients have recovered enough to participate in at least 3 hours of therapy each day and have the potential for return to their prior level of function. Physical therapists in acute care hospitals are predicting a patient's ability to meet these requirements in their discharge planning recommendations, as the admission committees of rehabilitation hospitals are reviewing these same plans to determine acceptance of patients for admission. The discipline and/or program managers in a rehabilitation center take part in these admission decisions that are made on a daily basis.

There is less of a focus on traditional nursing care and diagnostic testing in rehabilitation hospitals. The management of interdisciplinary services for the coordination of interventions among all members of the team—rehabilitation and nursing—are the focus instead. Managers shift their efforts to the development and performance of staff who establish longer-term professional relationships with patients than do therapists who work in acute care hospitals.

Subacute Care

A relatively new concept, subacute care has been developed to address the needs of a particular patient population—people who need goaloriented, rehabilitative care immediately after, or instead of, acute hospitalization because of the complexity of their conditions or the complexity of the care required. Examples are patients with head trauma or spinal cord injury or stroke; others whom are ventilator-dependent; people who need a course of intravenous antibiotics or another series of complex treatments for short periods.[13] Although most subacute patients are likely to be elderly, these settings provide care to patients across the life span.

Patients are candidates for subacute care when they are not dependent on the high-technology monitoring or complex diagnostic procedures only available in acute care hospitals, but they do need the services of an interdisciplinary team that is more intensive than can be provided in traditional skilled-nursing facilities. They may not be eligible for admission to an inpatient rehabilitation hospital because they are too sick to tolerate the required daily hours of therapy. It is best thought of as a program rather than a place because it can be provided in a variety of health-care settings from freestanding centers devoted entirely to subacute care or units in nursing homes and hospitals.[13]

The early development of subacute nursing as a specialty field is another indication of the growth and need for this level of care[14] which is increasingly perceived as filling an important gap in the continuum of health care. While receiving the same level and intensity of care that may be found in hospitals, costs may be reduced because the overhead of hospital emergency rooms and surgical suites are avoided.[13] See Sidebar 19.1.

Licensure, Certification, Regulation, and Accreditation

Regardless of the type of hospital or hospital system, The Joint Commission is the accrediting agency not only of each type of hospital but other types of health-care organizations, including subacute care regardless of the setting. Licensure and accreditation are intertwined with many jurisdictions deferring to The Joint Commission's accreditation of an organization as evidence of meeting state licensure requirements. The Centers for Medicare and Medicaid (CMMS) also rely on The Joint Commission evaluations of health-care organizations as a requirement for certification as a Medicare/Medicaid provider.

As organizational changes have occurred in hospitals and health systems, so has the process of accreditation, which used to depend upon a "snapshot" of an organization at regularly scheduled intervals. Currently, The Joint Commission has shifted to program accreditation and standardized, patient outcome performance measures that can be used for comparison of organizations by interested parties. The focus of their review processes has shifted to unannounced site visits with a focus on direct

> *Sidebar 19.1*
>
> **Hospital Resources**
>
> Other information about contemporary hospital issues can be found on the Web pages of:
> American Hospital Association: http://www.aha. org/aha/about/
> Hospital Connect: http://www.hospitalconnect. com/
> Association of Academic Health Centers: http://www.aahcdc.org/
> National Association of Subacute/Post Acute Care: http://naspac.net/faq.asp#Q2

observation of patient care and interviews of patients, family members, students, and all levels of staff in the organization.

Rehabilitation hospitals (and rehabilitation units of hospitals) also may seek accreditation from the Commission on Accreditation of Rehabilitation Facilities (CARF). This accreditation process is based on an on-site survey of the hospital with a consultative partnering rather than an investigative approach to improve the quality of patient care. In all program areas in which accreditation is sought (e.g., stroke, spinal cord injury, traumatic brain injury, pediatrics), the organization is asked to demonstrate to a survey team conformance to standards highlighting the organization's values and approaches in these areas:[15]

+ Core values and mission
+ Input from the persons served and other stakeholders
+ Individual-centered planning, design, and delivery of services
+ Rights of the persons served
+ Quality and appropriateness of services
+ Continuity of care
+ Leadership, ethics, and advocacy
+ Planning
+ Financial management (including risk management)
+ Human resources
+ Accessibility
+ Health and safety
+ Outcomes management and performance improvement
+ Infrastructure management

CARF recently acquired the Continuing Care Accreditation Commission so that its accreditation now extends to organizations that provide aging services, behavioral health, employment and community services, child and youth services, vision rehabilitation, subacute care, etc.[15]

Workforce Issues in Hospitals and Hospital Systems

Downsizing of staff and reducing the number of staffed beds became the hospital management strategy of the 1990s as managers strived to control costs to maintain profits with the prospective payments for the care they delivered. Mergers and acquisitions to pool resources, increase purchasing power, and reduce competition are important to both nonprofit and for-profit hospitals as health systems continue to evolve.

Staffing Models

Hospital-management models have flattened mid-level positions to reduce the costs associated with wages and benefits for employees who do not contribute directly to the provision of patient services. Smaller hospital units have been combined and many managers, including those who are physical therapists, find themselves responsible for staff from a variety of disciplines, and perhaps responsible for some units unfamiliar to them. Managers have shifted from discipline-specific experts to efficiency and cost-reduction experts, regardless of the initials behind their names in these new, complex matrix models of management.

Even with these efforts, many newly formed multidisciplinary managerial units are small compared with the total number of nursing personnel. Nonclinical support services comprise the other large cadre of employees (i.e., housekeeping, maintenance, kitchen, etc). Combining physical therapy, occupational therapy, and speech language pathology services (and often psychology, electromyography, and other units) under one manager is a commonly used strategy. The clinical manager of the new unit is likely to be a rehabilitation professional, but nurses or other health professionals may also have responsibility for rehabilitation units.

Because the major responsibility of clinical managers has changed from discipline-specific revenue generation to interdisciplinary program management, the skills required for these positions have less to do with one's clinical expertise than it has to do with the skills needed to control and reduce costs while maintaining the quality of patient care to achieve expected patient outcomes. Doing more with less has become, perhaps, the most important skill for these managers.

Employees may have issues about organizational threats to their professional identity because of the consolidation of the duties of their managers. These concerns often fall on the deaf ears of upper-level managers. Their attention is directed, rightfully so, to profit margins and the declining resources available to achieve more stringent patient outcome expectations while sustaining the quality of patient care. Managers perceive advantages to meeting these challenges in mid-level managerial duties and responsibilities that are shared and blurred rather than clearly delineated. Assignment and utilization of human resources can be more quickly and effectively reorganized as demands change in this model.

Program Management

Another management strategy that is a result of the regrouping that has recently occurred in hospitals and health systems is program management. Interdisciplinary teams are assigned to programs to meet the needs of particular populations more efficiently and effectively. Clinical decision making becomes decentralized as responsibility in programs falls to a smaller, focused group of frontline providers. The roles of physicians in these programs may vary from ultimate authority to consultative. Program managers in this model typically are responsible for all fiscal and human resources needed to implement the program. The nonclinical hospital support services typically remain centralized in this model.

This simple example of a program management model may take on a variety of modifications depending on a several factors such as the number of different populations to be served by a particular organization, availability of staff to be distributed among programs, and the size of the organization. For instance, a large teaching hospital may have rehabilitation, pharmacy, and nursing managers with responsibility for staffing and assignments; who work with program managers who are responsible for the care and outcomes for the stroke, organ transplant, oncology, or cardiac programs.

Another mixed model example is one in which a program manager is responsible for inpatients and outpatients across the continuum of their care in a particular program (e.g., oncology). Other programs have managers who are responsible for inpatient units with a different manager responsible for all combined outpatient services. Coordination of the responsibilities and the distribution of accountability in these mixed models can be confusing and subject to frequent changes because they are often created by trial-and-error decisions or availability of personnel.

Support for program management is driven by the knowledge that groups whose members devote a higher percentage of their time to working with a particular patient population tend to develop stronger relationships (i.e., shared goals, shared knowledge, and mutual respect) and more effective patterns of interaction. These interactions and focus are believed to result in increased quality of care for the patient *and* reduced hospitalization costs for the payer.[16]

Program Management and Physical Therapists

Miller and Solomon identified several themes in their interviews with physical therapists who were deployed to different programs when the departments of physical therapy, and others, were disbanded with a merger of several hospitals and other units in a large health-care system. Among the conclusions were that the physical therapists experienced:[17]

+ A sense of loss of professional identity because the collegiality and informal friendships that were part of departmental interactions were gone. No longer having a department head felt as if professional representation in the organization was lost as well.

+ Low morale, which was expressed as a sense of giving up, lack of enjoyment, no job satisfaction, and expectations to do more with no change in salaries.

+ Additional administrative responsibilities without preparation to assume them. The need for strong communication skills became more important because there was no one person to rely on which forced the therapists to speak for themselves. The tasks and work of the director did not go away; rather it was redistributed with each physical therapist assuming those tasks within their program teams. Standards of practice were no longer monitored as a result, with a potential negative effect on the quality of care.

+ Less support for educational funds and opportunities including curtailment of in-services.

+ Inconsistent mentoring and orientation of new employees, which became dependent on the willingness of other therapists to volunteer rather than assigned responsibility.

Program management appears to be more problematic for new graduates who will be expected to be the experts on physical therapy for the programs they are assigned to with little room for learning as you go. Professional advantages to program management also were identified:[17]

✦ Increased interdisciplinary work resulted in greater recognition of the roles and skills of physical therapists.

✦ Program management provided opportunities to expand the scope of their responsibilities which they welcomed.

✦ More opportunities to learn from other disciplines.

This study was conducted a few years ago, so whether or not the same themes are prevalent among hospital employees today requires further investigation. Whether or not new graduates are now better prepared for these new responsibilities in direct and nondirect patient care is uncertain. Comparison of a physical therapist who is the only physical therapist in a program to physical therapists involved in many programs may also be needed.

Perceptions of both informal (effective relationships with others on the program team) and formal power (contributions to organizational goals) are equally important predictors of the empowerment of physical therapists in an organization. These sources of formal empowerment are often gone as professional networks in organizations are disbanded, support from physical therapist peers is reduced, and discipline-specific leadership positions as a researcher, department head, or clinical education coordinator are no longer available. On the other hand, in the program model, program-specific and patient-specific information is enhanced and opportunities for informal power may be improved within a coordinated interdisciplinary team approach to care.[18]

Shortages

Regardless of the type of hospital, the projected shortage of workers at all levels of care is likely to become the most critical management issue in hospitals. The attractiveness of health careers seems to have changed in the last decade or so from one of the most desirable to one of the lesser-favored places of employment. The Strategic Planning Committee of the American Hospital Association has drawn the following conclusions about these trends:[19]

✦ In an information economy, young people see health care as low-tech.

✦ In today's labor market, health care is seen as chaotic and unstable.

✦ In the past, health care provided one of only a few employment options for women who now have many choices.

✦ In today's short-stay hospital system, staff is focused on disease protocols, regulatory compliance, and documentation rather than establishing helping relationships with patients.

✦ The 24/7 demands of hospitals are seen as unacceptable and heightened by the short-stay, high-acuity patients who place continuous demands on hospital staff for their care and support.

✦ Hospital-based educational programs of the past that provided an ongoing supply of staff in-house have been replaced by community college programs whose graduates are presented with a wide range of employment opportunities in different types of health-care organizations.

✦ The baby boomer generation will be replaced by a relatively small pool of workers from which to recruit hospital workers.

✦ Many baby boomers have already retired or reduced to part-time positions because of the perceived increased stress of their hospital careers.

The AHA Strategic Planning Policy Committee urges hospitals to consider the following long-term implications of these trends:[19]

✦ While electronic and automated systems may change the nature of some work, they will not replace hands-on care.

✦ It is unlikely that hospitals will return to be the favorable employment environment it once was.

✦ Managers must recognize personnel as a strategic asset as important as adequate payment, capital acquisition, and market share.

✦ New work arrangements are required to build loyalty and create a sense of stability in hospitals. Permanent staff, both part-time and full-time, find the work environment increasingly hectic and uncertain. The expanded use of agency and temporary staff to create more flexibility in the staffing defeats this objective.

✦ Educational systems need hospital involvement to help identify skills and capabilities in demand in the labor market.

✦ New technologies that allow staff to emphasize the caregiving and care-supporting functions of their positions are essential for hospitals to attract, develop, and retain employees.

✦ The workforce will only expand if hospitals attract staff from the economy generally by increasing the attractiveness of health careers relative to other employment options.

Hospital managers at all levels will need to devote a great deal of attention to workforce recruitment, retention, and development. Increasing the satisfaction of both direct caregivers and supportive staff may need to rise to the level of top priority. The nature of hospital work needs to be re-examined to identify innovative approaches to reduce administrative duties so that employees can realize the value of their professional expertise and the satisfaction of helping others. Perhaps, like other industries, hospitals may need to take more responsibility for the development of employee skills and expertise specific to the needs of their unique organizations. Fair compensation for the advanced education they bring to the hospital, and their continual training requires serious planning that goes beyond bidding wars for employees when revenues are increasingly limited.

Inpatient Acute Care and Physical Therapy

The dramatic changes that have occurred in hospitals in response to the many economic and policy changes that have transformed health care in the last 25 years have affected the delivery of rehabilitation services in hospitals in several important ways. Some strategies for controlling costs of rehabilitation services in acute care settings have been:

✦ Eliminating centralized therapeutic gyms and treatment areas to reduce space and equipment costs and the need for staff to transport patients.

✦ Conducting therapy sessions at the patient bedside for increased efficiency (transporting

patients to a therapy department has essentially been eliminated) and effectiveness (functional training provided where hospital function occurs).

✦ Creating smaller, centralized staff offices for documentation and coordination of services.

✦ Shifting as much inpatient service as possible to outpatient settings (e.g., presurgical physicals, laboratory tests, intake interviews completed as outpatient services before the patient is admitted to the hospital for other than a medical emergency).

✦ Shifting the provision of durable medical equipment and other supplies to patients postdischarge to reduce the inpatient cost/patient.

✦ Dischargeing of patients as soon as possible to less intensive and less costly settings.

Many older physical therapists have been surprised about the professional role they now play in acute care settings because care has shifted to meeting the immediate functional needs of patients and facilitating discharge, typically in a few days. Currently, patients are moving in and out of hospitals faster, and their therapy sessions are shorter and more focused on function at the bedside to meet the demands of caring for more patients with fewer staff. Providing interventions other than functional training has become more of an exception rather than the rule for many patients. Teaching other caregivers and making recommendations about the coordination of care become important professional roles in hospital settings.

The fast pace and immediate decision making required to meet productivity and quality of care goals in hospitals has raised the question of whether it is the most suitable setting for new graduates. Planning for discharge as they are conducting their initial examination and evaluation, often with limited information, has become a new challenge for physical therapists. Rather than determining appropriate goals for a patient and establishing a plan of care to reach them, physical therapists are faced with meeting pre-established discharge days within the limits set by prospective payments for patients.

It may be difficult for some novice therapists to predict the ability of the patient to function safely in the least restrictive setting when there is limited time to gather the data to reach those decisions. Other new graduates thrive on these expectations. They enjoy the fast pace of decision making in acute care. They relish the excitement of positively affecting the function of people who are critically ill or who have suffered traumatic injuries, and delight in being at the cutting edge of new medical advances.

Mentoring

Managers may find it necessary to establish formal mentoring or coaching programs to assure that new graduates, or experienced physical therapists who are new to acute care, are prepared for these important responsibilities. In many hospital situations, although therapists are all in the same inpatient settings, they function as a field operation. Therapists are scattered about the hospital to take care of patients at the bedside with little interaction with each other during the day.

This lack of ongoing peer interaction creates another issue for the new graduate. Unless deliberate efforts are made, the mentoring of new therapists by more experienced staff is difficult and time-consuming. Although important for all new graduates in any setting, having someone to turn to as they develop clinical decision making skills in the fast-paced, unpredictable acute care setting may be essential because of the profound affect these decisions may have on a patient's recovery and discharge placement.

Discharge Planning

Physical therapists share their information about the patient's current status and potential for rehabilitation with other members of the clinical team (hospital case managers, discharge planners, and admission screeners from potential facilities for patient placement) who contribute information on social and financial resources affecting discharge decisions. For many patients, physical therapists with the knowledge and skills to contribute to this multidisciplinary, consultative discharge process may be more important than those who provide direct interventions to improve their functional status.

These role changes have raised broader practice questions about acute care physical therapy within the profession, which include:

- ✦ Is physical therapy a core or supplemental service in general acute care settings?
- ✦ What is it that physical therapists do in acute care that no other professional can do?
- ✦ Are the typical patient care services provided by physical therapists in acute care considered skilled services?
- ✦ Should, and how should, physical therapy practice in acute care be reinvented?
- ✦ Is discharge planning in acute care an advanced skill?

Practice challenges also may be reflected in the results of the American Physical Therapy Association's 2007 survey of 45,000 physical therapists. Only about 16.6% of those physical therapists held positions in acute and subacute settings compared with 60% who held positions in outpatient settings.[20]

Subacute Physical Therapy

Physical therapy in subacute care more closely resembles the model of physical therapy practice that dominated general hospital care 30 or 40 years ago. Patients are in subacute centers for longer periods and receive more intensive rehabilitation while there. The model of physical therapy continues to evolve in subacute centers, particularly if a center has a particular focus (e.g., care of patients who are ventilator-dependent).

Rehabilitation Hospitals

Physical therapy practice in rehabilitation hospitals has probably changed the least over the years, although access may be more limited. The teamwork in neurological rehabilitation units has been investigated and a number of benefits have been identified, which include:[21]

- ✦ Sharing of knowledge and expertise or skills.
- ✦ Managing gaps in knowledge by assisting each other.
- ✦ Integrating and coordinating treatment across disciplines.
- ✦ Sharing of information and sharing of responsibility.
- ✦ Taking on different roles of team members.

- Everyone working toward the same common goals.
- Sharing the load to achieve patient goals.
- Dealing with individual holistic needs of each patient.
- Communicating each person's expertise to increase effectiveness.
- Limiting repetition of services that improves efficiency.
- Delegating tasks to the right people to improve efficiency.
- Eliminating the inappropriate jobs or tasks of team members.

See Sidebar 19.2. Figure 19.1 summarizes some of the differences in physical therapy practice across the three levels of inpatient care. The work in subacute care is mix of the two other settings and falls somewhere between them on each continuum.

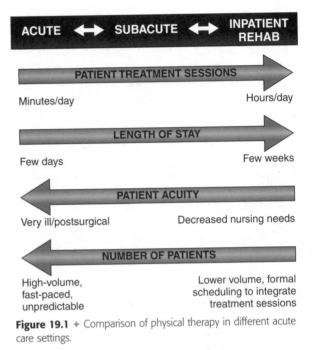

Figure 19.1 ✦ Comparison of physical therapy in different acute care settings.

Sidebar 19.2

Characteristics of the Work in Acute and Rehabilitation Hospitals

In acute care:

- Experience with a variety of patients with complex problems if able to rotate among hospital units, or an opportunity to specialize clinical practice with assignment to a single program or unit.
- Decreased interaction with other physical therapists in larger hospitals and systems unless deliberate efforts are made for meetings, etc. Less opportunity for informal mentoring.
- Fast-paced and unpredictable schedule that is individually controlled by each therapist.
- Independence in the content of work and solving problems.
- Opportunities for interaction with specialists on the cutting edge of practice, researchers in large medical centers, and the newest technology.
- Decreased opportunity for establishing professional relationships with patients.
- Possibility of assignment to specialty units that is not consistent with professional goals or interests.

- Patients too ill or unwilling to participate in rehabilitation sessions.
- Develop ability to think quickly for important patient care decisions.

In rehabilitation hospitals:

- Central gym and patient care conferences allow constant interaction with other physical therapists and rehabilitation providers that leads to joint team decision making.
- Establishment of longer term professional relationships with patients.
- Work schedule is assigned or negotiated with other members of the team.
- Typically assigned to a specialty team. Opportunity to develop specialty practice, but risk of assignment of an area of practice that is of less interest.
- Little interaction with referring or specialty physicians. Team lead by physician who chairs meetings, etc.

Part 2
Overview of Management in Hospital-Based Practices

Contemporary Hospital Management and Physical Therapy

The size of the hospital or health-care system is the key factor in determining the role of rehabilitation managers and their responsibilities. Some potential models include:

+ In a relatively small community hospital, the physical therapy manager may also be the primary provider of patient care—both inpatient and outpatient—using support staff or other therapists as necessary.
+ The physical therapist may be the manager of an interdisciplinary program or programs.
+ In larger hospitals, several unit supervisors and/or program managers may report to a rehabilitation manager or director.
+ In a large health-care system that includes several hospitals and outpatient centers, there may be several managers who may function relatively independently of each other, or they may function as a team that coordinates personnel assignments and other management decisions for consistency throughout the system.
+ There may be a systemwide vice president of rehabilitation services, who centralizes the efforts of supervisors in several centers who have less responsibility for management decisions and more responsibility for implementation of policies.
+ A national chain of hospitals may have a regional manager of rehabilitation services with directors in several freestanding hospitals who report to him or her with little interaction with each other.

Management Responsibilities

Mission, Vision, and Goals

Probably more than any other health-care setting, mid-level managers may struggle with upper-management decisions that may seem contradictory with the missions of many hospitals—to be of service to the community. Offering an acceptable level of quality at the least cost, in a more transparent system, first requires agreement among the members of an organization on what their goals mean, and how they are to be put into operation and measured.

Although individual therapists may have a great deal of independence in their patient care decisions, managers may feel more limited in their ability to try new approaches or ideas without permission of upper management. With decreased time and effort for orientation and mentoring of employees, managers may need to be alert to employees who find themselves in program boxes rather than disciplinary silos. An employee's relationship to the organization may be limited to the team they are assigned. Managers may take extra effort to assure employees' understanding or commitment to the larger organization and its goals. Managers may be redefining the mission, vision, and goals; or reasserting and reassuring staff that they have not changed as mergers and acquisitions take place.

Policies and Procedures

The larger the organization, the more likely managers are responsible for the implementation of, rather than the creation of, policies and procedures that may even be "packaged" to comply with accreditation and regulatory requirements. There may be specific professional issues that affect the quality of care that require additional policies and procedures. Evidence-based practice may be one example. Although important in all practice settings, the positioning of physicians in hospitals, the high level of patient care technology, and the desire for innovation to maintain a competitive edge may require formal policies and procedures to be certain evidence-based practice is the rule rather than the exception for rehabilitation professionals and physicians.

Evidence

In their recent survey Iles and Davidson[22] discovered that about 70% of all physical therapists said they read professional literature at least monthly, but only about 26% reported searching in online databases for new information, and about the same percentage of people critically appraised research reports. They found that the respondents in their study had a positive attitude toward evidence-based practice, but barriers to actually doing that included:

+ Time required to keep up to date
+ Access to easily understandable summaries of evidence
+ Journal access
+ Lack of personal skills in searching and evaluating research evidence

Although these barriers may diminish as academic programs better prepare graduates for these skills, managers may find it challenging to assure evidence-based practice. It may be implied (or assumed) in accreditation and other regulatory requirements, and even perhaps other policies and procedures, but managers may find that evidence-based practice may not be formalized as the foundation of patient care.

The development of policies and procedures may address an individual's efforts to practice based on evidence as part of job descriptions and evaluation of performance. Managers also may address the skill development needed for group identification of clinical questions to be posed, answers to be evaluated, and changes in patient care to be implemented.

Geyman, Deyo, and Ramsey[23] developed a modification of the traditional evidence-based medicine (EBM) process that they call information mastery. This approach may be valuable in all health-care settings, but it provides managers an opportunity to bring together their staffs scattered throughout a hospital-based practice. This process of information mastery relies on a search of secondary online databases, such as POEMs or InfoRetriever in which original resources have already been screened for validity and relevance to shortcut the EBM process to answer a clinical question that has been posed. For example, a clinical question might be: What is the effect of the use of continuous passive motion equipment on the functional performance of patients who have had knee surgery? Answers to questions about the information gathered are then directed to the specific patients who have had knee surgery that a

therapist or group of therapists actually see. The specific questions are:

+ Are the results of the review of the literature relevant to the patients I see?
+ Is the new information valid for my patients?
+ If it were true, would the new information require a change in my/our practice?

Action to be taken based on the answers to the questions makes evidence-based practice seem more practical and applicable for many professionals. Because the process directs attention to practical clinical questions in terms of patients actually cared for, physical therapists may be more eager and willing to invest the time in gathering and implementing new patient care strategies based on the evidence.

Electronic Medical Records

The other information issue important to managers is that staff has the technical skills to interact with electronic health records effectively, accurately, and legally. Spurred by the Health Insurance Portability and Accountability Act (HIPAA) of 1996 and The Joint Commission requirements, the electronic health record provides data to support operations, research, health-care policy, regulation, performance improvement, and patient care.

The use of the electronic health record in a variety of health-care settings by physical therapists has been investigated.[24] Based on this review of the literature, some conclusions were drawn. For instance, one of the advantages of electronic documentation is standardization of terminology and formats. A potential drawback is a system that does not reflect the workflow and practice demands of therapists. Efforts to develop a national physical therapy databank that merges with a health organization's existing system may not be possible because of confidentiality regulations and reluctance for competitors to share information with each other.

Policies and procedures related to implementation of HIPAA guidelines are a given. Managers also may need policies and procedures to assure the technical skills of therapists for the management of patient databases are acquired and adequate for accurate and thorough documentation. Providing information to software and systems developers so that the electronic health record reflects the work of physical therapists also is important.

Marketing

The trend in hospitals and health-care systems seems to be a customer focus to identify the expectations of key stakeholders, and to regularly determine their level of satisfaction with the organization. This approach means that marketing efforts focus on finding out what people want and design the service to meet it, rather than creating a service and then selling it. Collecting data through patient satisfaction surveys, focus groups, follow-up telephone calls after discharge, and community surveys now are common.

Managers need to assure that the information gathered by hospital-marketing departments, includes the person's experience and need for rehabilitation services. Without the traditional department head as the voice for physical therapy or rehabilitation, there is a risk that these services may get lost in the focus on nursing and physician interactions. Using the Internet to supply hospital customers and potential customers with information and choices is expanding rapidly and requires the same level of managerial attention.

Community Interactions

Hospitals and health-care systems are often the largest employer in an area. Managers need to consider the affect of their decisions not only on the health of the community but also on its economy. For instance downsizing staff, mergers, eliminating competition, relocating hospitals, negotiating third-party payer contracts all have an effect on the community that goes beyond measurement of health outcomes. Conversely, community businesses that change their health-care insurance contracts and coverage options for employees affect hospital finances. City and county development often depends on the reputation of its hospitals to attract new businesses and for those businesses to attract new employees.

Representing the hospital on the boards of corporations and community service organizations is an important role for hospital managers to keep their fingers on the pulse of the community. This community service becomes another source of information on a different set of customers—community leaders and organizations. Informal conversations and relationships that occur at board meetings are often the basis of trust and cooperation that is vital to the growth of the hospital and the community so that

trends and developments can be anticipated. Hearing what community leaders are really saying about the a hospital may be as important as the impressions of particular patients.

Staffing

Perhaps more than any other staffing issue, hospital-based rehabilitation managers need to consider the effect of nursing staff shortages on the provision of rehabilitation services. Therapists rely on cooperation and coordination with nursing personnel so that all components of patients' care are addressed. When nursing services are not working efficiently and effectively, it is difficult for therapy to work. Rehabilitation and program managers need to work with nursing in the development of staffing patterns and schedules that work best for everyone. Assuring that therapy sessions are included in a patient's busy schedule of diagnostic tests and nursing interventions may require a significant amount of a rehabilitation manager's time.

Job Satisfaction

Job satisfaction and burnout of physical therapists has received some attention because of the turmoil that has occurred in hospitals in recent years. It appears that physical therapists who see their work as controllable, with choices, and who can develop workable strategies to meet their productivity standards, not only survive, but thrive, in hospital-based practices. Seeing options and opportunities lays the foundation for developing time-management, assertive communication, delegation, discharge, and task-prioritizing skills.[25]

Lopopolo[26] also investigated the effect of hospital restructuring on physical therapist role behaviors, job satisfaction, stress, and commitment to the organization. The immediate supervisor of the majority of the 273 physical therapists in the study also was a physical therapist. Among the findings was that physical therapists:

+ Had moderately low levels of stress.
+ Had a strong sense of commitment to their occupation.
+ Were moderately satisfied with their jobs.
+ Were neutral in their commitment to their organizations.

✦ With more experience felt more role overload and greater organizational commitment.

✦ Who work in areas of their interest increase their job satisfaction.

✦ Continue to focus on their professional responsibilities while responding to organizational demands.

✦ Who have more interactions with others find that the interactions positively affect the negative effects of organizational change on job satisfaction.

✦ Rely on interaction among clinicians to feel comfortable with their work.

✦ With professional and educational activities outside of work have an enhanced sense of competence.

✦ Who have experienced decreased job satisfaction and commitment to the organization when work requirements encroach on professional autonomy.

✦ Do not correlate job satisfaction and organizational commitment with their occupational commitment.

✦ Who experience role conflict, role overload, or role ambiguity have less job satisfaction and organizational commitment.

Regardless of the discipline of the immediate supervisor or manager, attention to reinforcing and maintaining the strong sense of professional identity of physical therapists may be important to their recruitment and retention. Physical therapists may be willing to accommodate to organizational changes and demands as long as their ability to interact with other professionals and patients is preserved.

Contingency Workers

The importance of commitment of employees to an organization cannot be underestimated. Low absenteeism, less turnover of staff, higher job satisfaction, and high performance levels may be the result of commitment of full-time employees. The power of committed employees may be at risk with the rise in contingent employment arrangements which include in-house temporaries, floats, direct-hire or seasonal workers, lease workers, consultants and independent contractors.[27]

Both employers and employees are attracted to the flexibility offered in contingency work. Hospitals see an opportunity to cut costs associated with employee benefit packages. They are able to manage the absences of regular staff and patient load fluctuations that may be seasonal. Health professionals may see contingency work as improving their employment opportunities with a variety of short-term work experiences that give them more flexibility. They may choose the work they engage in at any point in time, they have the opportunity to try out a variety of employment settings or even locations before making permanent career decisions, and their hourly fees are higher than the wages per hour performing the same job.

When cost and flexibility are the primary reasons for managerial decisions to hire workers to meet short-term specific needs (a contingency situation), the use of temporary workers (temps) appears to be good business. It may not be such good business as a stop-gap staffing measure when temps are hired to fill ongoing personnel shortages. As the demand for particular workers increases, so do their employment opportunities. During these times, health professionals may prefer contingency work because of the freedom to select work assignments that are most attractive to them. This preference further contributes to shortages in full-time, traditional employees.

Physical Therapist Assistants

Managerial decisions about the utilization of physical therapist assistants and other support personnel are important in hospitals because the patients are medically unstable with complex conditions. Professionals who are prepared to meet the demands of quick turnaround discharge planning that begins with the initial evaluations of patients are vital. This need often excludes physical therapist assistants in the care of many patients.

On the other hand, when the actual physical therapy interventions for acute patients are routine and straightforward, physical therapist assistants may be directed to assume responsibility for established plans of care. Clinical pathways and other guidelines used to standardize plans of care also make the assignment of many patients to physical therapist assistants appropriate.

The need to reduce costs makes the utilization of the least expensive licensed personnel very attractive. Managers must be aware of state statutes that regulate practice of physical therapist assistants in acute care settings. They may not be permitted to work without the direct supervision of physical therapists in hospitals. Reimbursement requirements may define skilled care in such a way that nonlicensed personnel may not be utilized in direct patient care at all. This may be particularly true in rehabilitation hospitals.

Managers must be cautious in implementing blanket policies and procedures, such as the automatic turnover of patients to assistants after the initial session is conducted by the physical therapist. The judgment of the physical therapist about tasks and duties that are assigned to others should be made on a patient-by-patient basis, particularly in hospitals where the patient's medical condition may be fragile or unpredictable. Managers must clearly understand the expected responsibilities of physical therapists for the supervision and direction of physical therapist assistants and insist on staffing patterns that facilitate those relationships.

A physical therapist assistant who is assigned specifically to one physical therapist may significantly improve therapeutic time they each spend with patients. Either working alone with a patient, or with the therapist when a patient demands the support of two people to participate in a therapy session, physical therapist assistants have an important role to play. When they are working as partners on the same caseload, there is more opportunity to dovetail direct patient care and administrative tasks. While physical therapists are doing those things that only a physical therapist can do, the physical therapist assistant can contribute to direct patient care and many of the support tasks like scheduling, preparing patients for treatment, documentation, arranging for equipment delivery, etc.

Contrast this with a model in which the physical therapist assistant is assigned his or her own caseload composed of patients who have been examined and evaluated by several therapists, or a physical therapist who has assigned patients to more than one physical therapist assistant. Direction and supervision by whom and when becomes much less clear and risky.

An alternative is to relieve both physical therapists and assistants of as many administrative tasks as possible by assigning many of those tasks to unlicensed personnel—technicians or aides. Managers must carefully develop job descriptions and training programs for these duties.

Managers also may consider a physical therapist assistant in hospitals as the glue that holds contingency workers and students together as they address their nonpatient care responsibilities. A full-time physical therapist assistant with a long work history in a hospital may have a great deal of knowledge about the idiosyncrasies of the organization. They are invaluable as the go-to person as new staff and students navigate their new surroundings and learn to manage their time. As always, serving as the extra set of hands with complex patients is another important responsibility. Remembering that physical therapist assistants are extenders of all of the roles of physical therapists increases their value to organizations.

Weekend Services

Supervision issues are particularly important during holidays and weekends when reduced rehabilitation services may be provided. Identifying the physical therapist who is responsible for supportive staff becomes challenging because they are typically very busy with a patients who *must* be treated for one reason or another. These responsibilities leave little time for the supervision of the physical therapist assistant(s). Everyone working on a weekend or holiday may be a contingency worker. They may not know each other, which further complicates the communication and establishment of a supervisory relationship. Particularly when the work schedule and patient assignments are pre-established for the weekend, it is easy to become involved in direct patient care so that there is little interaction with coworkers, let alone time for supervision of others. Managers need to be alert to the risks inherent in these situations. Orientation to policies and procedures for these special days may be crucial in deterring errors and maintaining the quality of services.

Patient Care

Anecdotal reports have always suggested that the more physical and occupational therapy a patient receives, the better are the outcomes of care. Two studies confirmed the relationship between, and the frequency and duration of, therapy services and outcomes, such as discharge to home.[28,29] The challenge for managers is achieving the same results with fewer staff to provide the service and decreased contact time with each patient.

These studies both suggest that with more physical therapy, mobility scores of patients may have been improved and the discharge placement from hospitals may have been less restrictive for many patients.

How managers may affect other decision makers who are eager for early discharge of patients and rely on general guidelines rather than individual patient data in discharge planning is a major management concern.

Although conducted more than 10 years ago, a study by Curtis and Martin, identified perceptions of physical therapists about factors that affected acute care practice which included:[30]

+ Discomfort with patient medical complications, behaviors, and pain.
+ Lack of patient motivation and cooperation.
+ Ability to integrate a great deal of information—pathology, pharmacology, radiological and diagnostic reports—to, assess their patients' needs, and project realistic, achievable goals to effectively prepare the patients for the next level of care.
+ Difficulty in adding to or changing a patient's orders, and receiving appropriate referrals.
+ Scheduling of multiple required medical tests.
+ Inadequate time to work with patients to accomplish what they were capable of accomplishing.
+ Preparation for treatment sessions and failed attempts to see patients that is time-consuming.
+ Patient discharge frequently occurring within 1 or 2 days of referral without opportunity to coordinate with the family and with postdischarge providers.
+ Distinguishing between patients who require high-level, ongoing care by the physical therapist and those who could be seen by support personnel for treatment.
+ Increasing numbers of part-time and per diem staff and new graduates who may not be prepared to function effectively in the acute care setting.

Hopefully, during the last 10 years, new graduates have been better prepared for the acute care practice and current employees continue to demonstrate the expertise required to manage very complex, sick patients. Managers have opportunities to advocate for patients and their staff as they address factors like people who are too sick to participate in physical therapy, and scheduling conflicts that often place diagnostic tests and other procedures ahead of physical therapy. Managers who develop positive relationships with hospitalists also may reduce some of the tensions related to fulfilling physician orders in a timely manner rather than immediately.

Managers also may need to do a detailed job analysis to identify, at least, the direct patient care skills that therapists must have in acute care. Even a simple checklist of specific things to know and things to do during treatment sessions may be helpful, particularly for new graduates, new employees, and contingency workers who are coping with the complexity of hospital-based care. Updating this list as new technology and new procedures are introduced is an important management responsibility. Orientation to the nonpatient-care duties and responsibilities are equally important particularly because physical therapists often work independently from each other in hospitals.

Although physical therapists in acute care establish their own daily work schedules, managers who are available to assist with scheduling conflicts or unexpected tasks that arise contribute significantly to coordination of smooth, efficient patient care.

Managers may also find the instrument developed by Lopopolo valuable.[31] The Professional Role Behaviors Survey (PROBES) reflects five role behavior dimensions (evaluating and planning, productivity, interacting, information sharing, and administration/clinical) and includes the following 26 role behaviors of hospital-based physical therapists that may be used to determine changes (i.e., increase, decrease, no change) in these aspects of their responsibilities over time or as organizations change:

+ Focus on the functional needs of patients
+ Delegating and supervising of physical therapy treatment
+ Teaching of patients, families, and other health-care providers
+ Using critical pathways/care paths to guide care
+ Focus on efficiency/productivity in the performance of activities
+ Integration of physical therapists into multidisciplinary teams
+ Physical therapist's role as a consultant, specialist, or advanced clinician
+ Administrative activities
+ Work in more than one clinical area of the hospital or site
+ Work on weekends/holidays on a rotating schedule
+ Ability to plan and control how the work will be done

- Professional approach to patient care
- Interacting with and assisting other physical therapists with patient care
- Time spent doing care other than physical therapy
- Professional identity of the physical therapist
- Participating in the clinical education of students
- Participating in self-education
- Attending staff meetings
- Social interaction with other physical therapists in the facility
- Involvement in professional activities outside of work
- Teaching of groups in the community
- Assuming the formal responsibility of a case manager
- Documenting the results of patient care
- Communication/collaboration with other health-care professionals
- Time spent in patient evaluation and program planning
- Time spent in direct patient care (i.e., treating patients)

Asking managers and staff physical therapists to consider how they are spending their time provides valuable insight into assignments, productivity, and roles that may have an important effect on patient care. Opportunities to anticipate the effect of managerial decisions on these roles, and to identify which of these factors may be affecting the delivery of quality care and achievement of expected patient outcomes makes this a valuable tool, particularly for managers who are not physical therapists.

Fiscal

Mid-level managers may be far removed from the complex organizational budgeting and financial planning processes (e.g., borrowing and investing funds) in hospitals and health-care systems. In the broadest terms, financial information is *one* source of information that is used to accomplish the organization's purposes. Mid-level managers are more likely to rely on accounting (current and prospective) reports to plan and control the services they are responsible for, and to report the results of their

efforts and decisions. Because this level of information is for internal use only, each organization typically develops a reporting format and process that works for them. On-the-job training is usually involved in these responsibilities although some knowledge of budgeting, cost accounting, and operations research is helpful.[2]

Program and department managers are typically held accountable for, at the least, monthly and quarterly reports on staff productivity and the costs of the services provided in their units. Daily review of data may be conducted to assure prompt and responsive managerial decisions. Their responsibility and accountability for the appropriate use of resources in relation to the goals of the organization are typically discussed in terms of accounting reports.

Distinguishing variables that affect the use of resources that are within the control of the manager and those that are not is an important component of the financial accountability at the program or department level that includes a strong understanding of reimbursement policies. Depending on the organization's culture (i.e., top-down or bottom-up planning), the ability of mid-level managers to act on or only to report the facts and figures about the units of their responsibility is another important way that the roles of managers differ from one hospital to another.

Legal, Ethical, and Risk

Patient safety is perhaps the biggest risk issue for hospitals and health-care systems. The Joint Commission argues that accreditation itself is a risk reduction activity because compliance with its standards is intended to reduce the likelihood of bad patient outcomes. With that in mind, in 2007 The Joint Commission revised the National Patient Safety Goals for each type of health-care organization. For hospitals these goals are:[32]

- Improve the accuracy of patient identification.
  Use of at least two patient identifiers.
- Improve the effectiveness of communication among caregivers.
  Read back verbal or telephone orders, standardize abbreviations, improve timeliness of critical information, standardize "hands-off" communication.
- Improve the safety of using medications.
  Prevent errors involving interchange of look-alike drugs, label all medication containers, reduce harm in use of anticoagulation therapy.

✦ Reduce the risk of health-care–associated infections.

Comply with World Health Organization (WHO) or Centers for Disease Control (CDC) hand hygiene guidelines, manage sentinel events associated with infection.

✦ Accurately and completely reconcile medications across the continuum of care.

Process for comparing current medications with those ordered while in the hospital, a complete list of medications is communicated to the next provider of service and to the patient.

✦ Reduce the risk of harm resulting from falls.

Implement and evaluate the effectiveness of a fall reduction program.

✦ Encourage patients' active involvement in their own care.

Establish the means for and encourage patients and families to report their concerns.

✦ Identify safety risks inherent in its population.

Organization identifies patients with emotional or behavior disorders.

✦ Improve recognition and response to changes in a patient's condition.

Have a method that enables staff to directly request additional assistance from specialty trained individuals if a patient's condition worsens.

The shortage of hospital personnel adds to the risks as fewer people attempt to do more with less for patients who are older, more vulnerable, with complex medical conditions. This increases the risks for negligent acts and medical errors. All managers in hospitals must be constantly alert for hospital-wide opportunities to increase the safety of patients and their employees, while attending to the risks in the provision of services for each patient.

Treatment Cancellations

At the same time, managers need to be certain that staff have guidelines and communication skills necessary to sort out patients who are too ill or unstable to participate in rehabilitation sessions from those who simply prefer not to participate. Understanding that patients have the right to refuse treatment for a life-threatening condition is not the same as patients having the right to refuse therapy because they have visitors or simply do not want to be disturbed. Managers have to analyze cancellation of treatment sessions to determine if these clinical decisions are appropriate, particularly for staff who may be overwhelmed and inadvertently fail to encourage patient participation.

Communicable Diseases

Another related management issue is assignment of staff to patients who are perceived to place the therapist at risk. Managers may decide to assure that the same therapist does not consistently draw the "short straw" to care for patients with contagious diseases (e.g., severe acute respiratory syndrome, tuberculosis) or uncontrollable behavior. Alternatively, they may decide to prepare some staff to specialize in the care of these patients with special needs to avoid these safety and assignment issues while improving the care of these patients through staff consistency.

Ethical Issues

Rehabilitation managers are often faced with difficult ethical decisions when resources are limited. Deciding whether to see every patient once before treating any patient twice, or establishing a triage system for identifying patients in greatest need of therapy becomes important. This choice is closely related to a manager's relationship with physicians and nurses, who are typically the first providers to identify the needs of patients.

In academic health centers, patients who are also subjects in clinical research studies may become priority patients although patients with safety risks may require more attention and time. Patients who may not receive therapy that they need because they are subjects in a study also present an ethical dilemma.

Receiving referrals only for patients who are appropriate for rehabilitation services requires that managers educate other professionals about patient goals that therapists can assist in meeting with their skilled services. Reducing inappropriate referrals for therapy increases efficiency and the best use of limited resources. Failing to be involved in the care of patients who would benefit from rehabilitation interventions is equally disturbing.

Ethical issues occur at every level of management of complex health-care organizations on a regular basis. It is not unusual to have available full-time in-house legal counsel, a risk-management staff, and an ethics committee to resolve the many possible things that can go wrong when an organization is responsible for the care of people who are acutely ill or severely injured. Managers must be familiar with the reporting requirements for the hospital to be proactive rather than reactive to legal and ethical dilemmas.

Communication

Sorting out what information needs to be immediately disseminated, and what information is better left unshared often leads to difficult decisions in communication with upper management, and with staff and managers in similar positions in the organization. Formal policies and procedures for the content, distribution, and approval of both internal and external messages are often in place in large organizations to decrease some of these concerns and to assure consistency in the messages that organizations wish to send.

One-on-one interactions with staff often require managers to be on the move in a hospital. With staff conducting treatment sessions at patient bedsides, managers must go to them for informal meetings. Meeting over lunch breaks may also provide opportunities for chats as long as they do not lead to more work when personnel should be taking a break from their clinical duties.

Conclusion

The following activities provide some insight into the complex decisions that are made as managers of hospital-based services are held accountable for the performance of their staffs and the outcomes of the care provided. Probably no other health-care setting continues to be as volatile and unpredictable. Because of this, hospitals provide many opportunities for professional growth and increased responsibility for people interested in health management careers. It may not be unreasonable to suggest that hospital-based rehabilitation may evolve as a specialty practice similar to that of hospitalists that requires knowledge and clinical expertise in a wide range of diseases, trauma, and postsurgical care.

Decisions about when and how to intervene with patients with unstable and unpredictable clinical pictures makes this setting demanding and exciting. Managers and the staff they supervise never know what the day will bring. This makes hospitals very attractive to people who seek variety and thrive on work that is never the same from day to day. They interact with a large number of professionals from many disciplines and patients with a range of psychosocial issues and complex diagnoses. Influencing the recovery of people with severe medical problems to achieve what seem to be impossible functional goals contributes to their job satisfaction.

Activities 19.1 to 19.27 provide the opportunity to address inpatient hospital and health system management issues.

ACTIVITY 19.1
PATIENTS OR CLIENTS?

Are the people who receive hospital-based services more like patients or clients as defined by the American Physical Therapy Association? Defend your answer in a group discussion.

ACTIVITY 19.2
TRENDS

Take each of the facts listed below and discuss the effect of these trends on mid-level hospital managers in hospitals and hospital systems.[1]

- Of the 5,756 hospitals in the United States, almost 2,716 are in a health system (a corporate body that may own or manage health provider facilities or subsidiaries) and 1,455 are part of health networks. In 2005, 51 deals involving 88 hospitals were added to the 59 mergers and acquisitions involving 236 hospitals in 2004.
- 60% of hospital systems also offer home health services, 60% offer hospice services, and 45% have skilled nursing facilities.
- The average hospital length of stay decreased from 7.6 days in 1981 to 5.6 days in 2005.
- Payment-to-cost ratios for private insurance were 130%, for Medicare 95%, and for Medicaid 86%.
- Costs of employment in hospitals increased 4% in a year.
- 39% of hospital costs are related to Medicare, 37% private insurance, and 6% of hospital costs are uncompensated.
- Hospitals employed 4 million FTEs. 60% of the costs of hospitals were wages and benefits.
- 11% of hospitals had fully integrated electronic health records and 57% had partially implemented systems. Hospitals with more than 500 beds in urban settings that were part of systems were furthest ahead in implementation of electronic health records.

ACTIVITY 19.3
NEW HOSPITALISTS

Bentley Health Care has contracted with Physicians for Hospitals, Inc. to staff their three general hospitals in Broadmoor County. Sylvia Tallarino, the rehabilitation director for Bentley Health Care, has been invited to the first meeting of the hospitalists assigned to the three hospitals. They have invited her to give a 5. to 10-minute presentation about rehabilitation at Bentley. She will have the opportunity to ask the hospitalists questions. What should Sylvia include in her presentation? What questions should she ask?

ACTIVITY 19.4
CLINICAL EDUCATION

Antonio Sorranto, rehabilitation director for Van Husen Medical Center has been invited to meet with the Vice Dean of the School of Physical Therapy and Rehabilitation Sciences and the Director of Clinical Education for the School. The only agenda item is to develop a strategic plan to meet one of the mutual goals established by the new Dean of the Medical School of Van Husen University and the chief executive officer (CEO) of the medical center. The goal is: Beginning with the next class of physical therapy students, each student is to be placed for at least 50% of their required clinical education hours in Van Husen Medical Center.

Each of the 50 students must complete 36 weeks of full-time clinical education, spaced throughout the curriculum as 6 weeks in year 1, 12 weeks in year 2, and 18 weeks in year 3. Antonio has 12 full-time physical therapists and a pool of about 20 contingency staff (who primarily work weekends and as vacation relief). They are all assigned to general medical/surgical, orthopedics, neurology, inpatient rehabilitation, outpatient rehabilitation, inpatient/outpatient pediatrics, and a satellite outpatient center.

His staff is reluctant to give up their affiliations with other schools, and Antonio feels this plan will decrease recruitment of new graduates from other schools. He also is concerned that the staff will be overburdened. Currently, being a clinical instructor is voluntary and the policy has been that a therapist only supervises one student/year. Role-play this meeting.

ACTIVITY 19.5
A CHILDREN'S HOSPITAL

Ron Fleming, the director of rehabilitation at one of the Shriners hospitals (see http://www.shrinershq.org/ Shrine/ and click on list of hospitals for more information), is concerned that his small staff of 10 physical, occupational, and speech therapists is torn in two directions. The hospital has received several research grants over the years related to the care of children who have congenital limb absences and children who have had amputations. The treatment of children with these conditions is considered the specialty of the hospital.

Because of concerns about funding and controlling costs, marketing efforts have been directed to building and increasing philanthropic funding for outpatient services. The efforts have been successful. Ron is concerned, however, that this success has resulted in a patient population with a much broader range of diagnoses that are challenging for his highly specialized staff. The staff report they need extensions on their grant renewal deadlines because they are spending more time treating patients. What actions should Ron take?

ACTIVITY 19.6
OUTCOMES

Rodney Williams, the rehabilitation manager at Osakee Rehabilitation Hospital is concerned. For the third consecutive quarter, patient outcome measures have fallen below the average of outcomes for all 80 hospitals in the Rehabilitation Hospitals of America chain that includes Osakee. He is meeting with the vice president of Osakee and the director of nursing to identify the causes for these disappointing outcomes and to identify action for improvement. Role-play the meeting.

ACTIVITY 19.7
STAFFING IN SUBACUTE CARE

Jerry Weiss is the rehabilitation manager for the newest subacute hospital in the National Hospital Corporation chain. His first task is to staff the six new positions in rehabilitation services. He has a meeting with the director of human resources who wants to brainstorm some recruitment strategies. What are some ideas Jerry might present?

ACTIVITY 19.8
A NEW ASSIGNMENT

For the past 2 years, Jocelyn Ramos has been the supervisor of the inpatient rehabilitation team at Twin Cities Regional Hospital, a 250-bed hospital. In addition to her patient care duties in this position, she has been responsible for scheduling staff and monitoring productivity goals. The position of rehabilitation manager for the 100-bed rehabilitation hospital in the same system has become available. The vice president of clinical services has asked Jocelyn to accept the promotion. What should she consider in making her decision?

ACTIVITY 19.9
THE BIG OPPORTUNITY

Their move to the brand new, state of the art Carrollville Regional Medical Center from the old Carrollville Community Hospital was long awaited by Rosemarie Raddison and her rehabilitation staff. Along with the new hospital came a new upper-management team from the corporate offices of the All American Hospital Corporation that had purchased the old hospital and immediately began construction on the new one. Unhappy with many of the new management team's decisions, Rosemarie, who has been the rehabilitation director at Carrollville for more than 20 years, resigned as soon as the move to the new hospital was completed. The rest of her staff followed and within a month, there was no one left on the rehabilitation staff.

Since then, the hospital has been relying on intermittent services of a few physical therapists who work in other practices in the community. They have been willing to provide a few hours of care to patients in the evenings and on weekends while Carrollville continues to recruit a new rehabilitation director and staff.

After 4 months of searching, none of the rehabilitation positions has been filled despite a state-of-the-art rehabilitation center in the hospital and the attractiveness of Carrollville as one of the fastest growing communities in the state. The fill-in staff are becoming concerned that this is a longer than expected commitment to the hospital.

A recruiter has approached Daniel Steinman, an experienced rehabilitation manager in another state, to consider becoming a candidate for the director position. The salary offer is almost twice what Daniel currently makes, so he is interested in the position and Carrollville is an attractive location. What are the list of questions and issues that Daniel should prepare in his consideration of this opportunity? Role-play Daniel's interview with the vice president of clinical services at Carrollville Regional.

ACTIVITY 19.10
A SHIFT IN MANAGEMENT

After only 2 years at Clara Barton Medical Center, Daniel Steinman has submitted his resignation to accept a new position in Carrollville. The rehabilitation staff has been advised that the vice president for clinical services has decided to take the opportunity of his resignation to eliminate Daniel's position—rehabilitation manager. Ron Abelson, the respiratory therapist who is also the cardiopulmonary program manager will manage all of inpatient and outpatient rehabilitation services. Identify all of the stakeholders in Clara Barton's rehabilitation services. Determine the effect of this decision on these stakeholders.

ACTIVITY 19.11
INFORMATION MASTERY

In a small group, develop a policy and procedure(s) to incorporate a plan for ongoing information mastery for the staff of the rehabilitation services in a large teaching hospital. First, decide if the policies and procedures will address individuals or the staff as a whole—or both.

ACTIVITY 19.12
SAFETY GOALS AND PHYSICAL THERAPY

Discuss which of The Joint Commission's safety goals apply to physical therapists. What policies and procedures should be in place for physical therapists to contribute to these goals? Outline these policies and procedures.

ACTIVITY 19.13
PRODUCTIVITY

Robyn Latimer, the rehabilitation manager for Holy Family Health Center is distressed to learn that the average productivity rate for her staff is down. To help her determine where the problems may lie, she decides to use the PROBE role behaviors to identify possible things that may be adjusted so that her staff is spending more time on initial evaluations and direct patient care. Which behaviors might Robyn focus on? What would be her plan of action?

ACTIVITY 19.14
SUPERVISON OF A PHYISCAL THERAPIST ASSISTANT

Phyllis Ames is a physical therapist assistant who has worked at Dellano Community Hospital for almost 20 years—longer than anyone else in the department. She has enjoyed the management responsibilities she has assumed over the years, particularly when the director's position has been unfilled. She has recently completed a master's degree in health services administration because of these interests. The director's position is again vacant and she is applying for the position. Consider all of the stakeholders in the decision to have Phyllis as the director of rehabilitation services. What will be the effect of this decision on them?

ACTIVITY 19.15
WEEKENDS

Riverside Rehabilitation Hospital contracts with Quality Staffing Services to provide rehabilitation services on Saturdays and Sundays. This arrangement is the result of assuring full-time staff that weekend coverage was not an expectation. This promise has been a great recruitment tool to fill full-time positions.

However, recently, several of the physical therapy and occupational therapy staff who are full-time employees of Riverside, also are contracting with Quality Staffing Services for additional income, much to the surprise of Debra Watson, Riverside's rehabilitation manager. Sometimes they are assigned to other organizations in the area, and, even more surprisingly to Debra, they have reported to work at Riverside on weekends as employees of Quality Staffing Services.

She had already voiced her concern about her lack of input into the staff that Quality Staffing Services assigns to Riverside. They have been inconsistent in the people assigned and unpredictable in the numbers who appear to work each weekend. Debra has asked to discuss those issues and this new development with her staff appearing to work on weekends with Rhonda Smith, the Human Resources director at Riverside.

During the meeting, Rhonda advises Debra that there is no policy about concurrent employment with other companies. She would obviously prefer that Debra arrange for overtime pay for Riverside staff who work weekends at Riverside than be paying the very high rates that Quality Staffing Services charges for weekend services. What else should they discuss during their meeting?

ACTIVITY 19.16
WORKING IN MULTIPLE UNITS

Sanderson Community Hospital has reduced its inpatient staff to just one physical therapist and one physical therapist assistant. There are days when the inpatient census increases unexpectedly and there is a need for another physical therapist to meet the demands for initial evaluation of several patients within the 24-hour window required. As rehabilitation supervisor, Jonathan Martin's solution to this staffing need has been to ask the three outpatient physical therapists to see inpatients when they have patient cancellations or patients who do not show for their appointments during the day. They have refused. Role-play a staff meeting that Jonathan calls to resolve this issue.

ACTIVITY 19.17
CHARTING AREA

Rajiv Patel heads the interdisciplinary rehabilitation staff at Roosevelt Medical Center. The charting room for his 30 full-time staff has been moved 3 times in the last year because of new construction and renovations of the hospital. These changes have been disruptive and demoralizing—the last move was to a former laundry room in the basement without enough space for everyone to have a designated desk and storage space. The staff leaves early and often fails to complete their documentation and other tasks because the room is noisy and disruptive. Because he is afraid this issue is driving therapists away, Rajiv has persuaded the vice president for clinical operations to include a new state of the art rehabilitation planning room in the next phase of hospital remodeling. In groups, determine the purpose of the room and submit a proposal for its design and furnishings. What other issues does this upper management decision making suggest? What other issues might Rajiv need to address with upper management?

ACTIVITY 19.18
RELUCTANT PT

Annemarie Watson has been a physical therapist at the hospital for more than 20 years. She has not taken well to the series of changes in the hospital's organization. Her favorite expression is "there's nothing new under the sun." She tends to be unimpressed with the progress the hospital has made, and frequently voices her dissatisfaction to anyone who will listen. There has been some concern about her clinical skills although patients love her and she is effective in meeting their goals. Her documentation is very weak, and she has been resistant to learning the new electronic-documentation system.

Rose Evans, the rehabilitation manager, is about to meet with Annemarie to share her impressions of her behaviors, when Annemarie submits her resignation. The reason for resigning, she says, is because she is worn out. However, she indicates that she is willing to work intermittently for vacation coverage, or to provide weekend coverage one or two weekends a month. What should Rose say?

ACTIVITY 19.19
SUBACUTE CARE TASKFORCE

Eliot Emerson has worked his way up to be the regional rehabilitation manager of eight subacute hospitals. When the American Physical Therapy Association asks him to join a taskforce to develop guidelines for physical therapy services in subacute care, he is flattered and agrees. What issues should he make sure are addressed by the taskforce?

ACTIVITY 19.20
WEEKEND COVERAGE

Tom Bradford, contract PT, who has been working most weekends at Cramwell Rehabilitation Hospital is very upset when he meets with Mary Strickland, the rehabilitation manager. Tom reports that Bette Shannon, another contract therapist, has been documenting and reporting seeing patients whom she has not seen. Tom learned this yesterday when one of the patients that Bette has been scheduled to see the last few weekends asked Tom why he had not been getting therapy on weekends before. The records show that Bette documented seeing the patient the two previous weekends. Tom was embarrassed by the patient's question and is furious with Bette. What should Mary do?

ACTIVITY 19.21
PRODUCTIVITY

The weekly staff meeting has degenerated into angry expressions of frustration. It began with the rehabilitation manager, Jean Holmes, giving a report on productivity goals that were not met. The reaction of the staff again was to ask Jean to do something about revising the goals that are impossible to meet due to things beyond their control, such as patients who are unavailable because they are in x-ray, receiving some other treatment, or simply refusing treatment because they are sick or tired. Jean has suggested in the past that the staff stagger their hours into later in the evening to decrease these conflicts and give patients some rest during the day. They refuse. What is the next course of action?

ACTIVITY 19.22
PATIENT REFUSAL

James Hunter, a rehabilitation manager, is concerned about Val Morres. She has significantly more patient cancellations due to patient refusal than any other person does on staff. When James meets with Val to discuss this, Val reports that she strongly believes a person has a right to refuse treatment—it is what she learned in school. Cancellations also give her more time to spend with patients who want therapy so she really does not understand why it is a problem. What should James do?

ACTIVITY 19.23
PRIORITY PATIENTS

James Hunter has to do something. He seems to be spending most of his time responding to complaints that patients have been referred for therapy and are not scheduled in a timely manner. The nursing shift managers are angry because several patients have been discharged without a physical therapist seeing them as was ordered. What actions should he take?

ACTIVITY 19.24
PATIENT ASSIGNMENT

Bonnie Bradman feels that Sid Bleekman, the rehabilitation manager, has ignored her concerns that she is always assigned the most difficult patients. Although this was flattering at first, she feels these assignments make her look bad because her productivity numbers are down as a result. A memo from Sid advising her to bring up her numbers has angered her. She is meeting with Sid today. Role-play this meeting.

ACTIVITY 19.25
EFFICIENCY

Helene DuPrise, the rehabilitation manager in a large teaching hospital, has good news and bad news. The good news is that referrals for physical therapy are more appropriate and timely because of her efforts to educate physicians and nurses about physical therapy. The bad news is that physical therapists often are completing examination and evaluation of patients before diagnostic test results are known and a medical diagnosis has been established. The physical therapists are concerned that they are intervening too soon in many cases. They are making many assumptions about patient status when there may actually be contraindications and precautions that have not been identified because diagnostic reports are not yet available. Concerned about these risks, what should Helene do?

ACTIVITY 19.26
TECHNOLOGY

Helene DuPrise uses her high-tech environment as a recruiting tool. However, after they are hired, staff members have complained that they feel that rehabilitation is an afterthought in the selection of new technology for the hospital and that they are second-class citizens in training for the technology that is available. What should Helene do?

ACTIVITY 19.27
PRIORITY PATIENT LIST

John Butterworth has no choice. The time has come to develop a priority list for rehabilitation patients in the hospital. The resignation of another physical therapist was the last straw. He simply does not have enough staff to treat the number of patients who are referred for physical therapy. He had already announced to the nurses that all patients would be seen only once a day, so referrals to see patients twice a day could not be accepted. He does not want to discourage referrals, which he may never build up again. What should be his criteria for sorting referrals into a priority list? Patients with orthopedic postsurgical needs before patients who are on the general medical/surgical wing? Patients of a particular physician before those of another? First-come, first-served?

REFERENCES

1. American Hospital Association. Trendwatch chartbook 2007: Trends affecting hospitals and health systems. Chicago, IL: American Hospital Association; 2007. Available at: http://www.aha.org/aha/trendwatch/2007/cb2007chapter2.pdf. Accessed October 23, 2007.

2. Nowicki M. *The Financial Management of Hospitals and Healthcare Organizations*. 3rd ed. Washington, DC: Health Administration Press; 2004.

3. Van Amerongen D. *Networks and the Future of Medical Practice*. Chicago, IL: Health Administration Press; 1998.

4. Society of Hospital Medicine. Information about SIM. Available at: http://www.hospitalmedicine.org/Content/NavigationMenu/AboutSHM/GeneralInformation/General_Information.htm. Accessed October 31, 2007.

5. Society of Hospital Medicine. Measuring hospitalist performance. Available at: http://www.hospitalmedicine.org/AM/Template.cfm?Section=White_Papers&Template=/CM/ContentDisplay.cfm&ContentID=13595. Accessed October 31, 2007.

6. Institute of Medicine. Academic health centers: Leading change in the 21st century. Washington, DC: Institute of Medicine; 2003. Available at: http://www.ion.edu/Object.File/Master/13/779/AHC8pgFINAL.pdf. Accessed October 31, 2007.

7. Wartman SA, ed. *The Academic Health Center: Evolving Models*. Washington, DC: Association of Academic Health Centers; 2007.

8. Langabeer JR, Napiewocki J. *Competitive Business Strategy for Teaching Hospitals*. Westport, CT: Quorum Books; 2000.

9. Medicare Payment Advisory Commission. Report to congress: Physician owned specialty hospitals. Washington, DC:2005. Available at: http://www.medpac.gov/documents/Mar05_SpecHospitals.pdf. Accessed October 31, 2007.

10. Cram P, Vaughn-Sarrazin M, Rosenthal GE. Hospital characteristics and patient populations served by physician owned and nonphysician owned orthopedic specialty hospitals. *BMC Health Services Research*. 2007;7:1472. Available at: http://www.biomedcentral.com/content/pdf/1472-6963-7-155.pdf. Accessed October 31, 2007.

11. Wisconsin Hospital Association. Summary of final rule on Medicare program: Changes to the criteria for being classified as an inpatient rehabilitation facility. May, 2004. Available at: http://wha.org/financeAndData/pdf/inpatientrehabclass.pdf. Accessed October 31, 2007.

12. American Hospital Association. Utilization trends in inpatient rehabilitation: Update through Q 2: 2007. Available at: http://www.aha.org/aha/content/2007/pdf/2007septmoranreport.pdf American Hospital Association. Accessed October 31, 2007.

13. American Health Care Association. Nursing facility subacute care: The quality and cost-effective alternative to hospital care. 1996. Available at: http://www.rai.to/subacute.thm. Accessed November 1, 2007.

14. De La Cruz P. Subacute nursing: Different stages of development. *MedSurg Nursing*. 1997. Available at: http://findarticles.com/p/articles/mi_m0FSS/is_n4_v6/ai_n18607507. Accessed November 1, 2007.

15. Commission on Accreditation of Rehabilitation Facilities. Who we are. Available at: http://www.carf.org/consumer.aspx?content=content/About/News/boilerplate.htm. Accessed November 1, 2007.

16. Gittell JH. Achieving focus in hospital care: The role of relational coordination. In: Herzlinger RE, ed. *Consumer-driven health care*. San Francisco, CA: John Wiley & Sons; 2004.

17. Miller PA, Solomon P. The influence of a move to program management on physical therapist practice. *Physical Therapy*. 2002;82:449–459.

18. Miller PA, Goddard P, Laschinger Spence HK. Evaluating physical therapists' perception of empowerment using Kanter's theory of structural power in organizations. *Physical Therapy*. 2001;81:1880–1888.

19. AHA Strategic Policy Planning Committee. Workforce supply for hospitals and health systems issues and recommendations. 2001. Available at: http://www.aha.org/aha/issues/Workforce/workforceB0123.html. Accessed November 1, 2007.

20. American Physical Therapy Association. PT demographics: Type of facility. 2007. Available at: http://ww.apte.org/AM/Template.cfm:Section=Demographics&CONTENTID=41549&TEMPLATE=CM/ContentDisplay.cfm. Accessed October 24, 2007.

21. Suddick KM, De Souza L. Therapists' experiences and perceptions of teamwork in neurological rehabilitation: Reasoning behind the team approach, structure and composition of the team and teamworking processes. *Physiotherapy Research International*. 2006;11:72–83.

22. Iles R, Davidson M. Evidence based practice: A survey of physiotherapists' current practice. *Physiotherapy Research International*. 2006;11:93–103.

23. Geyman JP, Deyo RA, Ramsey SD. *Evidence Based Clinical Practice: Concepts and Approaches*. Woburn, MA: Butterworth-Heinemann; 2000.

24. Vreeman DJ, Taggard SL, Rhine MD, et al. Evidence for electronic health record systems in physical therapy. *Physical Therapy*. 2006;86:434–449.

25. Donohoe E, Nawawi A, Wilker L, et al. *Factors associated with burnout of physical therapists in Massachusetts rehabilitation hospitals. Physical Therapy*. 1993;73:750–761.

26. Lopopolo RB. The relationship of role-related variables to job satisfaction and commitment to the organization in a restructured hospital environment. *Physical Therapy*. 2002;82:984–999.

27. Van Breugel G, Van Olffen W, Olie R. Temporary liaisons: The commitment of 'temps' towards their agencies. *Journal of Management Studies*. 2005;42:3.

28. Kirk-Sanchez NJ, Roach KE. Relationship between duration of therapy services in a comprehensive rehabilitation program and mobility at discharge in patients with orthopedic problems. *Physical Therapy*. 2001;81:888–895.

29. Roach KE, Ally D, Finnerty B, et al. The relationship between duration of physical therapy services in the acute care setting and change in functional status in patients with lower-extremity orthopedic problems. *Physical Therapy*. 1998;78:19–24.

30. Curtis KA, Martin T. *Perceptions of acute care physical therapy practice: Issues for physical therapist preparation. Physical Therapy*. 1993;73:581–598.

31. Lopopolo RB. Development of the professional role behaviors survey (PROBES). *Physical Therapy*. 2001;81:1317–1327.

32. The Joint Commission. 2008 national patient safety goals hospital program. Available at: http://www.jointcommission.org/PatientSafety/NationalPatientSafetyGoals/08_hap_npsgs.htm. Accessed January 18, 2008.

Chapter 20

Commentary on the Physical Therapist as Manager

What We Know

Official documents of the American Physical Therapy Association (APTA), such as *The Guide to Physical Therapist Practice* and the Normative Model for Physical Therapist Professional Education describe the administrative and managerial roles of physical therapists in general terms that are consistent with traditional perspectives of management. The consensus processes that led to the development of these documents reflect the broadest common denominators of physical therapist practice. The APTA Standards of Practice for Physical Therapy also address some organizational components of physical therapy practice that have been addressed in this text. See Sidebar 20.1.

Sidebar 20.1

APTA Standards of Practice

The Criteria for Standards of Practice for Physical Therapy may be found at: http://www.apta.org/ AM/Template.cfm?Section=Policies_and_Bylaws& CONTENTID=25762&TEMPLATE=/CM/ ContentDisplay.cfm.

Although these resources have provided a long-needed clarification of the responsibilities of physical therapists, including a managerial role, they lack specificity and consideration for different requirements for managers in different settings. They also continue to reflect only one model in which a physical therapist is the manager of other physical therapists. Except perhaps for private physical therapy practices, this model of management does not seem to reflect current interdisciplinary health-care trends. The clinical discipline of a manager seems less important to upper-level managers in organizations with program management models of health care.

In response to some of these limitations, recent research efforts have been directed to more clearly and narrowly defining the health-care managerial skills required of new physical therapist graduates. In one study, hospital-based, private practice, and academic physical therapists were asked to rank 75 managerial activities. All groups identified communication, financial control, resource allocation, entrepreneur, and leader as the five most important categories of skills of physical therapists in managerial positions. They identified technical expert and figurehead as the least important skills. The groups differed significantly in their ranking of the activities however, and the identified managerial skills were consistent with those of managers in nonhealth-care settings.[1]

More recently, the **F**inance, **I**nformation management, **N**etworking, **H**uman resource management, **O**perations, and **P**lanning and forecasting (FINHOP) model of administration and management has been defined. The model was derived from previous work that detailed the administrative and managerial skills important to physical therapy practice, called the leadership, administration, management, and professional (LAMP) model,[2] and the six categories of administration and management identified by Luedtke-Hoffman.[3] The FINHOP model was used to determine the level of importance of 121 administration and management skills for new physical therapist graduates in 2010.[4] Respondents were physical therapists in academic programs and those in hospital-based and private clinical practices. There were no statistical differences among the responses of these subgroups.

They concluded that new graduates would be expected to be independent in the FINHOP skill groups of self-management, compliance with rules, ethics and culture, and insurance coding. Graduates in 2010 are expected to be moderately independent in the management of human resources, information, operations, and networking. Marketing and strategic planning, financial analysis and budgeting, and environmental assessment were the expected managerial skills projected to require the greatest development in new graduates. The expected levels of independence move from those managerial skills that are related more to direct patient/client management responsibilities, on to those related to organizational management, and finally those related more to the management of the organization within the larger environment.[4]

This study seems to suggest that the expectations for doctoral-prepared physical therapists in 2010 reflect the typical physical therapist career ladder of the past. New graduates have traditionally practiced managerial skills on a small scale within their zone of safety of direct patient care, were then promoted to line supervisory positions with responsibility for small units in organizations, and some moved to mid- and upper-level management positions with broader responsibilities. Perhaps the only differences over the years have been the result of changes in health-care organizations. Even line supervisory positions are more likely to include responsibility for interdisciplinary

teams, and nonclinical managers have joined clinicians who have come up through the ranks in mid-level and upper-management positions in health care.

Although the FINHOP model and hierarchy may reflect expectations of graduates in the next few years, whether or not this picture of the future will advance the profession as a whole may be questionable. The focus of the vision of the APTA lies with patient care, perhaps as it should be, at this stage in the development of the profession. The individual physical therapist interacting with the individual patient remains the heart of the profession, so it is reasonable that managerial expectations for new graduates also lie with direct patient care. Anecdotally, however, it appears that even within a year of graduation, new physical therapists face challenges that demand an understanding of the importance of a broader vision and expanded viewpoint of physical therapy practice within health care.

Without the knowledge and skills necessary to meet these challenges, physical therapists who are entrepreneurs developing their own independent practices, or those who hold managerial positions at all organizational levels, may be disadvantaged individually, which places the profession at a potential disadvantage. Unless physical therapists hold managerial positions in which they can influence decision making in organizations, the broader impact of the physical therapy profession on the business of health care may be lost. It may be shortsighted to find comfort in the 2010 expectations revealed in the FINHOP study for new graduates that seem not to have changed significantly over the years, although our health-care system has changed, and will continue to do so.

What We Need to Know

Although these studies and the intentions of the APTA are a start in the right direction, we do not know a great deal about physical therapists who are currently managers in health-care organizations, and we know even less about managers of physical therapists who are *not* physical therapists. With the development of the FINHOP model, there may be opportunities to track changes at many levels of management in health care across the range of health-care settings that go beyond the skills of new graduates.

A starting point may be to have novice physical therapists who may actually face managerial challenges early in their careers serve as subjects in a study of the FINHOP model. What they consider as the skills they will need in 2010 may differ from those that more experienced physical therapists have speculated. Important questions remain unanswered as the dynamic nature of health-care challenges managers and the physical therapy profession, such as:

✦ At what point do physical therapists identify more with their managerial roles than their clinical roles?

✦ What is the most effective means for preparing physical therapists for managerial responsibilities?

✦ When should physical therapists prepare for managerial responsibilities?

✦ Are the knowledge and experience of health-care managers transferable from one physical therapy setting to another?

✦ What is the effect of having a non–physical-therapist manager on the professional duties of physical therapists?

✦ What is the effect of non–physical-therapist managers in organizations on the profession?

✦ Should there be parallel tracks for preparing entrepreneur physical therapists and physical therapists who seek managerial roles in other health-care organizations?

✦ What should be the relationship between managers in private practices and those in other health-care organizations?

✦ How do the managerial roles of physical therapists impact the vision of the profession?

✦ What technical, economic, social, and political trends impact the management of physical therapy services?

These potentially serious issues may require the profession to take a broader perspective of the management of physical therapy practice, and a closer look at preparing physical therapists for these positions.

Career Development

As a general rule, physical therapists begin their careers in staff positions with a focus on refinement of clinical skills and getting to know the "system."

After this initiation period, physical therapists are often ready to move on to new responsibilities. Some may choose a clinical track of career development that may lead to certification as a specialist. Some may choose an academic research track, and others may elect a managerial track. Still others may opt for some combination of these roles. Because the career tracks for clinical and academic growth are more formalized, they find wide acceptance as career options. Both options lead physical therapists to careers with a more narrow view of the profession.

Physical therapists also link these career paths more easily to direct patient care than they link management to direct patient care. More often they consider managers an intrusion rather than support for clinical services. Many coworkers may feel somewhat betrayed when physical therapists leave patient care to pursue managerial roles.

A negative impression of management is enhanced in organizations in which the employee/employer relationship is adversarial. Physical therapists who were recruited reluctantly from the ranks to fill these positions may also resent being taken away from patient care to perform what are often considered unwelcome chores to be avoided whenever possible. Physical therapists in private practice may feel guilty as they are torn between time for patient care and time for management of their businesses.

Therefore, many students and graduates may see a managerial career track in a less than positive light, especially if they are already convinced that they do not have a mind for business. Coupled with the lack of a clear picture of a management track for physical therapists, these opportunities become less and less desirable to many of them. Some physical therapist assistants with less opportunity in academic and clinical specialist tracks, however, have found opportunities as managers because of the shortage of physical therapists to fill these positions.

Although it may seem awkward for physical therapist assistants to manage physical therapists, it may not necessarily be so if professionals really do not rely on their managers for assistance with their clinical decision making. The argument is often made that if others who are not physical therapists at all may supervise physical therapists, so may physical therapist assistants who meet the requirements of those positions. If physical therapists assistants in these positions are not providing direct patient care that requires the supervision of the physical therapist, confusion about who is in charge of clinical decisions is clear.

This apparent lack of interest in management is unfortunate because management is the career path that broadens the view of the profession through the eyes of the physical therapist manager. It increases the visibility of the profession as physical therapists join the management table for important decision making in health-care organizations. In many organizations, the profession may need a strong voice for physical therapy services to remain viable. The profession may need to direct as much attention to the importance of physical therapists in managerial positions as it does to evidence-based practice and autonomous clinical decision making in specialty practices.

Management as a Career Track

Physical therapists who are interested in a management career track in a health-care organization or in a private practice must take the initiative to identify graduate programs, in-house training programs in larger corporations, mentors, continuing education programs, etc. to prepare them for managerial responsibilities. This preparation often begins after the fact—they are already in managerial positions that they feel unprepared for.

Many of these formal educational opportunities address universal managerial skills. They are often extremely well done, and they provide physical therapists with the knowledge and skills to carry out new roles. Others may require physical therapists to "cut and paste" course content to meet the unique needs of the management of physical therapy or rehabilitation services. For example, an MBA degree with a health-care focus typically emphasizes the medical rather than the disability model as a foundation for the degree. Programs for entrepreneurs typically focus on products rather than services, and they rarely address health-care businesses.

One of the problems with this current approach to the development of managers in the profession is that there has been no model for a management career ladder for guidance. The profession relies on individual physical therapists to pull all of this together in contexts that are often foreign to them.

For many people, it becomes easier to shift away from physical therapy to other non–physical-therapy management opportunities than it is to incorporate new management skills into their profession because these links must be self-generated.

The Growth of the Profession

Physical therapists tend to *plan for* careers in academia or as clinical specialists and *fall into* careers as managers in health care. A more clearly defined structure for planning a management career might shift the balance of these three career tracks in the profession. New graduates might feel differently if there was a more formal managerial career path in physical therapy so that it might be more easily compared to other career paths. If they want to become a clinical specialist, they know how it is done, or if they want to be a researcher, they know what it takes. If management is even considered a possibility, it is more difficult to know where to start.

The APTA currently gives only cursory attention in its official documents to the responsibilities and expectations of physical therapists who are managers. The lack of attention is evident in its failure to address changes in managerial models as health care has changed. It often seems that many physical therapists fell out of health-care management as the system flattened by reducing the number of mid-level management positions. These organizational changes were missed opportunities for physical therapists to secure a prominent role in new management models in all health-care settings.

Unfortunately, the profession leaves a great deal to chance in the managerial roles of physical therapists because of its focus on the patient–physical therapist relationship and its encouragement of private practice. By taking a broader view and devoting the same level of commitment to management as it has to other goals, the profession as a whole, and individual physical therapists, may find themselves at a significant advantage in influencing today's health care. For instance, if the APTA developed recommendations for possible curriculum models to enhance management tracks and dual business/physical therapy degrees, academic administrators might be more inclined to implement them.

Recommendations for Physical Therapy Education

Professional Education

A start in addressing the managerial skills of physical therapists, as has been suggested in the FINHOP study, is with their professional education. Traditionally, curricula for physical therapists include a professionalism course near the beginning of curricula and a management course somewhere near the end of courses of study. This suggests that management is something that is tacked onto the clinical roles of physical therapists. Determining instructional strategies for integrating the entry-level managerial skills into patient/client management courses rather than as freestanding courses may be a beginning.

For instance, if the management skill categories of self-management, compliance with rules, ethics and culture, and insurance coding, were introduced early in a curriculum, this content could be consistently reinforced in case studies and other problem-solving in patient/client management courses.

Another model may be one in which content in the professionalism and management courses that run concurrently with patient/client management courses are scheduled so that they are reinforcing the managerial aspects of clinical decision making. For example, as physical therapist students are learning new clinical skills, it may be appropriate to expand those learning goals with managerial skills. Determining what components of a plan of care might be performed by physical therapist assistants, the charges that would be submitted for a particular treatment session, time management, possible ethical and legal issues, and self-assessment of performance may all be integrated into courses where clinical decision making and clinical skills are taught.

The problem is not all faculties have all content expertise, which is most likely how professionalism and management content became separate courses anyway. This separation is related to the perception, again, that patient care is the heart of the work of physical therapists and management detracts from it. Perhaps the nonclinical faculty need to serve as consultants to the patient/client management courses to develop course objectives, guest lectures, and activities in those courses that enmesh rather than tack on the development of these equally important managerial skills.

Like the research and education roles of physical therapists, management has levels of skills. There are some skill sets that are part of basic entry-level practice and other that are truly "other roles" of the physical therapists that go beyond patient care. Students need a strong orientation to these levels of responsibility and the career choices they have as a result. Clarifying the scope of managerial skills within patient care may be less overwhelming for many graduates who are often plunged into these responsibilities with a great deal of discomfort.

Clinical Education

The other component of professional education where managerial skills may be better addressed is clinical education. Rather than diminishing standardized performance requirements for managerial skills, or isolating them as separate categories of performance, they should be integrated into every patient encounter. Clinical instructors need to be deliberate in creating learning opportunities to develop nonclinical and clinical skills and measure that performance.

Learning opportunities in the later stages of clinical education, which focus on managerial responsibilities, is another possibility. Some students may focus on areas of clinical specialization or research while others focus on managerial skills. Some hard-held ideas about supervision of students may need to be relaxed so that students may have nonphysical therapists supervise managerial assignments that do not involve direct patient care. Preparing managers to provide expanded learning experiences and the tools to evaluate the performance of tasks and managerial decision making using the FINHOP model may be a step in the right direction. Balancing the learning of clinical and managerial skills may require more effort because the ways of doing clinical education are often deeply entrenched.

A Management Track

A move to a more integrative curriculum approach to management skills also calls for revision of the typical management course in a curriculum. What should it be? Freestanding management courses are an opportunity for curriculum planners to take interested students one step beyond entry-level expectations. Perhaps as independent study or through electives, students may pursue the other identified FINHOP skills of human resources, information, operations and networking, marketing, strategic planning, financial analysis, budgeting, and environmental assessment. This track could cover a range of possibilities that may culminate in a dual physical therapy/business or physical therapy/public health degree. An elective internship course that provides students the opportunity to work directly with a manager for an extended time may be another possibility that allows time for this study beyond clinical education courses.

Recruitment and Admissions

A link to a specific undergraduate degree program in business that includes a track for meeting the basic science requirements for admission may be a recruitment strategy for identifying potential applicants who have the potential for both clinical practice and management. Many people excel in both, so it may be important to overcome a bias toward applicants who excel only in the sciences as the basis for admission decisions. Consideration for prior managerial experience in other work settings, such as hospitality or retail sales may be another admissions strategy. Particularly if the college or university already has a strongly established history of interdisciplinary degrees, physical therapy programs have an opportunity to develop interesting degree programs that promote interprofessional models of practice in collaboration with colleges of business and public health.

Recommendations for the Profession

The importance of these efforts to formalize and increase the value for managerial skills of physical therapists may become critical in evolving health-care organizations. Many highly skilled and effective managers are physical therapists in a variety of organizations. Efforts to tap into this expertise may require that the APTA look to people who are not members of the association. Many health-care managers may be physical therapists who have moved on and away from the profession, and others may not be physical therapists. Keeping physical therapists current with a broader view of changes in health-care management may become critical in diminishing dissonance and dissatisfaction with their work.

Forming an expert study group that is assigned to conduct an environmental scan to determine the who and how of the management of physical therapy services across all health-care settings seems to be a desirable first step. Identifying models of management and the requirements to fill these managerial positions may be very revealing.

In addition, establishing the current positioning of physical therapy services in health-care organizations and private practices in communities is another important goal for the profession. Some measurement of the value and power of physical therapy services must be defined to determine its organizational or community impact. Positioning is not the same as demonstrating strong outcomes data with a focus on patient care. It is about the respect and importance of physical therapy services and the profession collectively in a changing health-care system.

The recent focus of the profession has been the efforts to assure autonomous practice. Although this drive for more professional autonomy may serve individual physical therapists well, an equal commitment to positioning the profession more strategically in health care may be necessary. Identifying the skills physical therapists in organizations need to possess to contribute to the positioning of the profession is as important as their ability to practice autonomously in those organizations.

Ongoing programs initiated by the APTA for the development of managers to secure the position of the profession in organizations are needed. Building on its success with its clinical specialization and evidence-based practice models, the APTA is well prepared to take on preparing and recognizing physical therapists with managerial expertise who will serve the needs of health organizations and of the profession.

Conclusion

The physical therapy profession is at a critical juncture for reviving the managerial opportunities for physical therapists in all aspects of contemporary health care. Inclusion of management with the current research and clinical practice goals of the American Physical Therapy Association, and thoughtful consideration of management content in professional curricula are timely considerations as the profession positions itself to meet the organizational demands that must be met to serve the needs of patients and clients.

REFERENCES

1. Schaefer DS. Three perspectives on physical therapist managerial work. *Physical Therapy.* 2002;82:228–236.
2. Lopopolo RB, Schaefer DS, Nosse LJ. Leadership, administration, management, and professional (LAMP) processes in physical therapy: A Delphi study. *Physical Therapy.* 2004;21. 137–150.
3. Luedtke-Hoffman KA. *Identification of essential managerial work activities and competencies of physical therapist managers employed in hospital settings* [doctoral]. Denton, TX: Texas Women's University; 2002.
4. Schaefer DS, Lopopolo RB, Luedtke-Hoffman KA. Administration and management skills needed by physical therapist graduates in 2010: A national survey. *Physical Therapy.* 2007;87:261–281.

Index

Note: page numbers followed by b, f, and t refer to Side Bars, Figures, and Tables, respectively.